PRISON HEALTH HANDBOOK

MIKE ENEMIGO

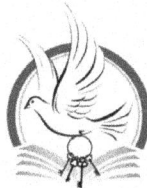

Freebird Publishers
www.FreebirdPublishers.com

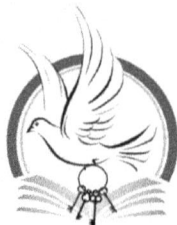

Freebird Publishers

221 Pearl St., Ste. 541, North Dighton, MA 02764
Info@FreebirdPublishers.com
www.FreebirdPublishers.com

Copyright © 2019
Prison Health Handbook
By Mike Enemigo

All Freebird Publishers titles, imprints, and distributed lines are available at special quantity discounts for bulk purchases for sales, promotions, premiums, fundraising, educational, or institutional use.

ISBN: 0-9980361-7-X
ISBN-13:978-0-9980361-7-5

Printed in the United States of America

CONTENTS

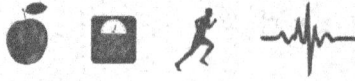

FORWARD: A LETTER FROM MIKE ENEMIGO

Prison is a filthy, depressing, dark, disgusting, even toxic place, both physically and mentally. It's bad for your health in every way. want some examples? Here, let me give you a few real titles of articles right out my PLNs ...

California Prisons Struggle with Environmental Threats from Sewage Spills, Contaminated Water, Air-borne Disease

Georgia Prison Doctor Rewarded for Cutting costs as Prisoners Died Under His Care

Seventh Circuit Dissent: "A Dog Would Have Deserved Better Treatment

Major Scabies Outbreak at Core Civic Facility in Tennessee

Deaths at North Carolina Jail Due to Lack of Medical, Mental Health Care

Lawsuit Alleges Four Oregon Prisons Served Food "Not for Human Consumption

Tennessee: High Cost of Drugs Cited as Reason to Deny Prisoners Hep C Treatment

Attica Medical Experiments Exposed

Do I need to continue? You get it, right?

After over 20 years of bouncing around from prison to prison in the state of California, I've experienced a number of unhealthy circumstances: having brown, dirty, rusty water coming out of my sink; I've been fed food that clearly says on the box "NOT FOR HUMAN CONSUMPTION"; I was denied surgery for two years for a torn rotator cuff, which allowed my shoulder to dislocate fourteen times during those two years; I once got a flu shot that made me sick for three months; I've been in a prison where guards and visitors are warned via posted signs to NOT drink the water because of high arsenic levels, yet it's the only water for prisoners to drink; I've been to prisons where inmates were actually dying from Valley Fever due to the contaminated land the prisons were built upon; and this doesn't even begin to get into the lack of nutrition, exercise, and the mental wear and tear I've gone through.

In an effort to survive, literally, I finally decided I'd have to take my health into my own hands, at least as much as possible, given my circumstances. So, though I'm no doctor, I began to collect information, read and educate myself, so I'd at least have a basic understanding and increase my odds at remaining healthy in such an unhealthy environment. I wasn't able to find one complete source -- one go-to source, if you will. I just began to gather all I could from doctors, gurus, therapists, experts and even prisoners, put it together and created my own go-to source that I could use as a reference when needed -- a guide for health success. And as a prisoner-author who specializes in self-help books and reports for prisoners, it was the natural next step that I share all I've learned and gathered with you, in the form of a one-stop book, so that you, too, can regain some power and control over your own health, both mentally and physically. Because, in prison, if YOU don't take care of YOU, who else will?

Sincerely,

Mike

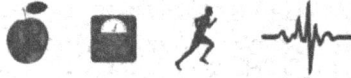

MENTAL HEALTH: THE SECRETS

Not only is it important that you stay physically healthy in order to survive prison, but it is as equally important that you stay mentally healthy. The prison experience/environment can easily take its toll on the minds of its men, so if you wish to survive, you must learn to overcome the challenges you are sure to face. No matter how strong your body is, prison will eat you alive if your mind is weak.

Despite what people on the outside may or may not think, it is important for you to understand that prisons are designed to mentally break its prisoners (you!) down. Once a man is broken down mentally, he starts to break spiritually. And one he's spiritually broken, he's as good as dead....

Furthermore, a mentally broken man is easier to control, as being mentally broken is to be tired. When he is tired, it's harder for him to resist. When it's harder for him to resist, it's easier for "them" to win. It is obviously to "their" benefit that you are weak; therefore, "they" have intentionally designed "their" system to exhaust you, and it is up to you to stand against falling a victim to that. In addition to the above, your psychological battle is not only with the depressing predicament that you find yourself in or the mental roller coaster designed by prison to suck out your energy and steal your spirit, but with your fellow prisoners, as well. Prison is a bloody shark tank full of Great Whites, and your fellow prisoners wish to suppress you just as much as anyone else. As explained in the mental warfare section of this book, you must learn to spot mental attacks from your fellow prisoners as well as defend yourself from them and, just as importantly, you must also learn to spot and defend yourself from the mental attacks/wars waged against you by prison itself.

Here are my tips to staying mentally healthy and strong while you are in prison.

KEEP YOUR CELL LIGHT ON:

For some reason, many prisoners like to keep their cell light off so that their cell remains dark all day. Why someone would want to live in the dark is beyond me, but it is an extremely common thing to do in prison.

Don't fall into this kind of program. Instead, keep your light on and live. Look at it like this: Light is life, and dark is death. When my celly wants to keep the light off all day I can physically feel a difference in my body. Too much darkness will bring upon depression. We are like plants: put us in sunlight, we will grow and thrive; put us in the dark, we will wither and die.

DON'T SLEEP TOO MUCH:

Another thing a lot of prisoners like to do is sleep all day. However, it's a mistake; don't do it. Sleeping too much will not only make you always feel sluggish and sleepy, but it, too, will bring upon depression.

EXERCISE:

Make sure you physically exercise at least a little bit each day. You have to keep yourself active. If you let a car sit too long without starting it, driving it around, etc., it's not going to run right. Well, the same thing goes for your body. A healthy body will help you keep a healthy mind, exercising will help you release tension and stress.

DON'T DWELL:

Know life isn't necessarily going your way right now. However, don't sit around and dwell on your situation all day. It won't change anything, it will only add to your misery.

Instead of dwelling, turn whatever injustice has been done to you into a reason to be strong and positive. Rather than dwell or get depressed, get angry and channel that energy into something positive and/or beneficial; let your situation fuel your fire. Rather than dwelling on your situation, change it.

STAY POSITIVE:

Despite your situation, you must remain positive. Too much negativity will kill you. Positivity (+) will add to your life; negativity (-) will take it away...

In addition to that, avoid negative people. They are like energy vampires; they will suck all the positive energy right out of you with their constant pessimism.

HAVE A SENSE OF HUMOR:

It's important and healthy to have a good sense of humor. No matter what your situation is, always try to look for the humor in things. Laughter heals.

HAVE A FOCUS:

Set goals for yourself and focus on them. Whether it's writing a book, studying something you're passionate about, or getting into something else that's time-consuming, escape prison by finding something positive and beneficial to do and focus on it. When you are focused on something, you will be too busy to dwell, stress, feel sorry for yourself, etc.

READ INSPIRATIONAL STORIES:

Another thing I think is a good idea is to read inspirational stories. Whether you're religious or not, I find that *Guideposts* (magazines) have a lot of stories that give me a good feeling each time I read them. *The Chicken Soup* for the Soul is a good series too. And they even have a *Chicken Soup for the Prisoner's Soul.*

Taking in good, positive, inspirational information is healthy. Whether it's reading books with these kinds of stories, or even watching TV shows like *Secret Millionaire* or *Home Makeover*, intake as much positive and healthy information as you can.

KEEP THE FAITH; REMAIN HOPEFUL:

Despite what your reality is today, you must remain hopeful. You'd be amazed how far faith and hope will take you. You must never give up. As long as you remain hopeful and continue to stay strong, you will have a chance of succeeding. If you lose hope and stop fighting, you will for sure not have a chance of succeeding. It's kind of like the concept, "you can't win if you don't play."

RELIGION:

I cannot say that I am a real religious man. However, as I get older, I have a much clearer understanding of the essence and concept of religion. It now makes sense to me why people find so much strength in religion, and it all comes down to keeping faith and remaining hopeful. If you have a religion, practice it. religion is a positive intake. Therefore, it will help you stay on a positive path and remain faithful.

MENTAL RELAXATION:

Finding time to relax your mind is crucial. You should dedicate at least 15 minutes a day to practicing some kind of relaxation technique-meditation, etc. In prison's chaotic environment, it is very important that you maintain peace of mind.

Note: I find calmative breathing to be a great, simply way to reduce anxiety, and it can be done anywhere, anytime. All you have to do is inhale through your nose, hold it for a count of four, and exhale slowly through pursed lips until you have expelled all of the air in your lungs. Try it; you will immediately feel more relaxed.

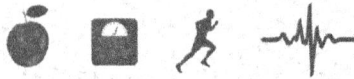

DEPRESSION

It is normal for everyone to feel down or sad sometimes. These feelings can occur after having a bad day at work, having an argument with a loved one, or getting a bad grade on an exam. In most cases, these feelings do not last, and a person's mood improves within a few days. But a person with depression has symptoms that interfere with his or her daily life for at least two weeks. Depression is a common and serious mental disorder. It can affect people in different ways. It can change how a person feels, thinks, acts, and handles daily activities, such as sleeping, eating, and working. People with depression may feel sad, hopeless, angry, irritable, and tired. They may have physical symptoms such as stomachaches, headaches, migraines, and muscle pains. They may have suicidal thoughts and suicide attempts.

Depression is sometimes called major depressive disorder or clinical depression. A person may experience depression only once in their lifetime; however, it often reoccurs. The following common and related disorders share symptoms with depression:

- √ **Persistent depressive disorder** (also called dysthymia) involves depressive symptoms that last for at least two years.
- √ **Adjustment disorder** causes many of the symptoms seen in depression, but occurs after a person goes through a stressful time in life, such as the death of a loved one, divorce or relationship problems, illnesses, unexpected catastrophes, or worries about money.
- √ **Postpartum depression** occurs in some women after childbirth and may make it difficult for new mothers to take care of themselves and their babies.
- √ **Psychotic depression** occurs in some people with depression, causing them to believe things that are not real (delusions) and hear or see things that others cannot (hallucinations).
- √ **Seasonal affective disorder** involves onset of depression during winter, when there is less natural sunlight, and generally lifts during spring and summer.
- √ **Bipolar disorder** involves shifts in a person's mood, alternating between depression and mania—feeling extremely "up," elated, and energized.

SIGNS AND SYMPTOMS

A person with depression may not realize it. The symptoms vary from person to person. Without proper treatment, the symptoms may get worse.

A person with depression will have some of the following symptoms for at least two weeks, as well as significant impact on their daily life functions:

- √ Sadness, anxiety, or feeling "empty" of any mood
- √ Feelings of hopelessness

√ Feelings of pessimism, expecting only bad things to occur.

√ Loss of interest or pleasure in previously enjoyed hobbies and activities

√ Neglecting care of oneself, such as not bathing, grooming, or eating

√ Fatigue or decreased energy level, moving or speaking slowly

√ Irritability

√ Feelings of guilt, worthlessness, or helplessness

√ Restlessness or having trouble sitting still

√ Difficulty concentrating, remembering, or making decisions

√ Difficulty following through with tasks, being unable to perform well at work, or ineffective parenting

√ Increase in pain sensitivity

√ Difficulty sleeping, waking very early in the morning, or sleeping more than usual

√ Increased or decreased appetite, large changes in the body weight

√ Aches or pains, headaches, cramps, or digestive problems without a clear physical cause or that do not ease even with targeted treatment

√ Thoughts of death or suicide, or suicide attempts

Not everyone who is depressed has all symptoms. The severity and frequency of symptoms and how long they last will vary depending on the person. A person who has had depression has an increased risk of having depression again. Some people may go many years without symptoms. The longer a person who has had depression goes without depressive symptoms, the lower the risk that the symptoms will come back.

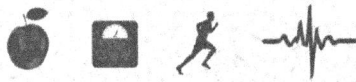

ANXIETY

Anxiety disorders are mental disorders that can occur at any age. Everyone feels worried and fearful at times. People with anxiety disorders worry a lot and are fearful and nervous. These feelings cause distress and impair daily life. The person may avoid situations such as work, school, and social activities.

There are several types of anxiety disorders. This summary focuses on generalized anxiety disorder, panic disorder, and social anxiety disorder.

SIGNS AND SYMPTOMS

Generalized Anxiety Disorder

A person with generalized anxiety disorder (GAD) has excessive feelings, thoughts, emotions, and actions. He or she has anxiety or worrying most of the time for at least six months. The worry may be related to job performance, money, health, and other activities. Sometimes the worry shifts from one focus to another. An adult with GAD has several of the following symptoms; a child may have just one symptom:

- √ Restlessness, or feeling wound up or on edge
- √ Being easily tired.
- √ Trouble concentrating, or feeling that their "mind goes blank"
- √ Irritability
- √ Muscle tension, aching, or soreness
- √ Sleep problems, such as trouble falling asleep or staying asleep, restlessness at night or unsatisfying sleep
- √ A person with GAD also may have a change in appetite and frequent sweating, nausea, or diarrhea

Panic Disorder

A person with panic disorder has unexpected or expected panic attacks. Panic attacks are sudden periods of intense fear, anxiety, or discomfort. The attack reaches a peak within minutes. It may cause an urge to escape or flee. During a panic attack, a person has several of the following symptoms:

- √ Pounding heart or fast heart rate
- √ Sweating
- √ Trembling or shaking
- √ Shortness of breath
- √ Feelings of choking

- √ Chest pain or discomfort
- √ Nausea or abdominal distress
- √ Dizziness or feeling lightheaded
- √ Chills or feeling overheated
- √ Numbness or tingling
- √ Feelings of unreality or being unconnected to oneself
- √ Fear of going crazy or losing control
- √ Fear of dying

After one or more panic attacks, he or she usually has one or both of:

- √ Worry that another panic attack might occur, and irrational fear that this will lead to loss of control of thoughts and feelings, a heart attack, or dying
- √ Trying to avoid panic attacks, such as by avoiding certain situations or places, or by stopping exercise or other activities.

Social Anxiety Disorder

Social anxiety disorder is sometimes called social phobia. The person fears being embarrassed or negatively judged by others in a social setting. This worry often causes him or her to withdraw or avoid certain situations. This causes problems at work, at school, or in relationships.

A person with social anxiety disorder often has the following symptoms for more than six months:

- √ Being afraid of or worrying about social situations, such as meeting new people or eating in front of others
- √ Feeling very self-conscious in front of others and worrying about offending others or being humiliated, embarrassed, or rejected
- √ Avoiding social situations that cause fear and anxiety, feeling dread or doom leading up to a feared situation, or being very uncomfortable if able to stay in the situation
- √ Feeling fear or worry about a situation greater than the actual threat and beyond what most people would feel
- √ Having problems at work, school, or in relationships due to the symptoms
- √ Changing the daily routine in response to the symptoms
- √ A person with social anxiety disorder sometimes feels nauseous. They may blush, tremble, sweat, or say their mind "goes blank" in feared situations.
- √ A small subgroup of people with social anxiety disorder fear having to perform, present, or talk in front of a group.

RISK FACTORS

There is no single cause of anxiety disorders. Genetics, brain structure and function, and environmental factors all seem to be involved.

General Anxiety Disorder

About 3% of adults and 1% of adolescents have GAD. Females are much more likely than males to have GAD. Most people with GAD develop symptoms between childhood and middle age.

Panic Disorder

About 3% of adults and adolescents have panic disorder. Females are more likely than males to have panic disorder. Most people develop panic disorder between ages 20-24. It can occur much earlier, but rarely starts after age 45.

About 25-50% of people with panic disorder also have agoraphobia. They start avoiding places such as crowded areas, buses, and elevators. Agoraphobia can occur without panic disorder.

Risk factors for panic disorder include having stressors in the months before the first panic attack. Stressors can include marriage problems, health problems, use of illicit drugs, misuse of medications, or death of a close family member.

Social Anxiety Disorder

About 7% of adults have social anxiety disorder in a given year. Children may have social anxiety symptoms. The rate of social anxiety disorder decreases with age. It is more common in women than in men.

All Anxiety Disorders

Genetics and biological factors. Anxiety disorders tend to run in families. A person who has a close relative with an anxiety disorder or depression is more likely to develop an anxiety disorder. It is unclear whether one or more genes are involved. In some people, an overactive thyroid can contribute to anxiety disorders. A person who tends to feel distress and withdraw from unfamiliar situations, people, and places may be more likely to develop an anxiety disorder.

Brain structure and function. Certain brain structures seem to play a role in anxiety disorders. The amygdala, the part of the brain that controls emotion, may be involved.

Environment factors. Environmental factors that may lead to anxiety disorders include:

- √ Smoking or using tobacco products, and nicotine withdrawal
- √ Having a parent with anxiety, depression, or bipolar disorder
- √ Having breathing problems, such as asthma, and fearing suffocation
- √ Withdrawal from alcohol or a medication such as a benzodiazepine
- √ Exposure to stressful life events in childhood and/or adulthood
- √ Physical or mental abuse, death of a loved one, desertion, divorce, or isolation
- √ Caffeine, prescription medications, and over-the-counter medicines such as diet pills and allergy medications that contain pseudoephedrine

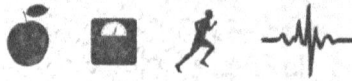

POST TRAUMATIC STRESS

Here are thoughts and feelings by two people who have experienced traumatic incidents:

"I feel terrible, very restless and irritable. This is not like me at all. The crash happened six months ago but I still can't feel safe in a car. Pictures of the accident come flashing into my mind, they won't go away, even at night. My dreams are more like nightmares with scenes of the crash happening again and again... I can't stop shaking when I think I could have died."

"Everything has changed, I keep thinking. Why us? I feel guilty thinking that I could have done more to save my friend. I re-live the experience all the time. I keep thinking, If only I had done this, if only I had done that... I am very low and depressed most of the time...

I think of the future... I feel helpless."

If you have suffered from a traumatic experience yourself, you may have had similar feelings. For example:

√ Flashbacks

√ Tension

√ Nightmares

The following was written by psychologists and people who have experienced prison. It aims to help you understand these reactions and offers some practical suggestions to help you cope.

What is a traumatic incident?

A traumatic event is something out of the ordinary that happens and is deeply distressing to someone.

Many things can have this impact. It could be a fire, an accident, an attack, being a witness or involved in a traumatic event such as a robbery or even a death. It can be on a large scale, such as a major disaster involving many people, or a personal event involving yourself, friends or family members. Being on trial and sent to prison can also be traumatic.

How do people react after a traumatic incident?

The following are some of the reactions you may experience after a traumatic event. In general, people's reactions will fall into the following five groups:

1. Reliving the trauma in your mind
2. Avoiding things to do with the trauma
3. Feeling more tense, irritable, or jumpy than usual
4. Feeling depressed, crying
5. Blaming others or self

It may help you to check to see if you are experiencing any of these symptoms.

Re-experiencing the trauma in your mind.

- √ Having unwanted pictures or images (often called flashbacks) of the distressing event appearing in your mind.
- √ Having upsetting dreams about the trauma or dreams about other things that frighten you.
- √ Feeling that the trauma is happening again—strong sensations or re-living the trauma.
- √ Feeling very distressed at coming across situations or feelings that remind you of the trauma.
- √ Experiencing distressing physical reactions, e.g. heart beating faster, dizziness, etc. when you are faced with memories of the trauma or situations that remind you of it.

Avoiding things related to the trauma and numbing

- √ Trying to avoid thoughts, feelings and conversations about the trauma.
- √ Avoiding activities, places or people that remind you of the trauma.
- √ Being unable to remember things about the trauma.
- √ Losing interest in life, feeling detached from others or not having your usual feelings.
- √ Feeling that you are living on borrowed time.
- √ Trying not to be seen as weak in front of others.

Feeling more tense and irritable than usual

- √ Feeling angry or irritable.
- √ Not being able to concentrate.
- √ Finding it difficult to fall asleep.
- √ Feeling over alert all the time and easily startled.
- √ Lack of tolerance, being unforgiving.

Post-traumatic stress reactions can affect us in at least four different ways:

- √ How we feel
- √ The way we think
- √ The way our bodyworks
- √ The way we behave

It may help you to identify the symptoms you are experiencing regularly:

How do you feel?

- √ Anxious, nervous, worried, frightened
- √ Feeling something dreadful is going to happen
- √ Tense, uptight, on edge, unsettled
- √ Unreal, strange, woozy, detached
- √ Depressed

What happens to your body?

- √ Heart races and pounds

- √ Chest feels tight
- √ Muscles are tense or stiff
- √ Feel tired/exhausted
- √ Body aching
- √ Feel dizzy, light headed
- √ Feel panicky
- √ Feel depressed, low, at a loss
- √ Feel angry-cry

How do you think?

- √ Worry constantly
- √ Can't concentrate
- √ Experience flashbacks—pictures of the trauma coming into your mind
- √ Blame yourself for all or part of the trauma
- √ Think it will happen again
- √ Unable to make a decision
- √ Feel regret, shame or bitterness
- √ Thoughts racing
- √ Feel jumpy or restless
- √ Stomach churning
- √ Have sleep problems/nightmares
- √ Easily startled

What you do

- √ Pace up and down
- √ Avoid things that remind you of the trauma
- √ Can't sit and relax
- √ Avoid people
- √ Avoid being alone
- √ Are snappy and irritable
- √ Spoil relationship
- √ Drink/smoke more
- √ Depends on others too much
- √ Use drugs

Common thoughts

- √ It was my fault-I'm cracking up
- √ I'm going to have a heart attack
- √ It's controlling me

√ I can' t cope

√ I'm going to faint

√ Why did it have to happen

√ I can't see the point anymore

√ If only I …

Why do we react so strongly to trauma?

There are many reasons why trauma leaves such a strong impact on us.

Firstly, if often shatters the basic beliefs we may have about life: that life is fairly safe and secure that life for us has a particular form, meaning and purpose. It may be that the image we have about ourselves is shattered, we may have responded differently from how we expected or wanted to behave.

Secondly, trauma usually occurs suddenly and without warning. We have no time to adjust to this new experience. It will usually be outside our normal range of experience and we are faced with not knowing what to do or how to behave. You may have felt you were going to die, people around you may have died, you are shocked. In the face of this danger our mind holds on to the memory of the trauma very strongly, probably as a natural form of self-protection to ensure you never get into that situation again. The result of this is that you are left with the post-traumatic reactions described above.

What can I do to help overcome the trauma?

It is important to understand that the reactions you are experiencing are very common following trauma, they are not a sign or weakness or going crazy. The following suggestions may help you begin to cope with the post traumatic reactions:

1. Making sense of the trauma
2. Dealing with flashbacks and nightmares
3. Overcoming avoidance
4. Overcoming low mood

1.   Making sense of the trauma...

Try and find out as much as you can about what really happened. This will allow you to piece together a picture and understanding of the event more clearly. This can help you in your recovery.

If others were involved, talk or write to them and ask them their views of events. Other victims, helpers from the rescue service, or passersby, may all be people who would help you gain a broader view of what happened.

It may help to think it through with other people. You may feel the trauma has altered your whole view of life. It is helpful to try and clarify how you now feel, and talking can help you do this. Some people talk to a friend, family member, partner, etc. Other people have found it helpful to write down their experience.

2.   Dealing with flashbacks and nightmares...

Many people try to put the experience of trauma behind them by attempting not to think about it. Although this may seem a natural thing to do, it does not always help them to overcome the problem. People may find that they continue to be troubled by unwanted pictures of the trauma in their mind (flashbacks) and by unpleasant dreams or nightmares related to the trauma. One of the approaches which has been found to reduce flashbacks and nightmares is to make time each day for reviewing and going over unpleasant memories or nightmares.

Many people have found that if they put time aside to calmly think over, talk over or jot down notes on the trauma, their unwanted flashbacks and nightmares will gradually become less powerful and less frequent. If you have nightmares, it may help to do this before you go to bed.

This can allow you to regain some control over these thoughts rather than them intruding upon you. It is important to try and keep calm and relaxed when looking back over the trauma you have experienced, if you possibly can.

Try the following approaches:

- √ Write down details of the flashbacks or nightmares you experience.
- √ Find a time of day when you could think over what has happened.
- √ Think of some positive things about your current situation: For example, "I survived it and I'm still here," "I can now begin to plan for a new future," "The worst is now over."

3. Overcoming tension, irritability and anger

Tension, irritability and anger are common aspects of a post-traumatic reaction. There may be physical symptoms, too, including breathlessness, heart racing, over breathing, dizziness and muscle tension. Try the following ways of reducing physical symptoms.

In order to reduce the severity of physical symptoms it is useful to nip them in the bud, by recognizing the early signs of tension. Once you have noticed the early signs of tension, you can prevent anxiety from becoming too severe by using relaxation techniques. Some people can relax through exercise, listening to music, watching TV or reading a book. For others it is more helpful to have a set of exercises to follow. Some people might find relaxation or yoga most helpful.

Relaxation is a skill like any other, which needs to be learned and takes time. The following exercise teaches deep muscle relaxation and many people find it very helpful in reducing overall levels of tension and anxiety.

Deep muscle relaxation

It is helpful to read the instructions first and eventually to learn them. Choose a time of day when you feel most relaxed to begin with. Lie down, get comfortable, close your eyes. Concentrate on your breathing for a few minutes, breathing slowly and calmly: in, two-three and out, two-three. Say the words calm or relax to yourself as you breathe out. This relaxation exercise takes you through different muscle groups, teaching you firstly to tense, then relax. You should breathe in when tensing and breathe out when you relax. Starting with your hands, clench one tightly. Think about the tension this produces in the muscles of your hand and forearm.

Study the tension for a few seconds and then relax your hand. Notice the difference between the tension and the relaxation. You might find a slight tingling; this is the relaxation beginning to develop.

Do the same with the other hand.

Each time you relax a group of muscles, think how they feel when they're relaxed. Don't try to relax, just let go of the tension. Allow your muscles to relax as much as you can. Think about the difference in the way they feel when they're relaxed and when they're tense. Now do the same for the other muscles of your body. Each time, tense them for a few seconds and then relax. Study the way they feel and then let go of the tension in them.

It is useful to stick to the same order as you work through the muscle groups:

- √ Hands-clench fists, then relax.
- √ Arms-bend your elbows and tense your arms. Feel the tension, especially in your upper arms. Remember, do this for a few seconds and then relax.
- √ Neck-tilt your head back and roll it from side to side slowly. Feel how the tension moves, then bring your head forward into a comfortable position.
- √ Face-there are several muscles here, but it is enough to think about your forehead and jaw. First lower your eyebrows in a frown. Relax your forehead. You can also raise your eyebrows, and then relax. Now, clench your jaw. Notice the difference when you relax?
- √ Chest-take a deep breath, hold it for a few seconds, notice the tension, then relax.
- √ Let your breathing return to normal.
- √ Stomach-tense your stomach muscles as tightly as you can and relax.
- √ Buttocks-squeeze your buttocks together, then relax.
- √ Legs-straighten your legs and bend your feet towards your face. Finish by wiggling your toes.

Don't try too hard, just let it happen.

To make best use of relaxation you need to:

- √ Practice daily.
- √ Start to use relaxation in everyday situations.
- √ Learn to relax without having to tense muscles.
- √ Use parts of the relaxation to help in difficult situations, e.g breathing slowly.

Remember, relaxation is a skill like any other and takes time to learn. Keep a note of how anxious you feel before and after relaxation, rating your anxiety 1-10.

Grounding techniques

If you are struggling with flashbacks and feeling detached, you can use grounding techniques to keep you in the present moment. Use the five senses—sight, sound, touch, smell, taste. The aim is to bring your attention on to the present moment.

- √ Sight-you could focus on things around you, the colors and textures.
- √ Sound-you could listen to loud music and focus on it.
- √ Touch-you could touch something soft and silky or something smooth and cold and focus on this.
- √ Smell-sniff a strong smell which can bring you in to the present—perfume or nice smelling oils can be a good choice.
- √ Taste-try something strong—a strong mint or chili or lemon can bring you into the here and now.

Controlled breathing

Over breathing is very common when someone becomes anxious, angry or irritable. This is sometimes called over breathing. People often begin to gulp air, thinking that they are going to suffocate, or they begin to breath really quickly. This has the effect of making them feel dizzy and therefore more anxious.

Try to recognize if you are doing this and slow your breathing down. Getting into a regular rhythm of in two-three and out two-three will soon return your breathing to normal. Other people have found breathing into a paper bag or cupped hands helpful. For this to work, you must cover your nose and mouth.

It takes at least three minutes of slow breathing or breathing into a bag for your breathing to return to normal.

Mindful breathing

This is a different approach to managing the symptoms of PTSD. The goal of mindful breathing is calm, non-judging awareness, allowing thoughts and feelings to come and go without getting caught up in them. The aim is to concentrate only on the present moment, not the past and not the future. Much of our anxiety is linked to thoughts and feelings about the past and the future.

Follow these instructions:

Sit comfortably, with your eyes closed or lowered and your back straight.

- √ Bring your attention to your breathing.
- √ Imagine that you have a balloon in your stomach. Every time you breath in, the balloon inflates. Each time you breathe out, the balloon deflates. Notice the sensations when the balloon inflates and deflates. Your chest and stomach rising with the in-breath, with the deflating out-breath.
- √ Thoughts will come into your mind, and that's OK, because when you notice those thoughts, then bring your attention back to your breathing.
- √ You can notice sounds, physical feelings, and emotions, and again, just bring your attention back to your breathing.
- √ Don't follow those thoughts or feelings, don't judge yourself for having them, or analyze them in any way. It's OK for the thoughts to be there. Just notice those thoughts, and let them drift on by; bring your attention back to your breathing.
- √ Whenever you notice that your attention had drifted off and is becoming caught up in thoughts or feelings, simply note that attention has drifted, and then gently bring the attention back to your breathing.

Thoughts will enter your awareness, and your attention will follow them. No matter how many times this happens, just keep bringing your attention back to your breathing. The more you can practice this exercise, the more it will help you to manage symptoms.

Distractions

If you take your mind off your symptoms, you will find the symptoms often disappear.

Try to look around you. Study things in detail: music playing, conversations, etc. Again, you need to distract yourself for at least three minutes before symptoms will begin to reduce.

Anger

It may be worth talking over your feelings of anger with those around you. Explain that your anger is not really directed at people around you even though at times it may seem like it. Ask for their patience until the anger and irritability pass, and ask people not to take it personally. Exercise, such as working out in your cell or the yard, can help, too.

4.   Overcoming avoidance...

Avoidance following a traumatic experience can take many forms. It can involve avoiding talking about the trauma, avoid becoming upset about the trauma, it can also be that you avoid anything, anyone or any situation that reminds you of the trauma. This avoidance prevents you from moving on from the trauma and in some cases it can prevent you from getting on with your life in a normal way. After recognizing the things you are avoiding, it may be helpful to write them down.

Set yourself very small goals to tackle these fears. We call this an anxiety ladder. Those situations that we only fear a little are at the bottom and our worst feared situations are at the top.

Here's an example:

Shortly before coming into prison, Mike was in a car crash where his friend was killed. Mike now avoids talking about life outside because he feels anxious that he will not be able to cope if anyone asks him about his friend. He avoids the television if he thinks anything about road accidents is likely to be shown. He has made the following anxiety ladder...

Most feared

    5.   Saying what happened to a group of people

    4.   Mentioning his friend's death to another person

    3.   Mentioning his friend's death to a more trusted person

    2.   Watching television, especially local news

    1.   Looking at local newspaper reports about car accidents

Least feared

It may help to try and make your own anxiety ladder to tackle avoidance. Remember that you may feel anxious at first, but if you are able to stay in the feared situation you will gradually begin to feel calmer.

5.   Overcoming low mood...

People often experience low mood following trauma. This can sometimes give rise to feelings of low self-worth, reduced confidence, helplessness and guilt. It is sometimes hard to recognize when your mood is low.

It is important not to let any gloomy or negative thoughts go unchallenged. Following trauma, people tend to think and expect the worst of themselves, their life and the future. Don't just accept these thoughts. Try to:

    √ Identify when your mood is very low.

    √ Jot down the unpleasant thoughts you are having during that time.

    √ Try and counter these thoughts by writing down arguments against them. Imagine what you would say to friends if they had such negative thoughts about themselves. This is particularly important if you are feeling guilt.

It may help to keep a diary of things you have enjoyed or achieved during the week. This can help you to concentrate on the good things rather than the bad things in your life.

Do something active

Physical activity is particularly helpful. Walk, run, do sit-ups, press-ups—anything that begins to increase your activity can help improve how you feel. Plan 15-20 minutes of activity every day, or every other day to begin with. This activity is possible even in a confined space like a prison cell. Physical activity can actually begin to make you feel less tired and can lift your mood.

Find something that interests you and spend some time on it. Plan to focus on things you usually enjoy and build some time into each day for these activities. You might find it helpful to take a new interest. Some people find that creative activities that help them to express their feelings, such as painting, writing or playing music, can help them feel better.

Look after yourself

Resist the temptation to cope with your low mood by drinking alcohol, misusing medication or turning to illicit drugs. These may give some immediate relief, but quite soon it will create further health and psychological problems for you to cope with.

Try to eat well; choose a healthy option from the prison menu if possible. A good diet can help keep you in good health and recovery is easier.

When should I ask for further help?

We hope the suggestions here have been helpful to you. Distress following trauma usually fades with time. However, if you feel that you are making little progress, then you may want to consider asking for extra help. Especially if you feel like you can no longer cope, or have thoughts of harming yourself. Antidepressants could also be considered to treat PTSD.

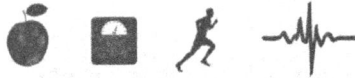

BREATHING TO RELIEVE STRESS

By James Fox

Exercise (10-15 minutes)

Sitting in a cross-legged seated position or upright in a chair, back supported and feet flat on the floor, allow your eyes to close. If you wish, you can also do this exercise laying down on your back.

Feel the weight of your body seated or lying where you are. Breathing in and out of the nose, place your right hand on your belly below the navel with your left palm covering it. Tighten the belly then release it three times, taking a couple of breaths in between doing so. Then let the belly relax becoming soft and feel it rising and falling under your hands as you breath. Be aware that the lower belly about 2 inches below your navel represents the center of your body. Make sure that you exhale slowly and completely before inhaling.

Do this for 10 breath cycles.

Then allow your eyes to open, and taking some full breaths in through your nose and out of your mouth, make an audible sigh upon exhaling (ahhh). Do this 8-10 times. Do not lift your shoulders as you inhale. Notice any area (throat, chest, diaphragm, belly) where you may be holding, gripping or where there is heaviness, and release it as you exhale.

Be sure to exhale completely as you sigh ahhh.

After you have completed this, close your eyes, return to your normal breathing, hands in your lap and just scan the internal energy of your body remaining aware of the natural movement of your breath. Do this for one minute before opening your eyes and completing the exercise.

You can repeat this exercise if desired.

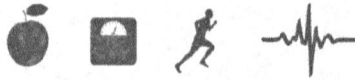

MEDITATION
By Bo Lozoff

It's easy to get so wrapped up in the spiritual "search" that we lose sight of the fact that it's an inner journey. Our greatest discoveries are gained simply by learning how to sit still. That's all meditation is when you get right down to it: Sitting perfectly still—silence of the body, silence of speech, and silence of mind. The Buddha called this *The Noble Silence*. It's just a matter of STOPPING.

Meditation practice has been a central focus of every religion and spiritual tradition, but because it takes place in silence, alone, it's always been set aside in favor of more social/religious practices like preaching and singing. For most of us it'd be easier to slice bread with a sledgehammer than to sit quietly and do "nothing" at all. When we first try a meditation technique, we think "Maybe other people can do this, but not me; I guess it's just not my nature."

But that's a crock. Meditation is hard for everybody, because we've all allowed our minds to run wild for many years. It takes time and effort to regain our rightful control, but it's well worth the discipline. An uncontrolled mind— no matter how much it knows, how smart it becomes, or how many pleasures it experiences—will never find peace or satisfaction. As soon as we fulfill one part of it, it'll hit us with another demand, another question, another passing thought. No wonder we spend about a third of our lives sleeping!

The mind can be a great servant, but a cruel and exhausting master.

Because meditation practice is so hard to get into at first, many different methods have been handed down through the ages so that we can find one that feels best to our individual needs. It's important to understand that meditation itself is a state of mind; it's not a method or exercise. Meditation is beyond words; it's our deepest natural state, which we open into once our mind stops being busy.

Another way of looking at it: Meditation practice is learning how to use our key in the Holy Trinity; meditation itself happens when we finally use our key in harmony with Grace and Spirit. It's also important to remember that just about any meditation method is as good as any other; we just have to choose one and then stick to it with a lot of patience and self-discipline.

Many people spend tremendous amounts of time and energy looking for a Guru or a master who can reveal to them the deepest secrets of the Universe. Such beings do exist, and it's wonderful to meet them, but the desperate search for them is usually just one more way of avoiding doing what we really need to do. There aren't any shortcuts on this path.

Besides, the very best that such a being can do is inspire us to look within ourselves for the "secrets". Wisdom can't be put into words; it has to be experienced. That's the main difference between wisdom and knowledge.

The secrets of the Universe are only secrets of the noisy mind. So, meditation practice is simply about making enough quiet space inside to allow all the wisdom of the ages, all the peace that surpasses understanding, to flow through us freely. It's a slow, steady process of opening and emptying, in the faith that when we make ourselves ready, our own completeness will be right here—and has been here with us all our lives.

Of course, it's not an easy process. Besides all the noise of our conscious minds, we also have some pretty heavy subconscious baggage we carry around with us.

Meditation practice is like turning on a light with a dimmer switch in a big room filled with furniture and clutter. At first we can only see a few things right around where we're starting from, but as the light brightens, we begin to see many vague shapes and shadows that may frighten us. Or we may get depressed when we realize just how far we have to go before this big room is empty—before the mind is really quiet, even for a moment.

But in order for us ever to get quiet, we have to begin right where we are. We may have to sit through intense periods of terror, lust, perversion, fantasy, grief, guilt, greed, pride, loneliness— whatever furniture happens to be stored away in here, collecting cobwebs and taking up our peace.

In order to clear it all out, we have to learn the delicate art of allowing a thought or feeling to be whatever it is, but without getting sucked into it; we can't let it control us. We have to be able to switch the movie of our minds without getting too lost in what's happening on the screen.

That's why all the various meditation methods have a similar approach: By having one point of attention, no matter what comes up in our minds, we can notice it honestly and then get back to the one-point. Then something else comes up, we notice what it is, and get back to the one-point. That's meditation practice.

The process sometimes gets frustrating, but frustration is just one more thought; one more type of noise to notice and then let go of.

There's an old story about Milarepa, one of the great ancient Tibetan masters. Before his enlightenment, he once moved into a secluded cave to do some intensive meditation practice.

But no sooner did he get settled, than he discovered that the cave was also home to a bunch of little demons—little creatures who enjoyed disturbing his meditations.

So the first thing he did was try to get rid of them by preaching the Dharma (the Gospel).

He preached and did all the customary exorcism rituals and then sat back down to meditate; but they were still there.

After a few more unsuccessful tries at preaching and scolding, he changed his strategy: He would completely ignore them. Maybe this would get rid of them. He tried this for a few days; no matter how loud or obnoxious they got, he sat firm and still, resisting them in his silence. But that didn't work either.

Finally, in total frustration and defeat, he screamed "All right, I give up! I can't force you out of here! But I'm not leaving either; I'll just have to share this cave with you!"

Then he sat down once again, his resistance completely gone. And so were the demons.

How To Sit

It's well worth our time to pay attention to the actual physical part of sitting to meditate. Nobody gets spiritual brownie points for looking like a great yogi, or enduring unnecessary pain in the knees and back. On the other hand, we won't gain much control over our minds if we slump over into a half-sleep every time we try to meditate.

What's important is a sitting posture which keeps the back, neck, and head in a straight line, yet is so balanced that there's no tension required to hold ourselves in place.

For most of us this takes a lot of practice. Try sitting on pillows or folded blankets, and see what the best height is for you to be able to sit straight with no effort. The knees should be down, not up, when your butt is at the right height. When the knees are down, the back is naturally straight.

Another sitting position is called "seiza" in Japanese. We sit slightly higher, but straddling the pillows like a saddle, and with our feet behind us. This is very comfortable for many people who can't sit the other ways. Just be sure to get up high enough that the feet don't fall asleep and the knees don't ache.

Sitting in a chair is also all right, although a tendency is to lean against the back of the chair, and that usually isn't very straight. If you do sit in a chair, don't lean; also make sure your feet and legs are symmetrical: legs crossed at the ankles or both feet flat on the floor a few inches apart.

In all of these sitting postures, the hands should be placed either on each leg or in the lap in such a way that you don't feel your shoulders being pulled down by the weight of the hands. Hands can be loosely clasped or held separate. Traditionally, they're kept sort of closed, since and open hand is a gesture of going outward, and meditation is a time to go inward.

Just Sitting Still

It's not a bad idea to use the posture itself as a meditation method for a few days or even a few weeks.

For 20-30 minutes at the same time each day, get as straight and balanced as possible, and then simply pay attention to the body sitting perfectly straight. After the first minute or two of minor shifting and scratching, keep the body in one straight position without moving at all. Pay attention to any feelings of muscle tension or imbalance so that you can learn to sit through the discomfort without moving. This is the first step in learning how to sit through the tougher mental/emotional stuff you may encounter down the line.

If you do use the body as a meditation method, don't be too concerned about what's going on in the mind. Even if the mind is running around like crazy, you're doing fine so long as you keep sitting perfectly still. For the moment, you're just working on "Silence of the body" and "Silence of speech." "Silence of mind" will come later.

Meditation on the Breath

One of the most universal meditation methods is to use your own breath as the one-point of concentration. After getting the body silent, bring all the attention to one of these two points: The tip of your nose, where the breath automatically goes in and out, or the lower abdomen, where the diaphragm rises with each in-breath, and falls with each out-breath.

Whether you choose the nose or the diaphragm, keep the mind right there, feeling the whole movement of each breath in and out. Don't follow it in or out; just keep the attention in one spot, observing however it feels as it goes by.

The breath is a very good one-point for concentration, because it's fresh every second; it helps us bring the mind into the present moment. And the present moment is the only place that true meditation ever happens (in fact, it's the only place anything ever really happens).

Time and time again—maybe hundreds of times in a half hour—the mind will wander, and you'll forget all about observing your breath. But the instant you remember that you forgot, simply drop the chain of thoughts in mid-stream, and get right back to the nose or the diaphragm. As in the story of Milarepa, there's no sense being frustrated by distractions, because the frustration is just another distraction. Remember, this isn't really meditation, anyway; it's meditation practice. If we were already good at it, we wouldn't need to practice.

When using the breath as a meditation method, it's not necessary to breathe any special way, or try to control the breathing at all. The idea is to observe the breath however it is.

Sometimes it may be long and slow, other times short and fast; no matter. Sometimes it's interesting to notice that the breath may change as our thoughts change. This is part of the self-education process. No need to do anything but observe and learn.

It may be helpful to channel the mind into the meditation method by thinking breathing in... as you feel the breath go in, and breathing out... as you feel the breath go out.

But try to make sure that you feel the breath the entire time; don't get stuck in the thought.

If the mind seems particularly wild sometimes, it may help to do this focusing exercise until it comes back under control: As you feel the breath come in, think breathing in and then count the breath as it goes out: Breathing in... one; breathing in... two; breathing in... three; and so forth up until ten, then start at one again. The only rule is, if you lose track of what number you're on—even if you're only slightly unsure—start over.

It's really amazing how our minds are sometimes so busy that we can lose count between one and two! It's happened to me many times. This exercise can be a good occasional indicator of how well or poorly our concentration is coming along.

Mantra Meditations

Mantra is a Sanskrit word that means mind-sound or mind protector. Using a mantra meditation simply means that instead of the breath or the posture, we try to concentrate on a particular sound or word (silently). The practice of using mantras goes back many thousands of years. AMEN and ALLAH are ancient, powerful mantras from the Western religious traditions.

OM, or AUM, is probably the most widely used mantra in the world. After getting the body still and straight, you would just think OM over and over, either along with each breath, or independent of each breath. Every time you get distracted, you simply come back to OM as soon as you remember.

A mantra works on various levels. The obvious one is, like the breath, a mantra provides a single point of attention so we can develop more powerful concentration and non-attachment to our steady stream of thoughts. The mantra becomes like an anchor as our minds toss about in stormy seas.

But at a deeper level, different mantras are said to have different subtle effects. OM helps to put us into harmony with the universe, while another—for example, OM AHH HUMMNN—may bring a more devotional feeling than the other two (it means Dear God, Hail God, Hail Hail God).

There may be many meanings and powers of mantras which we find through our own experiences, but for general purposes, anyone can use these mantras by trial-and-error and trust their own gut feelings to guide them further. If you do try one, try the same one daily for at least a month or two to be able to see how it feels.

Other Meditation Practices

Since the aim of all meditation practices is to bring the mind to one point, anyone should feel perfectly comfortable trying out any methods that feel useful. There are devotional methods like using the word ALLAH or CHRIST, or an image of Jesus or Mother Mary for the mind to try to hold steady.

There are non-devotional methods using imagery too, like holding the vision of a clear sky, through which thoughts keep passing like clouds without stopping. Zen meditators practice meditation with their eyes open, gazing at a spot on the floor about a foot or two in front of them. Many people try to focus their eyes on a candle flame.

Whatever method you choose, it's a good idea to stick with it for at least a month or more at the same time every day (once or twice a day) before deciding to try a new method.

Meditation practice is slow and subtle; it takes a while to know whether the method you choose is working for you.

The busy mind will come up with all sorts of good reasons to drop one method after another, but that's just more noise. Every method really does the same thing. First we have to develop concentration and control, which just takes time. It's difficult to do no matter what methods we use. The key is not which method, but rather our persistence, patience, and good humor.

Ending a Meditation Period

The end of each meditation practice, regardless of which method we use, is a good time to deepen our peace and wisdom in several ways.

What deepens our peace is to spend just a few moments offering and receiving blessings of good will, or what the Buddha calls lovingkindness.

One way of offering these blessings is to focus your attention on the heart-space, right in the middle of the chest, and imagine the breath going in and out of that place, that seat of love. Then picture the faces of people whom you love the most, and the people you hate or fear the most. One by one, offer them all good wishes for their difficult journey through life. Even the people who've hurt us are just stumbling and fumbling through this world like we are; it doesn't help us to hold on to bitterness or anger. So in our mind's eye we see their faces, wish them well, and deepen our own peace and wisdom.

The way to receive blessings is to focus your attention on the heart-space, and begin feeling love from those who love you, anywhere in the world. Your children, parents, lovers, friends, even the great masters and saints whom you can't see—try to feel their love.

Then offer yourself the same loving feelings, the same understanding and kindness, that you would offer to others. Forgive your faults, even the ones you acted on this very day.

Picture yourself sitting here in silence, a sincere spiritual seeker just like millions before you since the beginning of time, and try to appreciate just how much you've already changed in order to be doing this.

Try to realize that what you have prayed for is slowly happening—it really is.

These simple practices can be done in a matter of minutes at the end of each meditation.

What we're doing is to finally begin taking responsibility for controlling our minds and opening up our compassion—for others, ourselves, and ultimately for God.

After these "lovingkindness" techniques, the end of a meditation period is also a ripe time for reading something and letting it sink all the way in to the depth and openness created by sitting still.

For example, you might just open the Bible, Koran, Ramayana or Bhagavad Gita, or even modern Dharma books like Jonathan Livingston Seagull, Be Here Now, or in this book. Open it wherever your fingers seem to choose, and let your eyes glance anywhere they like. Sit for a minute or two trying to comprehend whatever the message is, and then take that thought out into the day with you. Just walk around the prison or wherever you are and look at all the people—all the pleasures and fears, hopes and sorrows, all the countless complex situations we create for ourselves, and see it as Rings and knots of joy and grief, all interlaced and locking. Gradually we begin to see our own lives in this way too; and wisdom deepens...

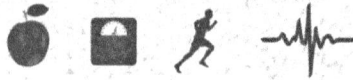

MEDITATION SECRETS

Jack Kornfield

Daily Meditation Practice

Exercise (20-30 minutes)

A daily meditation practice can help you to remain centered, connected to your authentic self, and allows for inner wisdom to arise.

First, choose a suitable space for your regular meditation. It can be wherever you can sit easily with minimum disturbance. Arrange what is around you so that you are reminded of your meditative purpose. You may want to make a place for favorite spiritual books, photos or cards.

Then select a regular time to practice that suits your schedule and temperament. If you are a morning person, sit before breakfast. If evenings fit your temperament or schedule better, try that first. Begin with sitting 10-20 minutes. Later you can sit longer or more often.

Daily meditation can become like bathing, a regular cleaning and calming for your mind and heart.

Sit in a posture that reflects dignity without being rigid. Allow your spine to lengthen, shoulders relaxed, palms of hands resting on your thighs, or placed in your lap with the top of the right hand resting in the open unturned palm of your left hand, allowing your thumbs to touch gently. Let the tip of your tongue rest on the upper ridge of your mouth, behind your teeth. Let go of any worries, concerns, habitual thoughts. Feel your body seated where you are. Feel its weight. Find any tension in your body—face, neck, shoulders, belly—and let it go.

Then tune into the natural movement of your breath. Feel the breath as it moves in and out of the body, and feel the sensations in the body that accompany the breath. The rise and fall of the belly, the chest, the expansion of the ribcage, the sensation of the air as it moves through the nostrils. Let the breath be natural. Feel the sensation in the breath, relaxing into the breath, noticing how the soft sensations of breathing come and go with each inhale and exhale. Take a few full breaths sensing where you feel the breath most easily.

You will notice that after a few breaths your mind will begin to wander. When you notice this, no matter how long or short you drifted off on thoughts, simply bring your awareness back to the next breath. If you wish to, you can mindfully acknowledge where your attention had been by softly saying a word, such as "thinking," "remembering," "hearing," etc. Gently and directly return to feel the next breath. One word of acknowledgement and return to the breath is best. As you sit, let the breath change its rhythm naturally. Calm yourself by relaxing into the breath. When you become distracted by thoughts, gently bring yourself back to your breath, a thousand times if necessary. Be patient and kind with yourself. Over the weeks and months of this practice you will learn how to calm and center yourself using the breath. You will experience many cycles in the process, difficult days and more easy ones. Stay with it. As you do, deeply listening and feeling, you will be able to disengage from constant thinking and connect deeply with your body and spirit.

Walking Meditation

Practice (20-30 minutes)

Walking meditation is a simple and universal practice for developing calm, connectedness and awareness. It can be practiced regularly, on its own, or before or after sitting meditation.

The art of walking meditation is to learn to be aware as you walk, to use the natural movement of walking to cultivate mindful awareness.

Select a place where you can walk comfortably back and forth, indoors or out, ideally ten to thirty paces in length. This can become an excellent meditation practice for walking on the yard if you can train yourself to let go of distractions and stay within yourself. You can also use this practice in your cell. Even though it is a small space with few steps from one wall to the other, you can walk very slowly, and deliberately using the practice to center yourself and practice being present in the moment.

Begin by standing with your feet firmly planted. Let your hands rest easily wherever they are comfortable. Close your eyes for a moment, center yourself and feel your body in touch with the earth. Feel the pressure on the bottoms of your feet and other natural sensations of standing. Then open your eyes and let yourself be fully present and alert.

Begin to walk slowly with a sense of ease and dignity. Pay attention to your body. With each step feel the sensations of lifting your foot and leg off the ground. Be aware as you place each foot on the earth. Relax and let your walking be easy and natural. Feel each step mindfully as you walk, particularly the soles of your feet as the contact they ground or floor. Pay attention to your breathing. You may wish to time your steps to your inhale and exhale.

If you are walking a straight path, when you reach the end of it, pause for a moment centering yourself. Carefully turn around and pause again so that you can be aware of your first step as you walk back.

If you are walking around the yard, simply stay focused on the bodily sensations of walking, the feeling of your feet contacting the ground and your breath. You experiment with whatever pace keeps you most present.

Continue to walk back and forth for 10 to 20 minutes, or longer. As with the breath and sitting, your mind will wander many times. When you notice that you can acknowledge it softly by saying to yourself: "wandering," "thinking," "hearing," "planning," etc. Then return with awareness to the next step. Whether you drift off for a second or a few minutes, simple acknowledge that you have and come back to a full awareness of your next step.

After some practice with walking meditation you will learn to use it to calm and collect yourself, and live more fully in your body. You can extend your practice in an informal way as you walk to various places throughout your day. You will learn to enjoy walking as a simple way to be truly present, bringing your body, heart and mind together as you move through life.

Meditation Reflecting on Difficulty

Practice (15 minutes)

Sit quietly, feeling the rhythm of the natural breathing, letting yourself become calm and receptive. Then think of a difficulty you are experiencing in your life. As you sense this difficulty, notice how it affects your body, heart and mind. Feeling it carefully, begin to ask a few questions, listening inwardly for answers.

How have I treated this difficulty so far? How have I suffered by my own response and reaction to it? What is this problem asking me to let go of? What suffering is unavoidable, and which is my measure to accept? What great lesson might this be able to teach me? What is the gold, the value hidden in this situation?

In using this reflection to consider your difficulties, the openings and understandings may come slowly. Be patient and kind with yourself. As with all meditations, it can be helpful to repeat this meditation many times, listening each time for deeper understanding and answers from your body, heart and spirit.

Meditation on Stopping the War Within

Practice (15-20 minutes)

You can engage in this practice for releasing the mental and emotional battles you have been waging inside of yourself.

Sit comfortably for a few minutes, letting your body be at rest, your breathing easy and natural. Bring your attention into the present and notice sensations in your body. In particular notice any tension, pain or sensations you may have been struggling with. Do not try to change them, simply notice them with interest and kind attention.

For each area of struggle in your life you discover, focus on relaxing your body and softening your heart. Open to whatever your experience is without resisting. Just breathe naturally and let it be.

Then after a few minutes., shift your attention to your heart and mind. Notice what emotions and thoughts are present. In particular notice any feelings or thoughts you are avoiding, going against or denying. Notice them with interest and kind attention. Let your heart be soft opening whatever you are experiencing without fighting. Let go of the battle; let it be.

Continue to sit quietly. Then bring your attention to all the battles that still exist in your life. Sense them inside of you. If you have an ongoing battle with your body, be aware of that. If you have been fighting inner wars with your feelings, been in conflict with your own loneliness, fear, confusion, grief, anger, despair or addiction, sense the upset that you have been carrying. Notice the struggles in your thoughts as well. Be aware of how you have been waging inner battles. Be aware of all that you have fought and been fighting within yourself, and how long you've been carrying on the conflict.

Gently and with openness, allow these experiences to be present, noticing them with kind attention. In each area of struggle let your body, heart and mind be soft. Open to whatever you are experiencing without fighting. Let it be present just as it is. Let go of the battle, the constant struggling. Breathe quietly and let yourself be at rest. Invite your mind, heart and body to be at peace.

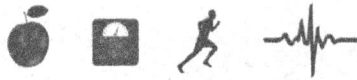

GROWING OLD GRACEFULLY

Today the average duration of human life in the United States is just about 70 years for women, and a little less for men. Conservative experts believe that man is really built to last about 100 years; and that medical advances and more healthful living habits could bring this about within a generation.

What good is it to add years to life if we do not also add life to years? In fact, unless people learn to enjoy life and grow old gracefully, the extra years may just be an additional burden.

From 18 to 30 years is roughly the period of highest physical and mental vigor. The experiences we accumulate from the day we are born help us to conserve and use our physical and mental abilities more wisely, so that for some time after 30 years we are able to perform increasingly well in spite of slowly slipping vigor. After age 50 the increasing accumulation of experiences is no longer able to offset the now more rapidly declining energy and therefore aging begins to assert itself noticeably and in many ways.

A number of things may come about gradually, such as people who have not used eyeglasses before may at some time in their forties need them for reading, and in their fifties they usually need bifocals.

Also in the forties, people are likely to put on weight because there is a general slowdown in the oxidation rate of the aging body tissue. Also we tend to do less strenuous work with no reduction in the amount of food consumed.

And in the fifties there is likely to be some loss of hearing. Usually the high-pitched tones go first, so words with the sounds of F, S, and TH are confused. A hearing aid may be needed in some cases.

Aging is generally accompanied by a loss in physical and mental flexibility. This is noticed in a tendency to become stiff in the joints; in slower comeback after a strenuous trip, excessive "partying," or hard work; in slower healing of wounds, sore muscles, and sprains; in slower recovery after an illness; and in greater difficulty to adjust to new people, new places, and new ideas.

Men, especially, will notice loss of muscular strength. There will be increased unsteadiness and delicate muscle movements will be more clumsy and the stride in walking will become shorter. The conclusion now is that the performance and ability of the elderly has long been underestimated and can be greatly improved by a proper diet, sleep and exercise along with rest and relaxation.

Most elderly people tend to lose their joy and will to live and chronic worriers may mope around and withdraw. Medical authorities say that laughter is one of the best medicines for the elderly. You can always keep your sense of humor tuned up by surrounding yourself with pleasant and interesting people. Just act your age and don't be afraid to laugh at yourself even when no one else is around.

Now that we all know the role that physical activity takes place in our lives, remember to do something physical every day. The joints must be used or quite simply they will tighten with age creating that stooped worn out appearance we often associate with getting old. Keep yourself flexible and fit on an exercise program consistent with your ability.

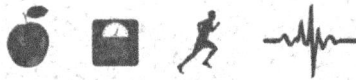

FACTS ABOUT ALZHEIMER'S DISEASE

Alzheimer's Disease is the term used to describe a dementing disorder marked by certain brain changes, regardless of the age of onset. Alzheimer's disease is not a normal part of aging—and it is not something that inevitably happens in later life. Rather, it is one of the dementing disorders, a group of brain diseases that lead to the loss of mental and physical functions. The disorder, whose cause is unknown, affects a small but significant percentage of older Americans. A very small minority of Alzheimer's patients are under 50 years of age. However, most are 65.

Alzheimer's disease is the exception, rather than the rule, in old age. Only 5 to 6 percent of older people are afflicted by Alzheimer's disease or related dementia—but this means approximately 3.3 million Americans (including prisoners) have one of these debilitating disorders. Research indicates that 1 percent of the population aged 65-75 has severe dementia, increasing to 7 percent of those aged 75-85 and to 25 percent of those 85 or older.

The onset of Alzheimer's disease is usually very slow and gradual, seldom occurring before age 65. Over time, however, it follows a progressively more serious course. Among the symptoms that typically develop, none is unique to Alzheimer's disease at its various stages. It is therefore essential for suspicious changes to be thoroughly evaluated before they become inappropriately or negligently labeled Alzheimer's disease.

Problems of memory, particularly recent or short-term memory, are common early in the course of the disease. For example, the individual may, on repeated occasions, forget to turn off an appliance or may not recall which of the morning's medicines were taken. Mild personality changes, such as less spontaneity or a sense of apathy and a tendency to withdraw from social interactions, may occur early in the illness. As the disease progresses, problems in abstract thinking or in intellectual functioning develop. You may notice beginning to have trouble with figures when doing math, with understanding what is being read, or with organizing what you're going to do for the day. Further disturbances in behavior and appearance may also be seen at this point, such as agitation, irritability, quarrelsomeness, and diminishing ability to dress appropriately.

The average course of the disease from the time it is recognized to death is about 6 to 8 years, but it may range from under 2 years to over 20 years. Those who develop the disorder later in life may die from other illnesses (such as heart disease) before Alzheimer's disease reaches its final and most serious stage.

The reaction of an individual to the illness and the way he or she copes with it also varies and may depend on such factors as lifelong personality patterns and the nature and severity of the stress in the immediate environment. As research on the disease continues, scientists are now describing other abnormal chemical changes associated with the disease. These include nerve cell degeneration in certain areas of the brain. Also, defects in certain blood vessels supplying blood to the brain have been studied as a possible contributing factor.

At the present time there's no way to determine who will get Alzheimer's disease. The disease has emerged as one of the great mysteries in modern day medicine, with a growing number of clues but still no answer as to its cause.

Because of the many other disorders that are often confused with Alzheimer's disease, a comprehensive clinical evaluation is essential to arrive at a correct diagnosis of any symptoms that look similar to those of Alzheimer's disease.

While Alzheimer's disease remains a mystery, with its cause and cure not yet found, there is considerable excitement and hope about new findings that are unfolding in numerous research settings. The connecting pieces to the puzzle called Alzheimer1s disease continue to be found.

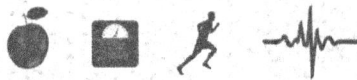

WORKING OUT: THE SECRETS

Just about everyone has heard the old adage "survival of the fittest." Well, that statement could never be more fitting than it is for describing life in the devil's playground. Not only is it extremely important to stay physically fit for physical health reasons, but for mental health and safety reasons as well.

It's true that your body is your temple. And in prison, unless you're on death row, the "authorities" can take just about everything from you but your temple. They can take all your personal property if they want to-justified or not. They can put you in the hole somewhere, by yourself, and even take your state-issued clothing, mattress, etc.; leaving you in a dark, cold cell with absolutely nothing. Trust me, I know; I've been through it.

So, being that they can't take your temple and, in the end, you are all you really have, no investment is as important as the one you invest into yourself.

Furthermore, prison is an extremely dangerous place; it is ruled by violence. Prison is full of brutes, beasts and bullies, who often want to prove themselves as the strongest, toughest, and most savage. If you want to increase your odds of surviving among such men, then you need to be in the best physical shape you can be in. You can bet that the prisoners around you are exercising and building their bodies as much as they can, so if you aren't, what are the odds you will be able to hold your own if and when it comes time for battle?

Prisoners are known for having a particular build (often referred to as a "prison build" big on top with skinny legs. A lot of prisoners focus on upper-body workouts because, in prison, we often have our shirts off, and guys want to look as big and buff as possible. It is also a defense mechanism, the bigger you are, the more intimidating you look; the more intimidating you look, the less people will want to challenge you. I know plenty of big boys who are pussies; however, not too many people want to take the chance of finding out for themselves.

Working towards achieving the "prison build" is an unintelligent way to work out. In order to work out properly, you must work your legs as well; they are your foundation. If you're top- heavy with the itty-bitty broomstick legs, you leave yourself open for a smart person-one who may even be smaller than you-to sweep them out from under you. And unless you're a trained MMA fighter or something, once you're on the ground, it will be easy for even a small guy to take advantage of your vulnerable position.

Working out/exercising/body building is not something you can master by reading a chapter or two out of a book or even by reading a book or two, for that matter. The art and science of "body building" is something that takes years and years of practice and study in order to really learn and master. Furthermore, I have read many muscle magazines over the years, and each one has had a different philosophy regarding what will get you the "best" results.

In the end, what it boils down to is that everybody is different, and you need to learn what works best for you and your body type. What works for one man may not work very well for you and on the flip side, what one man may think is ineffective may be what gets you your best results.

However, to get you started on becoming the man you're meant to be so better learn to be if you intend on surviving prison, I'm going to explain to you some of the more popular prisoner muscle-building exercises, as well as some techniques you are not likely to see the average prisoner doing on the yard, because they are the secrets told to me by some of the biggest, most powerful prisoners I've ever met.

Not all prisons have "weights" these days. Therefore, most of the exercises I'm going to explain to you are ones you can do without weights. However I'm also going to explain to you how we make our own weights in prison.

Here are some great exercises that will help you get in tip top shape.

BICEPS:

If you want to turn your biceps into solid rocks, you're going to have to do a lot of curls. In order to do a lot of curls, you're going to need something to curl, right? Well, since prison doesn't typically provide dumbbells, you're going to have to make your own.

Mattress Dumbbell

More than likely you have one of those 3-4-inch thick mattresses that are hard as hell and weigh about 30 pounds. And while it's a worthless provider of a good night's rest, it can easily be turned into a 30-pound dumbbell.

It is simple to make a curling weight out of your mattress. First, take your sheet, roll it up so that it forms a long strip, and lay it in the center of your floor. Then, roll your mattress up as tight as you can. Once your mattress is rolled into a tight roll, set it in the middle of your sheet "strip," and tie your sheet strip around your mattress so that it remains tightly rolled.

Once you have tied your sheet around your mattress, you will be able to grab the excess sheet strip and use it as a handle (for curling).

If curling your mattress is something you plan to do regularly, and you don't want to use your entire sheet, you can make "customized" ties by braiding 3-inch thick strips of sheet together, and instead of tying one strip around the middle, some prisoners prefer to use two ties and tie both ends of the rolled-up mattress. They then take an additional strip and tie it across the mattress, from one end-tie to the other, and use that as a handle. This gives it more of a dumbbell feel, and it also makes it easier to balance.

Once you have your mattress dumbbell, you are officially ready to start curling. You can do one arm curls for your "bulk weight" sets and two-arm curls for your burnouts. You can also do hammer curls and reverse curls for a more thorough arm workout.

I've explained to you how to make a dumbbell out of your mattress and sheet because those are items you will usually have access to. They're items provided to us, unless you're on some kind of discipline status where your stuff has been taken, you will always be able to utilize this method. However, there are many other ways prisoners make dumbbells when the materials are available, including ones that are much heavier.

Water Bag

When the materials are available, a lot of prisoners would rather curl a water bag than their mattress; curling a water bag is a lot less awkward. Furthermore, it's easier to customize the weight of a water bag so that it suits you best.

To make a water bag, you will need a large, thick trash bag. (Usually you can get one from the building porter(s).) Fill the trash bag with the amount of water that will give you the weight you want. Once you have put the amount of water you want into your bag, squeeze all the air out of your bag and tie the top into a knot by twisting the excess bag, looping it around itself and pulling it through.

Once you have made your water weight, get an old T-shirt and tie off the bottom. Then, put your water weight inside of the T-shirt, and take the sleeves of your T-shirt and tie them together as tight as you can.

Now that your shirt sleeves are tied together, you can use them as your handle. If you want you can put a separate piece of sheet or towel through the tied sleeves and use that for a handle. You can do one-arm, two-arm, hammer, and reverse curls; the shirt will prevent the bag from busting open.

Weight Bag

No access to a large, thick trash bag? Then you can always make a weight bag out of magazines. All you need to do is stack up about 8-inches of magazines and tie them together real tight with a shoestring or sheet strip-so that you have a "block" of magazines. You can make a few of these block weights, put them inside of a T-shirt and do the same thing you'd do with a water bag. Block weights are a little more awkward to curl than a water bag but they still work extremely well.

Note: Correctional Officers usually confiscate water and weight bags. However, if they find yours just make another one; it's nothing.

Sometimes, especially when you are in the hole, you will have to find other ways to work your biceps. When you don't have the materials to build a bag and you don't feel like curling your mattress, or your mattress isn't heavy enough, you may want to try this next exercise.

Body Weight Curls

Do you have a top bunk in your cell? If so, is there a space between the bunk and the wall (somewhere)? If there is, you can always wrap your sheet around the part of the bunk that's bolted or welded to the wall (usually the comer of the bunk), hold onto the sheet, lean back as far as you can, and then curl your own body weight. This method also allows you to do a variety of curling exercises-one-arm, two-arm, hammers, reverse, etc., and you can make your weight more difficult to curl by leaning further back.

TRICEPS

Tired of having noodle arms as skinny as your finger? Well, then you're going to have to put a lot of work into building your triceps also known as back-arms. Triceps make up 2/3 of your arm size; a triceps is a much bigger muscle than a bicep.

There are several ways for you to work your triceps, and here are a few of the more popular ways prisoners do it without the use of weights...

Nose-breakers

Nose-breakers can be done just about anywhere. All you have to do is grab the edge of your table, sink, toilet, etc., with an overhand grip, and take a step or two back. Once you are in position, lower your nose down to the edge of whatever it is you're grabbing, and using only your arms, push yourself back up. Repeat the up and down process until you fall forward and break your nose.

Depending on what you're grabbing, you can adjust your grip from narrow to wide. And you can adjust your weight by stepping farther back to make it more difficult.

Modified handstand triceps push-ups

Another great way you can work out your triceps is by doing modified handstand triceps pushups. These, too, can be done in just about any prison cell, and they are a bit more difficult than nose-breakers.

To do a modified handstand triceps push-up, place your hands on the floor (palms down) so your index fingers and thumbs make a triangle. Then, plant your feet on your toilet or stool behind you, push your hips up high, and bend your knees slightly. Lower your body straight down until the top of your head touches the floor. Keeping your back aligned, push back up; repeat the up and down process as many times as you can.

Note: You should brace your abs throughout this move.

Plank triceps extensions

Get into a plank position with your forearms on the floor—basically a push-up position with your palms and forearms flat on the ground. Your elbows should be directly below your shoulders. Push through your palms to straighten your arms, keeping your abs tight throughout.

"Bench" triceps extensions

This exercise is similar to a nose-breaker, but it will give you a slightly different stretch, and it is a little more difficult.

Get into a push-up position with your hands gripping the edge of your toilet, stool or desk. Bend your elbows and drop your head down until it's slightly under what it is you decide to grab. Push yourself back up, and then repeat the up and down process. This is good because the triceps respond well to exercises that overload the stretch portion of the movement.

Incorporate these triceps exercises into your workout plan and you should do all right. And remember, some of the other exercises you do, such as push-ups and dips, will also work your triceps.

CHEST

Now it's time to pump your chest up a little bit. Nobody in prison is going to take you serious if you're walking around with negative chest-the kind that is not even flat, it goes in.

Here are some of the more popular ways prisoners bulk their chest up...

Push-ups

Hopefully you already know how to do a push-up and can actually do one (and I don't mean on your knees). If you can't do a push-up then you're in serious trouble, and there isn't anything me or any book you read will be able to do to help you. In such a case, your best bet would be to get going and learn how!

So, assuming you already know how to do a push-up, the best advice I can give you is to do all variations of them: wide for your outer chest, shoulder-width for the middle portion of your chest, and diamonds for your inner chest.

You can also work the top portion of your chest by elevating your feet on your toilet, stool, or desk. This is equivalent to an incline bench press, and the higher you elevate your feet, the more weight it will put on your upper chest (and shoulders).

Many prisoners like to add weight to their push-ups by having their cellmate sit or lean against their back. For example, get into a push-up position. Then, your cellmate can put his butt and back up against your butt and back and lean his weight on you while you do your push-ups.

Fly Push-up:

Fly push-ups will also get you great results; it is equivalent to a fly press.

To do a fly push-up, fold two towels up and place one under each hand while you kneel on your floor with your hands under your shoulders-like a push-up position, but on your knees. Spread your hands apart and lower your chest to the floor, bending your elbows. (It should look like the down position of a wide-grip push-up). Push yourself back up while also pulling your hands together in a fly motion.

Note: This works best if your cell floor is waxed; it will help the towels slide easier. If necessary, you can also try soaping up the area of the floor where the towels will be sliding.

Scorpion Push-up:

Get into a push-up position and squeeze your butt cheeks. As you descend, rotate your upper body to your left while swinging your left leg across your right leg. Your left foot should touch the floor somewhere between your right foot and right hand (looking like a scorpion's tail). Push yourself back up and return the leg.

Dips are a great exercise that work a variety of muscles including your chest, triceps, and abs. Most prison yards have dip bars, so the opportunity to do dips is usually available.

If your yard doesn't have dip bars available or if you are on lockdown and don't have access to the yard, or if you'd rather just do them in your cell, there's usually a way that you can-depending on how your cell is designed.

Sometimes you can do dips between the top bunk and top locker. If one is a little higher than the other, you may need to place a book under the hand that is lower.

Some cells provide a place to do dips between your bottom locker and desk. However, if neither of these two ways are available, you can also do dips on a high, flat surface, such as a top bunk. All you have to do is balance yourself on the palms of your hands by leaning slightly forward, lower yourself down until your chest touches the bunk, and then push yourself back up. The stretch won't be as good as if dipping between two objects, but it still works.

ABS

Many prisoners like having ripped abs. The more defined your stomach is, the bigger your chest, shoulders, and arms look. Furthermore, if you are one of the lucky prisoners that will be getting out someday, the ladies will love it.

Crunches

Lie on your back with your legs bent and your heels close to your butt; put your chin on your chest and your hands behind your head. Then, raise your head up crunching your abs hard (you should only go about 1/3 of the way as compared to traditional sit-ups), lower, and repeat the movement as many times as you can.

Punch Plank

Get into a push-up position, balancing on your first two knuckles (of each hand), and with your feet no wider than shoulder width, lift one hand near your chin, resisting the urge to rotate your shoulders. Squeeze your pec on the side that's balancing and shift your weight on the opposite foot; hold it for as long as you can.

This exercise works your obliques really well. It also teaches you to bring your body's full strength together for things like push-ups and punching.

Full-contact Plank

Get into plank position. Have your cellmate shove your midsection or kick your thighs and soles of your feet to increase the challenge. Keep your body completely straight and resist any kind of motion.

Drop Plank

Get into a push-up position and lock your elbows. Push your palms into the floor so your shoulder blades flare out and your chest caves in closer to the floor. Tighten your body. Have your cellmate pick up both of your feet and then release one of them without warning. Now, prevent your leg from falling to the floor.

Note: When doing this exercise, always keep your shoulders parallel to the floor and look straight down.

Crunch Chin-up

Hang from a chin-up bar, and keeping your body rigid, pull yourself up. As you near the top, raise your knees to your chest, balling yourself up. Finish each rep by pausing for a moment in the up position.

BACK/LATS

Now it's time for you to learn how most prisoners build a big, strong, powerful back...

Pull-Ups

The best way for you to work your back and lats in prison is by doing pull-ups. Doing pull-ups will make you a lot stronger while adding bulk to your back and building your lats so that you get that nice "V" shape.

To do a pull-up properly, grab the pull-up bar with an underhand grip and hang down getting a good stretch in your lats. Then, pull yourself up until your chest hits the bar, lower yourself back down, and repeat as many times as you can.

Note: The concept of pull-ups is fairly simple, but actually doing them isn't that easy until you build yourself up. When you first begin, if you need some assistance, bend your knees, cross your ankles, and have your cellmate or workout partner hold your feet.

Do pull-ups with several grip widths. The wider you go, the harder it will be. You will also notice that pull-ups work your arms out as well.

Overhand Grip Pull-Up

These are done the same way as a standard pull-up but with your palms facing out (you should see the backs of your hands).

Overhand grip pull-ups should also be done in a variety of widths, and you should notice that when you put your hands together, it will work your forearms and biceps really well. When you grip the bar as wide as you can, the pull-up will be harder, but doing so is how you stretch your body wide and get the wings most prisoners want.

Behind the Head Pull-Up

Once you strengthen your back, shoulders and arms, you can do behind the head pull-ups. To do this exercise, grab the bar as wide as you can with an overhand grip and pull up, but, instead of touching your chest with the bar, tuck your head down and touch the back of your neck or top of your shoulders with the bar. This exercise will put a lot more strain on your back and shoulders than a standard pull-up.

Hyper-extensions:

It's important to have a strong lower back; not only so you have strong core muscles, but also because it will help you prevent back pain. And considering all the pain you're going to have anyway from sleeping on that hard prison mattress, you're going to need all the back pain prevention you can get.

The best way to strengthen your lower back in prison is by doing hyper-extensions. In order to do these, however, your prison yard will need to have long, parallel dip bars.

To do hyper-extensions, get in between the two bars, facing one. Grab the bar in front of you and push yourself up. Rest your lower stomach on the bar and lean forward, hooking your legs on the bar behind you to keep your body from flipping all the way over. Let go of the bar you're holding and place your hands behind your head. Then, bend forward at the waist as fast as you can, raise back up until your back is straight, and repeat the down-up motion as many times as you can.

SHOULDERS

If you're interested in filling up your prison shirt you're going to need to have big, strong shoulders.

Handstand Push-Ups

Pull-ups will work your shoulders, but only to a certain extent. If you really want to have big, strong, bulky shoulders, you will need to do handstand push-ups.

To do a handstand push-up, get into a handstand next to your cell well or door, and put your toes or heels–depending on which way you're facing against the wall door for balance. Once you are in a stable position, lower yourself until the top of your head touches the ground, push yourself back up, and repeat as many times as you can.

This is a difficult exercise for most people, so it may take a little bit for you to build up the strength in order to be able to do these. When you first start, ask your celly to hold your ankles to prevent you from falling forward. Falling forward in a little tiny cell isn't fun when there's metal bunks, toilets, and lockers to fall into.

LEGS

As I mentioned earlier in this section, in order to build your body properly, you must work out your legs. Your legs are your foundation; your foundation needs to be strong and rock solid. What good is a big, buff chest, if you get into an altercation and your opponent sweeps your skinny, weak legs out from under you and you fall to the ground? That will put you in a vulnerable and dangerous position.

Here are some of the popular leg exercises many prisoners do.

Squats

Squats work real well for building power and endurance in your thighs. To do a squat, stand with your legs about shoulder width apart. Stick your arms straight out in front of you for balance, and while looking up, slowly bend your knees and lower yourself until your butt is just about touching the floor. Using only your legs to lift you, slowly stand back up as straight as you can (keep your heels on the floor). Repeat the up and down squat process as many times as you can, and for variation you can place your feet wider apart or closer together.

Note: Once you build up your leg strength and you're ready to step it up a notch, you can do squats with your cellmate or workout partner on your shoulders. If you do this, do it under a pull-up bar so the person on your shoulders can hold on to the pull-up bar for balance, and when you're first beginning this exercise, can even pull himself up slightly to make it easier on you.

Harbor Steps

While they're typically called harbor steps, obviously nobody in prison is doing them on a harbor. Instead, we do them on our toilet or stool.

Harbor steps are good for working your thighs and calves, and they can be done in any cell.

To do a harbor step, place your left foot onto the edge of your toilet or stool, and using only the muscles of your left leg, stand all the way up straight. Lower yourself down, step off the toilet, and repeat with your right leg. Do as many as you can.

Note: If you really want a high step, try doing these on your desk. The higher you step, the harder it is.

Lunges

Lunges are also a great leg exercise you can do anytime, anywhere, and they work just about every part of your leg.

To do a lunge, start in a standing position with your hands on your hips. Then, with your left leg, step forward as far as you can, keeping your back straight in an up position, and touching your right knee to the ground. Without moving your right foot from its spot, step your left foot back so that it's side-by-side with your right and your body is standing back up completely straight. Do as many as you can, alternating between your left and right legs.

Calf Raises

Calf raises will build and strengthen your calves. You should do them on the edge of your toilet, and hold on to the wall for balance. While standing on the edge of your toilet, lower your heels to get a good stretch, then raise up on your toes as high as you can. Lower yourself back down and repeat the process as many times as you can.

Note: You can do these on the floor but you won't get the same stretch. However, when doing them on the floor, you can do different variations by pointing your toes in or out. Doing so will ensure you work all sides of your calf muscle.

Secrets

Now that I've explained to you the most popular and effective exercises done by prisoners, it's time to let you in on a few secrets on how to maximize your gain from doing them. If you ever wonder why these exercises seem to work better for some prisoners than others, it is because they are utilizing the following techniques.

Work to failure

This first technique is to just do the exercises in their traditional manner, but instead of doing a specific amount of reps during your sets, do each exercise until you no longer can. Doing this might not get you a lot of size, but it will definitely build up your endurance, and endurance is extremely important for later, heavier workouts.

Flex Hard and Hold It

Flex the muscle(s) you are about to work as hard as you can and hold it for 10 seconds, thus, pre-fatiguing them. For example, flex your triceps and chest muscles as hard as you can and then do a set of push-ups. This makes doing something as basic as push-ups much more difficult and produces much better results.

Reduce Rest Time Between Sets

Another technique is to reduce the rest time between sets. Start with resting for 60 seconds, then 50, 40, 30, 20, 10, etc. If you do a set of pull-ups and go until your muscles are really tired or even to failure, wait only a few seconds then do another set. How many reps were you able to do in your second set? Only 4 or 5, right? That's about what you'd do if you were doing some heavy pull-downs.

Supersets

This is one of my favorite techniques. It's what gets me a real good pump.

To do a superset, alternate exercises between two "opposite" muscles–biceps/triceps, chest/back, etc. For example, do a set of curls and then, without resting, do a set of nose-breakers. Going back and forth between these two exercises will have all the blood rushing to both your biceps and triceps and give you a great pump; your arms will feel like they are going to explode!

Slow Motion Reps

Slow motion reps are really good, especially when you don't have weights. To do these, try taking a full 12 seconds for the positive phase and 6 seconds for the negative phase of each rep. Don't lock out in the top position and don't rest in the bottom position-transition smoothly from the positive to the negative. Using slow continuous tension will make your exercise much more intense.

Flex While Doing Your Reps

For this last technique, try flexing your muscles as hard as you can while doing your exercise. For example, flex your pectorals, shoulders, triceps, biceps, and lats as hard as you can while doing very slow push-ups. Or, when doing pull-ups, flex your lats, shoulders, biceps, triceps, chest, and forearms as hard as you can.

Keep the tension hard and steady when using this technique. It may take some practice to get it down, but the incredible pump and muscle growth you will get from it will be well worth it.

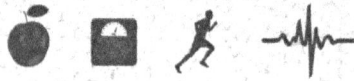

EXERCISE TIPS

Get Comfortable

Wear loose, comfortable clothes, and layer your clothes so you can add or remove layers to stay comfortable as you exercise. Wear shoes that have good support and soles made out of non-slip shock-absorbent material. Consider wearing shock-absorbent insoles to help cushion your joints.

Get A Drink

Drinking water throughout the day helps keep your body functioning properly, flushing toxins from your vital organs and carrying nutrients to your cells. It's especially important to drink water when exercising, as your body loses water through sweat and a faster breathing rate. If you don't drink enough fluids you could become dehydrated draining your energy and making you feel tired.

Try to drink the recommended eight (8 oz.) glasses, of water each day. It's important to be hydrated before exercise and replenish fluids afterwards. You may want to have a bottle of water with you while you exercise.

Warm Up

No matter what exercise you're doing, take five to 15 minutes to warm up before you begin your routine to reduce your chance of injury. To warm up, walk slowly for a few minutes or do a slow version of the activity you plan to do, then do gentle stretches. Simply move toward the end of your full range of motion (ROM), hold for five seconds and relax. Make sure to stretch all the muscles you'll be using during your exercise routine.

Stretching should NOT hurt. Move only until you feel a gentle stretch, then hold. Don't push so hard it hurts.

Don't Do Too Much Too Fast

Slight muscle pain is a normal part of starting a new exercise program. If you have more joint pain after you exercise than you did before, however, you've probably done too much and should cut back a little. Don't stop exercising completely—that could cause your pain to feel worse. Instead, reduce the number of times you do each exercise or do them a little more gently.

Don't Hurry

Rushing through your exercise routine doesn't make it more effective. Instead exercise at a comfortable, steady pace that allows you to speak to someone without running out of breath. Exercising at this pace gives your muscles time to relax between each repetition.

Do your ROM and flexibility exercises slowly and completely rather than doing many repetitions at a fast pace. If the exercises become too easy you can gradually increase the number of repetitions you do in each set.

Breathe

Don't hold your breath while you exercise. Instead, breathe out (exhale) as you do the exercise, and breathe in (inhale) as you relax between repetitions. Counting out loud during the exercise will help you breathe deeply and regularly. If you develop muscle pain or a cramp while exercising, gently rub and stretch the muscle. When the pain is gone continue your exercise with slow easy movements.

Cool Down

It's important to cool down after exercising to reduce your chances of injury. Cooling down simply means to slow down your exercises, not stop them completely. To cool down, simply repeat the exercises you did for warm-up. Be sure to cool down for five to 15 minutes, allowing: your heart rate and breathing to return to normal. End with gentle stretches to prevent muscles from becoming too sore.

Exercise can deplete your energy, and you may need to refuel your body to recover, repair tissue and get stronger. Ideally, you should try to eat something high in lean protein or with complex carbohydrates within 60 minutes of completing your workout, such as a handful of almonds, or fruit such as an orange, apricot, or plum.

Overcoming Obstacles To Exercise

Although you'll see the best results if you exercise on a regular basis, it can be difficult to keep up a routine day in and day out. There may be times when you feel too busy or too tired to; do your exercise routine. Instead of skipping a day just reduce the number of sets or the length of time you exercise.

Try to do ROM and aerobic exercises daily and your strengthening exercises every other day.

If you miss a day, don't be discouraged. You can pick up again where you left off. If you miss a few days, you may need to start again slowly to avoid injury and muscle soreness. Just don't give up completely. Inactivity can lead to muscle atrophy and further decrease joint stability.

If you're having trouble making time for exercising, try exercising at different times of the day to see what works best for you. There may be a time of the day when you learn works best for you. Some things you can try:

- √ Exercise in the morning before work to get the day started.
- √ Avoid strenuous exercises just after you eat; wait to exercise at least two hours after a meal.
- √ Do gentle ROM exercises before bed; this can help make you feel less stiff in the morning.
- √ Don't do any aerobic exercises before going to bed as it could make it hard to fall asleep

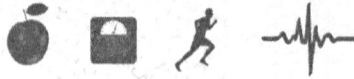

HOW TO DO PROGRESSIVE MUSCLE RELAXATION

Progressive muscle relaxation teaches you how to relax your muscles through a two-step process. First, you systematically tense particular muscle groups in your body such as your neck and shoulders. Next you release the tension and notice how your muscles feel when you relax them. This exercise will help you to lower your overall tension and stress levels, and help you relax when you are feeling anxious. It can also help reduce physical problems such as stomachaches and headaches, as well as improve your sleep.

People with anxiety difficulties are often tense throughout the day that they don't even recognize what being relaxed feels like. Through practice you can learn to distinguish between the feelings of a tensed muscle and a completely relaxed muscle. Then you can begin to "cue" this relaxed state at the first sign of the muscle tension that accompanies your feelings of anxiety. By tensing and releasing you learn not only what relaxation feels like but also to recognize when you are starting to get tense during the day.

Helpful Hints:

- √ Set aside about 15 minutes to complete this exercise.
- √ Find a place where you can complete this exercise without being disturbed.
- √ For the first week or two, practice this exercise twice a day until you get the hang of it.
- √ The better you become at it the quicker the relaxation response will "kick in" when you really need it!
- √ You do not need to be feeling anxious when you practice this exercise. In fact, it is better
- √ to first practice it when you are calm. That way it will be easier to do when feeling anxious.

Getting Ready

Find a quiet comfortable place to sit then close your eyes and let your body go loose. A reclining armchair is ideal. You can lie down, but this will increase your chances of falling asleep. Although relaxing before bed can improve your sleep, the goal of this exercise is to learn to relax while awake. Wear loose, comfortable clothing and don't forget to remove your shoes. Take about five slow, deep breaths before you begin.

How To Do It

The Tension—Relaxation Response

Step One: Tension

The first step is applying tension to a specific part of the body. This step is essentially the same regardless of which muscle group. For example, your left hand. Next take a slow, deep breath and squeeze the muscles as hard as you can for about 5 seconds. It is important to really feel the tension in the muscles, which may even cause a bit of discomfort or shaking.

In this instance you would be making a tight fist with your left hand.

It is easy to accidentally tense other surrounding muscles (for example, the shoulder or arm), so try to ONLY tense the muscles you are targeting. Isolating muscle groups gets easier with practice.

Be Careful! Take care not to hurt yourself while tensing your muscles. You should never feel intense or shooting pain while completing this exercise. Make the muscle tension deliberate yet gentle. If you have problems with pulled muscles, broken bones, or any medical issues that would hinder physical activity, consult your doctor first.

Step Two: Relaxing The Tense Muscles

This step involves quickly relaxing the tensed muscles. After about 5 seconds let all the tightness flow out of the tensed muscles. Exhale as you do this step. You should feel the muscles become loose and limp as the tension flows out. It is important to very deliberately focus on and notice the difference between the tension and relaxation. This is the most important part of the whole exercise.

Note: It can take time to learn to relax the body and notice the difference between tension and relaxation. At first it can feel uncomfortable to be focusing on your body but this can become quite enjoyable over time.

Remain in this relaxed state for about 15 seconds and then move on to the next muscle group. Repeat the tension-relaxation steps. After completing all of the muscle groups take some time to enjoy the deep state of relaxation.

The Different Muscle Groups

During this exercise you will be working with almost all the major muscle groups in your body. To make it easier to remember start with your feet and systematically move up (or if you prefer, you can do it in the reverse order from your forehead down to your feet). For example:

√ Foot (curl toes downward)
√ Lower leg and foot (tighten your calf muscle by pulling toes towards you)
√ Entire leg (squeeze thigh muscles while doing the above)
√ (Repeat on other side of body)
√ Hand (clench your fist)
√ Entire right arm (tighten your biceps by drawing your forearm up towards your shoulder and "make a muscle" while clenching fist)
√ (Repeat On other side of body)
√ Buttocks (tighten by pulling your buttocks together)
√ Stomach (suck your stomach in)
√ Chest (tighten by taking a deep breath)
√ Neck and shoulders (raise your shoulders up to touch your ears)
√ Mouth (open your mouth wide enough to stretch the hinges of your jaw)
√ Eyes (Clench your eyelids tightly shut)
√ Forehead (raise your eyebrows as far as you can)

It can be helpful to listen to someone guide you through these steps. There are many relaxation

CDs for sale that will take you through a progressive muscle relaxation (or something very similar).

Quick Tense & Relax

Once you have become familiar with the "tension and relaxation" technique and have been practicing it for a couple weeks, you can begin to practice a very short version of progressive muscle relaxation. In this approach you learn how to tense larger groups of muscles which takes even less time. These muscle groups are:

1. Lower limbs (feet and legs)
2. Stomach and chest
3. Arms, shoulder, and neck
4. Face

So instead of working with just one specific muscle group at a time (e.g., your stomach), you can focus on the complete group (your stomach AND chest). You can start by focusing on your breathing during tension and relaxation. When doing this shortened version it can be helpful to sat a certain word or phrase to yourself as you slowly exhale (such as "relax", "let go", "stay calm", "peace", etc.). This word or phrase will become associated with a relaxing state eventually saying this word alone can bring on a calm feeling. This can be handy during times when it would be hard to take the time to go through all the steps of progressive muscle relaxation.

Release Only

A good way to even further shorten the time you take to relax your muscles is to become familiar with the "release only" technique. One of the benefits of tensing and releasing muscles is that you learn to recognize what tense muscles feel like and what relaxed muscles feel like.

Once you feel comfortable with the tension and relaxation techniques you can start doing "release only" with involves removing the "tension" part of the exercise. For example instead of tensing your stomach and chest before relaxing them, try just relaxing the muscles. At first, the feeling of relaxation might feel less intense than when you tensed the muscles beforehand but with practice the release-only technique can be just as relaxing.

Final Note: Remember to practice progressive muscle relaxation often whether you are feeling anxious or not. This will make the exercise even more effective when you really do need to relax! Though it may feel a bit tedious at first, ultimately you will gain a skill that will probably become a very important part of managing your anxiety in your daily life.

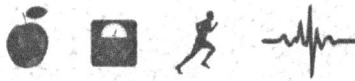

PRISON YOGA PROJECT
By James Fox

"The memory of trauma is imprinted on the human organism. I don't think you can overcome it unless you learn how to have a friendly relationship with your body." Bessel van der Kolk, M.D., Professor of Psychiatry, Boston University School of Medicine, and pioneer researcher in the field of trauma.

Prison is a breeding ground for mental, emotional and physical distress. Experiences of anxiety, depression, fear, distrust, agitation, hopelessness, grief, and violence can be greatly increased under incarcerated conditions. Psychiatrists, psychologists and clinical social workers acknowledge that embodiment practices such as yoga can greatly help people alleviate the symptoms that lead to both reactive behaviors and stress-related disease. So learning a practice in prison for Mindful Awareness and embodiment is not only important for supporting behavioral rehabilitation, it is also critical for physical and emotional well-being.

Dr. Van der Kolk's quote above illustrates that to heal from the emotional and sometimes physical pain of trauma requires establishing a meaningful connection with our hearts and bodies. Most people in prison have become dissociated from their feelings and bodies as a result of backgrounds of trauma including neglect or abuse, violent behavior, and/or the overuse of drugs and alcohol. The convict code can further distance one from a meaningful connection with his body, emotions and deeper self. Yoga helps to become more sensitive to yourself because it is a practice of self-awareness and self-control that promotes nonreactivity and self-acceptance. A regular yoga practice can help free the mind from confusion and the body from distress, allowing one to be at peace and receptive to learning new ways of thinking, feeling and being. Yoga emphasizes discipline of the mind and body for developing positive behavioral habits and impulse control.

The most often reported benefits from students involved in Prison Yoga Project classes are:

- √ Reduction of stress
- √ "More able to focus on the positive rather than the negative"
- √ Support in addiction recovery
- √ Greater mental clarity
- √ Pain relief
- √ Improved sleep
- √ "Better able to deal with the mental and emotional strain of prison"
- √ Greater access to inner peace

Raja Yoga

Raja yoga involves disciplining the mind, body and emotions to disengage from identification with the ego (the personal self), and achieve a state of higher consciousness for the specific purpose of self-realization, i.e. realizing one's true nature of Self. It includes the practice of postures (asanas), conscious breathing (pranayama) and meditation (dhyana).

One of the original purposes for practicing raja yoga was to prepare the mind and body for periods of prayer or meditation. Another was to develop the mental, emotional and physical discipline as well as spiritual values required of traditional warriors. In most tribal communities, warriors have always been those the community could count on for protection, and unlike today, their focus was on developing defensive skills rather than offensive ones, using force only as a last resort.

While there are currently many approaches to yoga, most embody a sophisticated system of exercises and stretches, or postures (asanas) combined with conscious breathing (pranayama) that can create strong sense of physical, mental and emotional well-being. The practice improved physical balance, flexibility and stamina while mentally and emotionally generating self-awareness and a sense of calmness. Unlike other forms of exercises that can strain muscles and bones, the intention of yoga is to rejuvenate the body and free the mind from tension brought about by the stress of life.

Mindful Awareness

Mindful awareness (also known as mindfulness) is at the very core of a yoga practice.

Mindful awareness involves using the mind for a different purpose than thinking thoughts.

Rather it focuses the mind on feeling sensations in the body and the movements of the breath. It is a practice of keeping the mind steady by paying close attention to what's going on moment-to-moment. It involves being present in each moment allowing the mind to observe rather than interpret what is going on. Mindful awareness can be practiced in seated meditation and while actively engaged in asana practice. The main components that constitute mindful awareness are:

- √ Learning to relax into a state of awareness and connecting with sensations in the body.
- √ Releasing involvement with thoughts and instead focusing on the movement of the breath while breathing through the nose.
- √ Practicing simply observing or witnessing one's moment-to-moment experience.

Thanks to research at the University of Massachusetts Medical Center, UCLA's Mindful Awareness Research Center, Harvard University and other prestigious institutes, mindful awareness has scientific support as a means for reducing stress, improving attention, boosting the immune system and promoting a general sense of psychological and physical well-being. Case studies have also shown that mindful awareness is effective in increasing self-esteem and holds great promise for both adolescents and adults with ADHD, depression, anxiety and other mood disorders.

Postures (Asanas)

The postures or asanas that are employed in the practice of raja yoga are what most people in America think of as yoga. However in actuality they only represent one of the Eight Limbs. The stretches, twists, bends, inversions and other postures that comprise the asana practice, along with conscious breathing (pranayama), are intended to cleanse and purify all the systems of the body removing obstructions to the flow of life force energy. While appearing to deal with the physical body alone, asanas and pranayama actually influence the nervous system and the chemical balance of the brain. So practicing yoga not only restores strength and stamina to the body but also can help improve one's mental and emotional states.

Conscious Breathing (Pranayama)

Pranayama the practice of conscious and control of breathing is another main component of Raja Yoga. Prana is the yogic word for the life force energy that permeates the individual, all life beings and life forms, as well as the air we breathe. Ayama is the storing of movement of that energy. So pranayama is the practice of influencing the flow of life force energy in and through the body using breath.

Our main source of prana comes from the air we breathe and the amount of prana we circulate through our bodies greatly impacts our overall vitality. The very basics of pranayama involve focused awareness on both inhale and exhale, breathing through the nose, and relaxing and stabilizing the breath to support the asana practice. Exhalation becomes consciously connected to letting go or releasing. Depending on the specific practice, engaging in pranayama can increase energy or provide calmness and clarity.

Prison Yoga Project offers two FREE yoga manuals written especially for people in prison. A Path For Healing And Recovery offers physical practices (asana), breathing practices (pranayama) and meditation (dhyana) to improve mental, emotional and physical well-being. The book also serves as a powerful resource for anyone trying to break free of negative behavioral patterns. A Woman's Practice: Healing from the Heart offers a simple and clear guide for women who wish to use yoga to help heal themselves from trauma, stress, or addiction. Write to them and request your FREE copy today!

Prison Yoga Project
PO Box 415
Bolinas, CA 94924

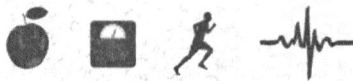

HATHA YOGA
By Bo Lozoff

Hatha Yoga is a system of mind/body/spirit development which is thousands of years old. It's not just a system of exercises like calisthenics or aerobics. It's more like the martial arts—a true meditation-in-action. In fact martial arts have sometimes been called "combat yoga".

The various positions in hatha yoga are called asanas—Sanskrit for "pose," or "posture". The idea is to get better and better at assuming each pose, which will bring a great number of benefits besides toning the body. These include better sleep, circulation, digestion, respiration, less illness, and so forth. Hatha Yoga also works on the non-physical "energy body" in many subtle ways.

This chapter isn't intended to make anybody into a super-duper hatha yogi. To make hatha yoga your whole path in life, you would need to live in seclusion somewhere with a qualified master, and follow extremely rigid rules of diet, sleep, activity, and concentration. Like any other intense spiritual regime that's a 24-hour-a-day lifestyle.

But we have to pay some attention to the body; it comes with the territory. So instead of blindly pursuing every fitness fad that comes down the pike, it's interesting to try out a system which honors our larger spiritual quest as well.

With just a few basic ground rules, anyone can practice hatha yoga and experience how good it feels to open the body and mind up. Like many people, I never go beyond simple asanas like the ones given here. I do some basic asanas every morning and they give me all I need from hatha yoga.

Basic Ground Rules

1.   Pay attention every moment. Keep your mind focused precisely on what you're doing in each pose. Each day, develop more and more concentration. Otherwise it's just exercise—not yoga.

2.   Stretch, don't strain. Yoga is the opposite of the "no pain, no gain" idea. Move just up to your own edge—the place where you can feel the stretch, but can still hold the pose calmly for a minute or more. Don't let the competitive ego-mind push you to injure yourself.

3.   Coordinate your breathing with your movements. Breathe in whenever the body expands, opens, or reaches outward; breathe out whenever it contracts, closes, or folds. Bottom line is; Concentrate. The breathing is the most important part.

4.   Focus on the spine. The movements and postures are designed to bring length, flexibility, and strength to your whole back. Especially think of making your spine longer, no matter what position you're in.

5.   Keep up your concentration between poses. No slouching or sprawling. Notice each

movement, each breath, from start to finish.

6.   Backward bends, and twists for the spine. If you were learning directly from a teacher, the teacher would give you a practice especially for your body. No book can teach the right things for every type of body. So if anything here seems risky for you because of an injury or weakness, don't do it! You must be your own teacher. Be careful not to put stress on your joints (especially shoulders and knees).

7.   Hatha Yoga will prepare your body and mind for sitting meditation, so it's great to do just before meditation. It's good to do the whole routine, but if you don't have time, do the routine from the beginning through at least two rounds of the "Salute To The Sun".

Easy Sitting Pose & Abdominal Breath

Sitting on the floor, on a firm cushion or a blanket folded up many times, bend the legs, one foot in front of the other, hands resting on the knees. Sit with your back straight, head straight over the spine, chin slightly down. This may not seem like an "easy sitting pose" at first, but with practice it will become one. (This is also a good way to sit for meditation.) Always begin by sitting quietly, noticing what is going on with body and mind that day. How does your body feel? What state is your mind in (calm, agitated, somewhere in between)? Next, become aware of your breath, flowing in and out from the nostrils (always try to breathe through your nose). Now as you breath out, gently draw in the muscles of your abdomen that are around your navel. This will help you exhale longer. As you breath in, bring the air to your abdomen first, letting go of those muscles you just pulled in, and let the air fill your rib cage and chest. Take a few breaths this way, trying to make your breath as long and smooth as you can. Now notice what effect the deep breathing has had on you. Use this way of breathing in all the movements and postures that follow.

Sunbird

Start on your hands and knees, hands directly under your shoulders and knees directly under your hips, knees hip-distance apart. Do one long abdominal breath. On the next inhale, gently arch your back and look forward. As you exhale, sit back on your heels, placing your chest on your thighs and your elbows and forehead on the floor. Inhale and slowly come back up to your hands and knees, gently arching your back, and stopping when your shoulders are right above your hands. Repeat the whole sequence for 6-8 breaths, feeling your back stretch and your spine beginning to loosen. Make your arms and legs do the least work they possibly can and make your back muscles do most the work.

Thunderbolt

Sit on your heels with your forehead on the floor and the backs of your hands resting on your low back. As you inhale, stand up on your knees while sweeping the right arm sideways and overhead. Look forward, chin down toward the chest. On the exhale, fold back down to the heels sweeping the right hand to the low back and turning your head slowly to the left.

On the next inhale, stand up on the knees while sweeping the left arm around and overhead, looking forward, chin down. On the exhale, fold down, turning the head slowly to the right and sweeping the left hand to the low back. Keep alternating arms, always turning the head away from the arm that is moving downwards. Repeat 4-6 times with each arm. For both the Sunbird and the Thunderbolt you may want to use a blanket under your knees for padding.

Tree Pose

Standing straight gaze at a spot on the floor about 6-feet in front of you. Bring one foot up onto the other thigh or bring it up so that the bottom of the foot is pressed against the inside of the other thigh (whichever way is easier). Place hands in prayer posture in front of chest. Inhale deeply while raising the arms out to the sides and then over the head like the branches of a tree. If it's easy to hold the body steady, let your eyes move around the room or try focusing the mind at the bottom of your foot and close your eyes. Repeat on the other leg. Hold as long as you feel steady and come down smoothly.

Salute To The Sun

This is a series of 12 asanas, that when done in a smooth flow is called a vinyasa. It's actually only 7 different poses because five of them are repeated. Most of the positions put the spine in either a forward bend or backward bend, going back and forth between the two, so it's a great way to loosen up the back and spine. The series is traditionally done facing east to greet the rising sun. Do from 2-12 rounds.

Position 1: Get centered and balanced with fresh concentration before each new round—Stand up perfectly straight with hands at your chest in prayer pose.

Position 2: Raise your arms forward and up feeling the rib cage open and lift. Gently arch your back but be careful to keep the upper arms alongside your ears. Your hands should remain in prayer pose.

Position 3: Technically the knees should be straight but most people need to bend them a little. Just before going from 3 to 4, bend the knees as much as you need to, to put your hands down on the floor right in front of you.

Position 4: Put one foot in between the hands, fingertips and toes on an imaginary line, knee right about the ankle. With the back foot, reach as far back as you can comfortably go, with back knee on the floor. Your back should be gently arched, chest open, looking forward, chin down toward chest.

Position 5: Move your forward foot back to meet the back foot, feet hip-distance apart. Arms and legs should be straight, heels pressed gently toward the floor, with your face toward your knees. Lengthen the legs and the back, butt straight up in the air. Notice the spot between your shoulder blades. This position is called the downward-facing dog and has many benefits.

Position 6: If possible, go into this position after exhaling all the air out, and do not inhale until position 7. This pose is called the stick position because you try to get your body straight as a stick: Hands under shoulders arms bent; back, head, buttocks, and legs on the same level, like the down part of a push up.

Position 7: Move into this position on an inhale. Arch your back, pelvis to the ground. Chest lifts and opens, arms straighten. Look forward but don't tilt head back. This is called upward-facing dog. Note: Hands and feet are to remain in the same place during positions 5-8.

Position 8: Same as position 5. Remember these positions are to be changes seamlessly in a flowy-type motion.

Position 9: This is the same as position 4, but whatever foot you had in back in position 4, move forward for position 9. If you have trouble getting the back foot forward from position 8 to 9, scoot the front foot forward with your hand, so it gets all the way up between the hands (DON'T move hands back to foot—that's cheating).

Position 10: Go back into position 3.

Position 11: Go back into position 2. Be careful not to strain low back.

Position 12: Go back to position 1, exactly how you started.

Seated Spinal Twist

Sit straight with your legs straight in front of you. Bend the right knee and cross it over to the outside of the left leg, right foot next to the left calf and flat on the floor.

Inhale and raise your arms straight in front, to the height of your shoulders. On exhale, lean forward slightly from the hips and them twist to the right. Place your right palm on the floor behind you with your fingers pointing away from you. Bring the left arm around to the outside of the right knee, pressing the right knee gently to the left. Then bend the left arm and let the left hand rest on the upper right thigh. Hold for 6 or more long breaths. Try to lift and lengthen the spine on the inhale, and gently twist more on the exhale. Come out of the pose on an exhale, hug the knees to your chest a moment (to let the low back stretch), and then do the twist to the left, reversing all the rights and lefts in these directions. Getting twisted up can be confusing, so be patient.

Head To Knee Pose

Sit straight, with legs straight in front of you. Bend the left leg and place the bottom of the left foot next to the inside of the right thigh. As you inhale, raise the arms overhead. As you exhale, bend forward from the hips and bring the chest toward the right thigh. Keep the back straight for as long as you can on the way down. Hold onto the right leg with both hands, having the elbows bent and the shoulders relaxed. It's good to keep the right knee straight, but if the stretch to the back of the right leg feels too intense, or if the low back hurts, then bend the right knee a little. Hold the position for 10 or more breaths. As you inhale in the pose, gently lift and lengthen the upper back. As you exhale, allow the upper body to move a little closer to the right thigh. To come out of the asana, inhale and lift the arms first. When the upper arms come alongside the ears, begin lifting the upper back, and finally use the muscles in the abdomen and low back to bring you the rest of the way up. Repeat the pose on the other side, having the left leg straight and the right leg bent.

Boat Pose

Lie on your stomach with your head turned to one side. Place the backs of your hands on your low back. If your hands start to slide off the low back, hold onto one hand with the other. As you inhale, lift the chest and legs as high off the floor as you can, keeping your chin down toward your chest. As you exhale, lower your legs and chest back to the floor. Repeat the movement 6 or more times. When your bring your head back to the floor, always turn it to the side so that you are resting on your cheek. Be sure to take turns with the direction you turn your head, so that your neck gets and even stretch. Which way feels better for your head to rest—to the right or the left? The answer will tell you which side of your neck is tighter. Remember to think of lightening the entire spine as you lift up into the backward bend.

Cobra Pose

The boat' pose has prepared you to hold the next backward bend, the Cobra Pose. Lie on your stomach with your legs close together and your head turned to the side. Place your hands palms down directly underneath your shoulders, so that your finger tips are right under the tops of your shoulders. The elbows are bent, and your arms should "hug" the sides of your rib cage. Bring your forehead to the floor, and on an inhale lift the chest as high up off the floor as you can without using your arms and hands. Make sure you are using your back muscles, and are not pushing yourself up with the arms. Keep your chin down toward your chest. Hold for as many breaths as is comfortable, come down on an exhale, turn the head to the side and keep your hands in place. Take a short rest and them come up into the pose again on an inhale. Cobra pose is excellent for making the low back stronger. It also opens the chest and the heart center so it's good to do lots of it if you're working on opening your heart.

Extended Pose

Lie on your back with your knees bent in toward your chest and your arms down alongside of you. As you inhale, raise your arms all the way overhead so that the backs of your hands reach the floor above your head and straighten your legs up toward the ceiling—the bottoms of your feet should be parallel to the ceiling. As you exhale, lower the arms back to their starting position and bend the knees back in toward the chest. Feel how long your spine gets when your arms are overhead and your legs are straight up. Repeat the movement 6 or more times. This will prepare you for lying flat and it's also good for stretching out any tightness in your back.

Relaxation Pose

Lie on your back with your legs several inches apart, arms alongside you with your palms turned up. Notice how your body feels. What is the state of your mind? How do you feel now as compared to the way you felt at the beginning of the practice? Stay in this pose for about five minutes allowing every part of your body to deeply relax.

A Final Word About Hatha Yoga

Be patient in learning these asanas; give yourself time to feel each movement, each pose. The first few times you try hatha yoga, keep going back to read the beginning of this chapter. Especially the "Basic Ground Rules" so that right from the beginning you'll be remembering the important parts. Doing even a half-hour a day of hatha yoga can make a tremendous difference in your life. It's a good way to get the body prepared for meditation and higher states of consciousness.

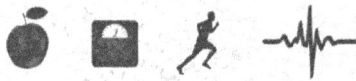

A DEEPER UNDERSTANDING OF YOGA

By Thomas Ryan

In the West, reasons for practicing yoga typically include: weight control, improved muscle tone, flexibility, coordination, stamina, restful sleep and inner well-being. While these benefits are real and undeniable, they are entirely secondary to the traditional aim of yoga. Yoga seeks to cultivate a focused awareness of one's deepest being, one's True Self. The physical exercises that prepare the way for the transformation of consciousness are an intuitive experience of the divine.

Yoga involves a systematic approach to attaining the highest level of consciousness by unraveling the obstacles that stand in the way of being centered, rooted, sensitized to the presence of God within the human person. Seekers of conscious union with the divine in various ancient civilizations discovered that by keeping the body still you can calm the mind; that by concentrating your attention, you settle the body; and that by certain methods of breath-control, the mind becomes quiet and focused.

Yoga facilitates contemplative prayer by quieting the mind and showing us into the mystery from within that our being springs. The physical exercises (asanas) simply prepare the body and the nervous system for the ensuing meditation. While yoga prepares one for meditation it is in itself meditation-in-motion. Asanas are correctly practiced only if they fulfill the central purpose of stilling the mind.

On the surface asanas look like a collection of stretching exercises coupled with breathing techniques, however the postures are to be performed with grace and control as a type of meditation. Their purpose is to bring one into a state of inner quiet, rebalancing the opposing forces within us to experience peace and inner harmony. As an example, during periods of stress when we experience discomfort in the neck, shoulders and back, the body is reacting to chronically distressed muscles. The first step to restoring inner peace is to relax the body. Stretching and lengthening muscles that are contracted helps to balance both the body and the mind. What happens in the body affects the mind, just as the mind affects the body.

There are two aspects to the practice of asanas: the external form that works through the body, and the internal form that works through the mind. It is often popular to stress the external form, the attitude or intention. In reality the physical postures are the external vehicle for the more important "inner posture"—the experience of stillness within. This "inner posture" can be maintained even while the external posture is constantly changing.

Practicing asanas is a vehicle for inner awareness, and therefore a way to practice a different attitude toward everyday life. It is not unusual that internal attitudes and perceptions begin to change within the practice of yoga and meditation. Focusing on dispersing inner tension leads to acceptance, integration and peace. Experiencing inflexibility in the body can shed light on inflexible attitudes and states of mind. Postures can serve as a gateway for encountering limitations and fear. When you intentionally encounter bodily limitations and resistance from stiffness in muscles and joints, holding the postures become a powerful vehicle to explore where you are in the moment—mentally, emotionally and physically. The way to progress at that point is to accept your limitations, your condition unconditionally.

In challenging life situations there are two divergent roads. You can say, "I've had enough of this; it's too difficult, uncomfortable and painful." In doing so you buy into limiting beliefs you hold about yourself and take refuge in regret, denial and/or escape activities.

Or you can say, "Even though this is uncomfortable, difficult and painful, I'm going to face this and work through it. By holding your posture, and releasing and relaxing into it as much as you can, you discover that you can actually extend beyond your preconceived limitations and fears.

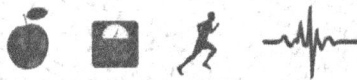

HOLISTIC EXERCISE SECRETS

The physical body is designed to move. We are born with 270 bones, several of which fuse during childhood to become 206 in adulthood. When movement is inadequate, many bones become increasingly less mobile, stiff, and uncomfortable. We have 700 different muscles with their respective tendons, and muscle mass makes up about half of body weight in a healthy body. These essential energetic functions need not only movement but also resistance to maintain optimal health and benefit. A healthy body contains 12 to 15 percent fat. All nonextreme movement is good, and in our modern relatively inactive life (especially when locked up in a prison cell), we need to provide a minimum of thirty minutes of modern exercise five days a week. This can consist of calisthenics, yoga, sports, jogging, Tai Chi, just bouncing in place, weight lifting or walking. Ideally, your heart rate should double for half or more of your exercise period.

Here are some morning and evening exercise routines suggested by holistic health guru Edgar Cayce.

MORNING CAYCE EXERCISES

Bend and Swing—An upper-body exercise that improves circulation, renews the air in lungs, and adjusts the spinal column.

- √ Stand with feet flat on floor.
- √ Bend forward and swing arms and upper body down and back up, with a rocking motion. Your fingertips should almost brush your toes on the downswing. Be careful of your balance until you're used to it.
- √ Exhale on the downswing.
- √ Some people combine this exercise with (2) "Reach for the Sky" (below), going straight up into it on the upswing.

Reach for the Sky—Improves circulation and arches, naturally adjusts the spinal column, and is famous as an outer hemorrhoids cure.

- ✓ In a standing position (without shoes) gradually rise up on the balls of the feet, raising your arms in front of you at the same time, until they are as high as you can reach. Again, breathe in as you go up.
- √ Still stretched out, slowly bend forward from the waist, with a clutching-the-air motion as you come down, until you can touch the floor. Breathe out as you go down.
- √ Repeat this as least 3-4 times at first, and work up to 10-12.

Swing Arms—Improves circulation to arm, and keeps joints limber and uncalcified—good for arthritis.

- √ Stand with feet apart.

√ Swing each arm slowly in a circle, like a windmill—first one direction, then the other. Increase speed to your comfort level. It may help to imagine a pitcher winding up to throw.

√ Keep your arms as relaxed as possible while you rotate them.

√ You should begin with 10 times each way, unless you're already in shape.

√ Rotate Legs—Good for the equilibrium and circulation, and keeps the joints limber.

√ Stand with spine straight.

√ Lift one leg at a time, and rotate with the toes pointing outward. See yourself drawing a circle with your toes.

√ Rotate each direction. Steady yourself by holding on to something, if you need to. Once you're used to it, try to balance yourself.

√ At first, do 5-10 each way, and work up to your comfort level.

√ Dr. Harold Reilly also suggests a variation with toes pointing up and heel down, while rotating.

Neck Rolls—Improves eyesight, hearing, circulation to the brain, and helps relieve stress. Cayce even said it would assist the thyroid.

√ In the morning, stand with feet spread slightly, and hands on hips.

√ Keeping the spine straight, bend the neck slowly—forward three times, back three times, left three times, right three times.

√ Next, roll the neck gently in a full circle, first one direction, then the ohter. Do this two or three times.

√ For all of you stiff necks out there, who have lots of tension, be careful! You can pull some muscles by going too fast or forcing. Relax... And if it hurts, don't push it—slow down even more and try to slide past it. (The rubberneck!)

√ The safest way I've found is to make the neck muscles follow the eyes. This is very natural, since the neck is designed to turn wherever the eyes look.

EVENING CAYCE EXERCISES

The evening exercises are done in a basically horizontal position, after being upright all day. It signals the body to relax for the night. Cayce gave them for insomnia, among other things.

Sitting Sit-Ups—Improves circulation and stretches legs

√ Sit on floor.

√ Touch toes repeatedly, rocking back and forth.

√ Do 5-10

Cat Walk—Clears up the sinuses, improves circulation and general mobility. Keeps you spry!

√ Get down on all four paws

√ Imagine that you are a cat, and try to walk fluidly like one. This takes some practice.

√ In addition to the daily routine, it's suggested you do this whenever congested, for quick relief. Cayce said this position was effective because early primates walked on all fours—and didn't suffer from colds.

Torso-Circles—Keeps the colon healthy, using centrifugal force to improve circulation in the colon, and strengthen its walls. This Cayce exercises is famous as an inner hemorrhoids cure, but is also very good for general health and longevity.

- √ Put your body in a push-up position, with the soles of your feet against a wall or other solid object.
- √ Rotate your torso, first in one direction, and then the other. Do equal numbers of these.
- √ It may help to hold your stomach in if you can, while pushing with your feet on the wall.
- √ Don't do very many at first, especially if you're out of shape or overweight—even two or three in each direction are adequate to begin with. You can gradually increase 5-10-20 each way (or more for severe cases of piles).

Bear Walk—Helps reverse the daily effects of gravity, improves circulation to the head, and loosens hip joints, in particular.

- √ Stand with feel flat on the floor.
- √ Lean forward and put palms flat on the floor as well. Try to keep the feet as flat as possible, with legs straight, not bent at the knees.
- √ Holding this position, walk forward and back across the room. This will be difficult, at first, since many people have trouble reaching their toes. But after daily efforts, you'll be able to amble around like a bear.

Neck Rolls—These are the same as described earlier, except that in the afternoon or evening, Cayce recommended a sitting position, either on the ground, legs crossed, or sitting on a bench or chair

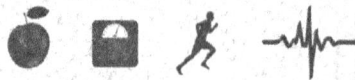

DECOMPRESS YOUR SPINE

All day long your spine is working to keep you upright. When you're sitting, your spine is engaged, keeping you torso from slumping over, and holding up your 10-pound head. It works extra hard when you pick up heavy objects.

So give your spine some love. The next time you're working out, in between sets, do a dead hang from a pullup bar. Here's why.

Between the vertebrae of your backbone are spinal disks that contain little sacks of fluid. When we load on pressure, the sacks spread and flatten. When we take off the pressure, the disks refill, or decompress.

A static hang creates even more space between the vertebrae, allowing the disks to expand with fluid more fully. If you want, make slow, small rotations, moving from the thoracic spine, which is the portion of your back behind your rib cage. (Don't simply twist your hips, which will engage the lumbar spine.) Do this between sets and at the end of a workout. All it takes is 30 seconds—and it feels good, too.

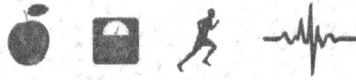

THE EFFECTS OF STRESS ON YOUR BODY

Stress is any change in the environment that requires your body to react and adjust in response. The body reacts to these changes with physical, mental, and emotional responses.

Stress is a normal part of life. Many events that happen to you and around you-and many things that you do yourself—put stress on your body. You can experience good or bad forms of stress from your environment, your body, and your thoughts.

How Does Stress Affect Health?

The human body is designed to experience stress and react to it. Stress can be positive (eustress) such as a getting a job promotion or being given greater responsibilities keeping us alert and ready to avoid danger. Stress becomes negative (distress) when a person faces continuous challenges without relief or relaxation between challenges. As a result, the person becomes overworked and stress-related tension builds.

Distress can lead to physical symptoms including headaches, upset stomach, elevated blood pressure, chest pain, and problems sleeping. Research suggests that stress also can bring on or worsen certain symptoms or diseases.

Stress also becomes harmful when people use alcohol, tobacco , or drugs to try to relieve their stress. Unfortunately, instead of relieving the stress and returning the body to a relaxed state, these substances tend to keep the body in a stressed state and cause more problems. Consider the following:

√ Forty-three percent of all adults suffer adverse health effects from stress.

√ Seventy-five percent to 90% of all doctor's office visits are for stress-related ailments and complaints.

√ Stress can play a part in problems such as headaches, high blood pressure, heart problems, diabetes, skin conditions, asthma, arthritis, depression, and anxiety.

√ The Occupational Safety and Health Administration (OSHA) declared stress a hazard of the workplace. Stress costs American industry more than $300 billion annually.

√ The lifetime prevalence of an emotional disorder is more than 50%, often due to chronic, untreated stress reactions.

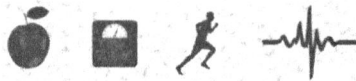

TAKE A DEEP BREATH...AND RELAX

As we all know, prison can be a very stressful place. And when you're under stress, your muscles tense and your breathing becomes shallow and rapid. One of the simplest (and best) ways to stop this stress response is to breathe deeply and slowly. It sounds simple, and it is. Most people, however, don't breathe deeply under normal circumstances, so it may help to review the mechanics of deep breathing and how it helps you to relax.

Breathing Under Stress

When prehistoric humans were in danger of attack, their muscles tensed and their breathing became rapid and shallow as they prepared to run or fight. Their high level of tension was a means of preparing their bodies for optimum performance. Today, the causes of our "stress" are different, but our stress response is the same. However, since we're not running or fighting, our tension has no release and our stress response builds. One way to counteract the stress response is to learn how to breathe deeply and slowly—the opposite of how we breathe when under stress.

How Deep Breathing Works

Deep breathing is not always natural to adults. Watch the way a baby breathes: The area beneath the chest goes in and out. Most adults breathe from the chest. This is shallow breathing, so less oxygen is taken in with each breath. As a result, the blood is forced to move through the system quickly so that enough oxygen gets to the brain and organs. Higher blood pressure results.

Deep breathing can reverse these effects. Take some time to practice this kind of breathing each day, especially when you're under stress. You can be sitting, standing or lying down, but it helps to wear loose, comfortable clothing. Begin by breathing in through your nostrils. Count to five, silently saying the word "in," and let your lower abdomen fill with air. Then count to five, silently saying the word "out," as you let the air escape through pursed lips. Do this deep breathing for two minutes or more each time. With practice, you'll be able to count slowly to 10 or higher. You can increase your relaxation if you imagine breathing in ocean air, the scent of flowers or forest air.

Effects Of Deep Breathing

By helping you let go of tension, deep breathing can relieve headaches, backaches, stomach aches and sleeplessness. It releases the body's own painkillers, called endorphins, into the system. It allows blood pressure to return to normal, which is good for your heart.

Deep breathing can allow held-in emotions to come to the surface, so your emotional health benefits from deep breathing, too. Use deep breathing anytime, anywhere. It's one of the best techniques for relieving stress.

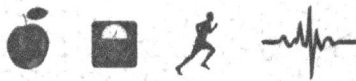

THE BETTER-SLEEP WORKOUT

Any exercise is good for sleep; this you probably know. But here is a special routine that combines two of the best kinds of workouts for sleep: high-intensity intervals, which make falling asleep easier, and yogic moves that can help improve sleep quality. Your heart rate ebbs and flows during sleep, dropping to its lowest point overnight, explains one fitness expert. This workout emulates that to help you sleep better. Go through the whole thing twice, doing as many reps of each move as you can for one minute before continuing. (Just don't do it right before bed—revving up your heart rate and body temp that can interfere with sleep.)

Squat

Stand with feet slightly wider than hip distance. Squat, keeping back flat and butt out, until thighs are parallel to floor. Return to stand.

Lunge Twist

Begin in a low lunge with right leg forward and hands on either side of right foot. Lift right arm overhead and twist open to the right, holding for a breath. Return to start. Switch legs as quickly as you can, and repeat.

Side-To-Side Squat Jump

Squat down. Jump back up and rotate right, swinging arms for momentum. Land in a squat, facing right. Jump back to start. Repeat to left.

Roll-Up

Lie on back, arms over head. Roll torso up off the floor into a C-curve, reaching for toes. Hold for a breath, and return to start.

Side Plank with Leg Lift

On left side, prop yourself up on your elbow with forearm flat on the floor under shoulder and feet stacked. Raise hips into side plank. Lift right leg as high as you can. Hold for 30 seconds. Switch sides.

Triangle

Stand with feet wide, legs straight, toes out. Extend arms at shoulder height and lean down toward right leg, ending with right hand on floor near right foot. Hold for 30 seconds. Switch sides.

Half-Pigeon

Sit cross-legged on floor. Extend left leg behind you. Walk hands out in front of right leg, resting torso over right shin, knee out to the side. Hold for 30 seconds. Switch sides.

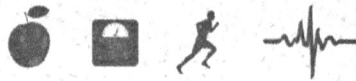

SLEEP TIPS

HOW TO TRAIN YOUR SLEEP

You probably spend lots of time thinking about, and constantly refining, your workouts.

And if you're going to spend all that time exercising, it's probable that your diet is dialed in, too. But when was the last time you gave the same kind of consideration to your sleep?

If the answer is, "Uh, never," that's a problem. Because lack of sleep not only makes you grumpy and drawn-looking, it jeopardizes your heart health, blood pressure, BMI, cognitive abilities, and more. And chances are you're not getting all the sleep you need. Sixty-nine percent of us are sleep-deprived, research shows. "The worse part about it is that you think it's OK," says Andrew McHill, a circadian-disorder researcher at Oregon Health & Science University. "You forget what being well-rested feels like."

You probably know a lot of this already. But what you don't know is how to fix the problem. This is about to change. You're about to be given advice from some of the top sleep experts in the world in order to create a systematic way to determine what's preventing you from getting the nightly rest you need (aside from the fact you're in prison). Think of it as kind of an elimination diet. After all, if you suffered from chronic digestive problems, you'd certainly go about finding the culprit—purging your diet of dairy, gluten, red meat, citrus—then reintroducing them slowly to find out what foods are tripping up your GI tract.

Read on to learn how to take the same approach to sleep, by learning the factors most likely to create sleep problems, and how you can go about fixing it.

How to Do It

First you'll need an idea of how much sleep your body needs. Go to bed early on Friday and sleep as late as you can on Saturday. Repeat the next night. You'll emerge with a rough idea of what a full tank feels like. Then set a goal of how many hours a night you'd like to get. (Most adults need from seven to nine hours.)

Now you're ready. Begin to institute these sleep rules, as many as you can, for two weeks. Track the hours of sleep you get. The idea of an elimination is a truth discovery.

Some rules are a hassle. After two weeks, ease up on those. But if your old ways make your sleep suffer, you might decide to change your habits.

Be diligent and you'll feel more energized, patient, and happier. It's hard to form new habits, but it's easier when you can feel the results.

Environment

Lights Out: If you can do so without getting a write-up, make sure your cell is dark—turn off your light, cover your window if possible, etc. If you can still see the stuff across the cell, it's not dark enough. Think cave-like conditions—which shouldn't be too hard since you basically live in one any way. Lights stop your brain from reaching the deepest level of shutdown, meaning that in a dim cell you won't get total rest. Don't leave your TV on—none of that. And if you can't cover all light sources without getting a write-up, such as your back window, fold up a shirt and sleep with it over your eyes. This will help you have NO light.

Keep it Down Over There: Unfortunately, loud neighbors, cops, etc., don't care about your bedtime. You might find instant relief from a white noise machine. Obviously you won't be allowed one of these in prison, but some inmates like to use a fan. In CA, we can buy personal fans from the package companies. Some provide enough white noise to drown out all the bullshit going on outside your cell; plus it circulates the air better which help gets rid of the funk. If you can't do this, it's likely you can come up on some ear plugs. Some inmates even know how to make their own.

Drop the Heat: Research suggests the ideal bedroom temperature is from 60 to 67 degrees, so try to accomplish this. I once had a clock that showed the temp and was able to know exactly what temp my cell was. Try to sleep in nothing more than your boxers and a T-shirt. Layer on sheets and blankets as needed. Your body changes temperature throughout the night, and it's less disruptive to adjust how much bedding is on top of you that to wiggle out of sweatpants.

Sleep solo: If you can go without having a celly, do so. You'll likely get better sleep. You won't hear any snoring, movement, or feel another man's energy. I can literally feel energy from another person, the light being on, or the TV being on. As soon as my celly leaves and I turn off appliances, I can literally feel the difference.

Night Habits

Eat Dinner Earlier: You can't control when the prison feeds you, but they likely feed you pretty early anyway. But if you're like me, you enjoy eating a fat meal at night—like burritos—after a hard day's work. I like to do this when I shut things down and watch my nightly TV shows, usually starting at 8pm. But this is not the best idea. Experts say to eat earlier, which will give your body enough time to fully digest. Plus, it could assist in keeping you trim. Research from Brigham and Women's Hospital in Boston finds that the later people eat at night, the higher BMI they   tend to have. When you eat closer to melatonin onset—the hormone that tells your body to go to bed—you're apt to have a higher body fat percentage. If you have the munchies, snack on some nuts.

Ditch All Devices: Don't listen to your CD player or radio to go to sleep. Turn everything off.

Day Habits

Try to Keep a Constant Schedule: Go to sleep and get up at the same time, weekends included. When your circadian clock is on a fixed schedule, you're not shaking off sleep when it's time to get up. Staying regular helps you perform better throughout the day. Research from Harvard shows students who keep an irregular sleep-wake schedule tend to have a worse GPA and cognitive performance, and adults who keep a scattershot schedule are prone to glucose intolerance—which can make you overweight. If you have to have a celly, try to be on the same schedule, so one's not up and making noise while the other's asleep.

No After-Work Workouts: Exercise raises your heart rate, ups your body temp, and makes you hungry, all of which are great—except if you're trying to sleep. in the evening is your only free time, try shifting your entire schedule up if possible.

Practice Stress Relief: If your cell is dark and pin-drop quiet and yet you still toss and turn, it could be stress. Quiet the inner noise with daily meditation. Whatever time during the day is convenient works. If your mind is still racing when you try to go to bed, write a list of what's keeping you up and the next steps for dealing with it. You'll declutter your thoughts and give yourself peace of mind in the form of tomorrow's to-do list.

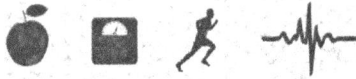

5 MEDICAL REASONS YOU SHOULD MASTERBATE

Taking matters into your own hands isn't just fun, it may actually have health benefits!

By Maridel Reyes

Science has shown that masturbating can provide plenty of health benefits. A study from adult product peddler Adam and Eve reveals that 27 percent of Americans admit to masturbating once or twice a week. That number seems low to us, especially since science has shown that being master of your domain can provide additional feel-great benefits.

"Masturbation is a part of a healthy sex life," says Gloria Brame, Ph.D., a clinical sexologist. "It's totally safe and harmless."

Just as brushing your teeth should be a regular occurrence, some people masturbate. Here are five health reasons to consider a self-pleasure routine.

It Prevents Cancer

An Australian study found that men who ejaculated more than five times a week were a third less likely to develop prostate cancer. Disease-causing toxins build up in your urogenital tract, and each time a man ejaculates he flushes the bad toxins out of his system, says Brame.

It Makes Better Muscle Tone

As you age, you naturally lose muscle tone... even down there. Regular sex or masturbation works out your pelvic floor muscles to prevent erectile dysfunction and incontinence.

"It keeps the angle of your dangle perky," says Brame.

Aim to (ahem) arrive three to five times a week for rock-solid results.

It Helps You Last Longer

"Masturbating an hour before a date will give you more control," says Brame. Train yourself by timing how long it takes you to orgasm, suggests Ava Cadell, Ph.D. If it usually takes two minutes solo, try for three next time. Or count how many strokes needed to get to your happy place. If you're spurting after 50, shoot for 60. "Most men can double the number of strokes and the time within one month," Cadell says.

It Ups Your Immunity

Ejaculation increases levels of the hormone cortisol, says Jennifer Landa, M.D., a specialist in hormone therapy. Cortisol, which usually gets a bad rap as a havoc-wrecking stress hormone, actually helps regulate and maintain your immunity in the small doses.

"Masturbation can produce the right environment for a strengthened immune system," she says.

It Boosts Your Mood

Masturbating boosts your mood and releases stress. An orgasm is the biggest non-drug blast of feel-good neurochemicals like dopamine and oxytocin that list your spirits, boosts your satisfaction, and activate the reward circuits in your brain.

Want to know where to get all the hottest non nude adult entertainment for prisoners? Order Kitty Kat today by sending $24.99 plus $7.00 S/H to: Freebird Publishers; POB 541; North Dighton, MA 02764. Kitty Kat is filled with companies that sell non-nude photos; magazines; page-turning books; must-see movies; strip clubs; porn stars; thought-provoking stories; photo spreads and much, much more!

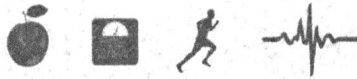

WALKING AND WEIGHT LOSS

Three universal goals most of us share are: to live longer, to live free of illness, and to control our weight. Interesting enough, normal walking lets us achieve all three.

In fact, walking may be man's best medicine for slowing the aging process. First, it works almost every muscle in the body, improving circulation to the joints and messaging the blood vessels (keeping them more elastic). Walking also helps us maintain both our muscle mass and metabolism as we age. It also keeps us young in spirit. For anyone out of shape or unathletically inclined, walking is the no-stress, no-sweat answer to lifelong conditioning.

All it takes is a little time, common sense and a few guidelines. Unfortunately, there's a lot of misinformation floating around regarding fitness walking, weight-loss and dieting.

Walking is one of the best exercises for strengthening bones, controlling weight, toning the leg muscles, maintaining good posture and improving positive self-concept.

People who diet without exercising often get fatter with time. Although your weight may initially drop while dieting, such weight loss consists mostly of water and muscle. When the weight returns, it comes back as fat. To avoid getting fatter over time, increase your metabolism by exercising daily.

To lose weight, it's most important to walk for time than speed. Walking at a moderate pace yields longer workouts with less soreness leading to more miles and more calories spent on a regular basis.

High-intensity walks on alternate days help condition one's system. But in a walking, weight-loss program, it's better to be active every day. This doesn't require walking an hour every day. The key is leading an active lifestyle 365 days a year.

When it comes to good health and weight loss, exercise and diet are interrelated.

Exercising without maintaining a balanced diet is no more beneficial than dieting while remaining inactive.

The National Research Council recommends eating five or more servings of fruits and vegetables a day. Fruits and vegetables are the ideal diet foods for several reasons.

They're relatively low in fat and calories, yet are often high in fiber and rich in essential vitamins and minerals.

Remember that rapid weight loss consists mostly of water and muscle the wrong kind of weight to lose. To avoid this, set more reasonable goals, such as one pound per week.

Carbohydrates are high-octane fuel. They provide energy for movement and help raise internal body metabolism. They're also satisfying. The key is not adding high-fat toppings to your carbohydrates.

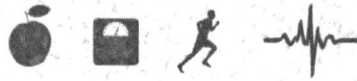

EXERCISE MELTS BODY FAT!

If you want to reduce your body fat, focus on increasing the amount of exercise you get, not just decreasing your food intake. A national study was done using two groups of sedentary men, one group in their 20s and the other over age 65. A lot was learned from this accumulated data and it is interesting to note that there was a significant relationship between lack of physical activity and body fat. Not surprisingly, the most sedentary men had the most body fat.

Leading experts recommend that people who want to lose weight start increasing their physical activity. Just being more active in general (such as moving around instead of sitting still, sitting up instead of laying down, as well as showing some excitement and enthusiasm instead of boredom), are things that more effectively burns calories and reduces body fat. Many people have seemed to have lost sight of the value of being active. Consider this, a half-hour aerobic workout accounts for far less energy expenditure than our minute-to-minute movement in our cells.

Millions of people are trying to lose weight. Americans spend approximately $30 billion a year on diet programs and products. Often they do lose some weight, but, if you check with the same people five years later, you will find that nearly all have regained whatever weight they lost. A national panel recently sought data to determine if any commercial diet program could prove long-term success. Not a single program could do so.

Being seriously overweight and particularly obesity predisposes individuals to a number of diseases and serious health problems, and it's a known fact that when caloric intake is excessive, some of the excess is frequently saturated fat.

People who diet without exercising often get fatter with time. Although your weight may initially drop while dieting, such weight loss consists mostly of water and muscle. When the weight returns, it comes back as fat. To avoid getting fatter over time, increase your metabolism by exercising regularly.

Walking is one of the best exercises for strengthening bones, controlling weight, toning the leg muscles, maintaining good posture and improving positive self-concept. To lose weight, it's more important to walk for time than speed. Walking at a moderate pace yields longer workouts with less soreness—leading to more miles and more fat worked off on a regular basis. Hight intensity walks on alternate days help condition one's system. But in a walking, weight-loss program, you are not required to walk an hour every day as some people would have you believe.

When it comes to good health and weight loss, exercise and diet are interrelated. Exercising without maintaining a balanced diet is no more beneficial than dieting while remaining inactive.

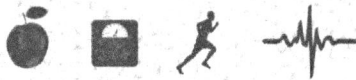

A POSITIVE WEIGHT LOSS APPROACH

Once you have made up your mind that you want to lose weight, you should make that commitment and go into it with a positive attitude. We all know that losing weight can be quite a challenge. In fact, for some, it can be downright tough. It takes time, practice and support to change lifetime habits. But it's a process you must learn in order to succeed. You and you alone are the one who has the power to lose unwanted pounds.

Think like a winner, not a loser. Remember that emotions are like muscles and the ones you must grow the strongest. If you always look at the negative side of things, you'll become a downbeat, pessimistic person. Even slightly negative thoughts have a greater impact on you and last longer than powerful positive thoughts.

Negative thinking doesn't do you any good, it just holds you back from accomplishing the things you want to do. When a negative thought creeps into your mind, replace it by reminding yourself that you're somebody, you have self-worth and you possess unique strengths and talents.

Contemplate what lies ahead of you. Losing weight is not just about diets. It's about a whole new you and the possibility of creating a new life for yourself. Investigate the weight loss program that appeals to you and that you feel will teach you the behavioral skills you need to stick with throughout the weight-loss process.

First you should look for help among family and friends. It can be an enormous help to discuss obstacles and share skills and tactics with others on the same path. You might look for this support from those around you who are also looking to lose weight, and you might seek guidance from someone who has successfully accomplished what it is you want to do.

There are success stories all over these days, TV, magazines, etc, about people who have miraculously lost untold pounds and kept it off. In all instances they say their mental attitude as well as their outlook on life has totally changed. You will notice that a positive outlook is one of the common denominators among just about all success stories, including those related to health. It is mentioned countless times throughout this very book.

You will probably need to learn new, wiser eating skills. You will want a weight loss regimen that gives you some control, rather than imposing one rigid system, especially since you are in prison and require some flexibility.

Keep in mind, too, that your weight loss program will most likely include some physical exercises. Look at the exercising part of your program as fun and recreation and not a form of grueling and sweaty work. The fact is that physical fitness is linked inseparable to all personal effectiveness in every field. Anyone willing to take the few simple steps that lie between them and fitness will shortly begin to feel better, and the improvement will shortly begin to feel better, and the improvement will reflect itself in every facet of their existence.

Doctors now say that walking is one of the best exercises. It helps the total circulation of the blood throughout the body, and thus has a direct effect on your overall feeling of health. There are things such as aerobics, jogging, etc. that will benefit a weight loss program. Ask your doctor for any advice, tips or "secrets" he or she can share.

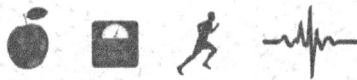

FROM SURVIVING TO THRIVING
By Intelligent Allah

"Stay away from gambling, snitches and trouble makers." While incarcerated on Riker's Island in 1995, that was the advice I received from an old timer who had done time Up North. I was 19 years old and he was teaching me cardinal rules necessary for me to smoothly navigate New York state prisons during my 19 year sentence. In 2011, after making my rounds at nine prisons Up North, I've seen the validity of those cardinal rules. But my ambition drove me beyond the need to survive. I had a desire to thrive. Health development and writing became the primary means through which I thrived in prison.

Health development for me is a physical process that encompasses exercise, diet and nutrition. I have been known to flirt with weight lifting, my standard exercise routine of crunches and sit-ups, plus an arm and chest regiment of pushups, pull-ups and dips. These exercises stimulate optimum blood circulation, increase stamina and enhance strength while keeping my body lean. The goal is to reduce my risk of contracting heart disease, hypertension and diabetes—diseases that have claimed the lives of a number of my family members and men I've known in prison.

Diet and nutrition are essential to health development. I learned this after intense self-study of diet and nutrition. Numerous studies have proven that a diet free of meat, meat byproducts and ingredients derived from meat increases the lifespan of human beings and contributes to a healthy lifestyle. While cholesterol levels above 150 elevates one's potential for contracting heart disease, my diet and exercise routine keep my cholesterol between 122 and 125. Lowering the cholesterol levels and other goals of health development are essential for incarcerated people. Because prisons are generally plagued with subpar care.

My diet helped me develop discipline, a focal characteristic I lacked while running the streets of East New York, Brooklyn as a reckless teen. Developing discipline is important for people in prison, because many of us have committed crimes to make fast money because we lacked the discipline required to pursue a job. Crime is generally the culmination of seeking the easy way out, which is a hallmark of a lack of discipline. Also, the volatile nature of crowded prisons packed with countless personalities of incarcerated men, officers and civilian staff often ignites the tempers of stressful men. Therefore, discipline is a trait which can prevent incarcerated people from uncontrolled emotional responses to potentially dangerous situations.

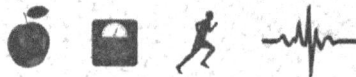

BUILD YOUR MIND, REFINE YOUR PHYSICAL
By Sha Be Allah

Besides staying away from the TV and phones begging for visits, one of the more important facets of my bids was rationing and planning my diet. The DOC in any given state feeds inmates the MINIMUM daily allowance of nutrition that is required to keep a person alive, and most facilities that I've had the experience of going through didn't even give the inmates that. In most prisons, one of the first budgets the administration will make cuts are from prisoner meals.

But I used this to my advantage. This was the first step in practicing and honing my discipline. Most people that end up behind the wall had terrible dietary habits in the streets. Excessive amounts of meat, candy, cakes, sodas, fried foods, salty snacks, and let's not forget the liquor and cigarettes that go along with feeding an obsessive compulsive mentality. So if you ate garbage on the outside, you'll be content with garbage on the inside. But that's bad news for you in the long run, so you can actually use this time to change your habits. After all, you have more time to consider what you put in your system because you're not on the street in between fast food spots.

Even though I had the fortune of having people in the free world who held me down financially, I tried my best to keep the sweets and treats to a minimum. Tuna fish and mackerel aren't the best meats for your system, but they're probably the best you can get on commissary.

Peanut butter and jelly on whole wheat bread, fruit, nuts, and massive amounts of water was a regular part of my daily diet.

Don't drink the Kool Aid! I never drink juice made by a correctional facility because it is alleged that some prisons add chemicals designed to suppress your sexual appetite. Who knows what else is in there? Needless to say, I've gone up to 6 months on strictly water to drink.

So it's not impossible.

To further enhance my body, I stayed on a twice a day exercise regimen consisting of pushups, sit-ups, jogging, weight lifting, and any other physically conducive moment I discovered.

Even if confined strictly to your cell, you can use your "furniture" to further modify your workout. From dips on the side of the bottom bunk, to exercises using the toilet and the sink, the variations are endless.

Not only did exercise enhance my strength, it eased the stress of my confinement. I also kept a balance by exercising my mind with a reading regimen. My reading list was critical to my emotional and mental health. Trust me, if you want to stay sane, you'll need to read and write REGULARLY.

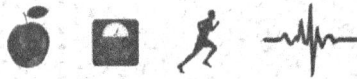

SENSIBLE DIET TIPS

Start your diet with a food diary, record everything you eat, what you were doing at the time, and how you felt. That tells you about yourself, your temptation, the emotional states that encourage you to snack, and may help you lose weight once you see how much you eat.

Instead of eating the forbidden piece of candy, brush your teeth. If you're about to cheat, allow yourself a treat, then eat only half a bite and throw the other half away.

When hunger hits, wait ten minutes before eating and see if it passes. Set attainable goals. Don't say, "I want to lose 50 pounds." Say, "I want to lose 5 pounds a month." Get enough sleep, but don't sleep too much. Try to avoid sugar. Highly sweetened foods tend to make you crave more.

Drink 6 to 8 glasses of water each day. Water itself helps cut down water retention because it acts as a diuretic. Taken before meals, it dulls the appetite by giving you that "full" feeling. Diet with a friend. Like with a workout partner, this can help keep you motivated.

Substitute activity for eating. When the cravings hit, go to the yard, or do a workout in your cell. This is especially helpful if you eat out of anger or stress.

If you're a late-night eater, have a carbohydrate, such as a slice of bread or a cracker, before bedtime to cut down on cravings. Keep an apple or a cup of water by your bed to keep quiet the hunger pangs that wake you up.

If you use food as a reward, establish a new reward system. Give yourself a nonedible reward. Write down everything you eat including small snacks. If you monitor what you eat, you can't go off your diet.

Make dining an event. Eat from your own special plate if possible, on your own special placement, and borrow the Japanese art of food arranging to make your meal, no matter how meager or simple, look lovely. This is a trick that helps chronic over-eaters and bingers pay attention to their food instead of consuming it unconsciously.

Keep plenty of crunchy foods like raw vegetables on hand. They're high in fiber, satisfying and filling. Leave something on your plate (or in your bowl). This is a good sign you can stop eating when you want to, not just when your plate is empty.

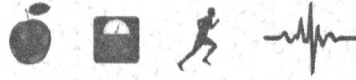

WHERE DIETS GO WRONG

When we discover that we are heavier than we want to be, we have a natural inclination to eat less food. We may skip lunch or eat only a tiny amount of our dinner in the hope that is we eat less our body will burn off some of its fat. But that is not necessarily true. Eating less actually makes it more difficult to lose weight.

Keep in mind that the human body took shape millions of years ago, and at that time there were no diets. The only low-calorie event in people's lives was starvation. Those who could cope with a temporary lack of food were the ones who survived. Our bodies, therefore, have developed this built-in mechanism to help us survive in the face of low food intake.

When researchers compare overweight and thin people, they find that they eat roughly the same amount of calories. What makes overweight people different is the amount of fat that they eat. Thin people tend to eat less fat and more complex carbohydrates.

Losing weight is not something one can do overnight. A carefully planned weight loss program requires common sense and certain guidelines. Unfortunately, there's a lot of misinformation floating around and lots of desperate people are easily duped and ripped off.

Every day one can open a magazine or newspaper and watch TV and see advertisements touting some new product, pill or something that will take excess weight off quickly. Everyone seems to be looking for that "magic" weight loss pill or solution. Millions of people in our country are trying to lose weight, spending billions of dollars every year on diet programs and products. Often they do lose some weight. But, if you check with the same people five years later, you will find that nearly all have regained whatever weight they lost.

A survey was done recently to try and determine if any commercial diet program could prove long-term success. Not a single program could do so. So rampant has the so-called diet industry become with new products and false claims that the FDA how now stepped in and started clamping down.

Being seriously overweight and particularly obese can develop into a number of diseases and serious health problems, and it is now a known fact that when caloric intake is excessive, some of the excess frequently is saturated fat.

The myth is that people get heavy by eating too many calories. True, calories are a consideration, but overall they are not the cause of obesity in our country today. Americans actually take in fewer calories each day than they did at the beginning of the century. If calories alone were the reason we become overweight, we should all be thin. But we are not. Collectively, we are heavier than ever. Partly, it is because we are more sedentary now (especially when locked in a small prison cell). But equally as important is the fact that the fat content of the American diet has changed dramatically.

People who diet without exercising often get fatter with time. Although your weight may initially drop while dieting, such weight loss consists mostly of water and muscle. When the weight returns, it comes back as fat. To avoid getting fatter over time, increase your metabolism by exercising regularly.

Select an exercise routine that you are comfortable with and remember that walking is one of the best and easiest exercises for strengthening your bones, controlling your weight and toning your muscles.

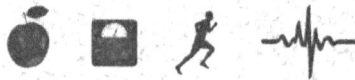

NUTRITION INFO YOU PROBABLY DON'T KNOW, BUT SHOULD

By C. Norman Shealy, MD, PhD

Water

As an adult you should drink half your body weight in pounds in ounces of good water. For 150 pounds of weight, that means 75 ounces of water! If you live in a city, I strongly recommend a good filter to remove chlorine and fluoride, at least from your drinking and cooking water. Obviously this is not likely to be an option while in prison. Ideally, you would remove it from your bathing water as well. Coffee and tea do not count as water, although any caffeine-free herbal tea will count as water intake. Fruit and vegetable juices also do not count as water, as they have many other substances that require the water content for metabolism.

Antioxidants

There are many natural antioxidants in nature, and if you eat at least 80% of your food as fresh fruits and vegetables, you will probably get enough. A list of important antioxidants follows:

Anthocyanins these great red, orange, and blue colored fruits and vegetables—are tremendous and should be part of every diet.

Ascorbic acid the essential in vitamin C—was discovered by the great scientist, Szent-Gyorgyi, who took 10 grams daily. For adults, I recommend 2000 mg, best taken with 1000 mg of methyl sulfonyl sulfate, 60 meg of molybdenum, and 3 to 6 mg of beta 1 3 glucan.

This combination helps restore DHEA. For serious illnesses such as bad viral infections or cancer, I recommend up to 100 grams of Vitamin C IV in a Myers cocktail. Of course, that requires a physician prescription and administration!

Vitamin A the best known vitamin A comes from fish liver oil, most commonly cod liver. However, larger doses of vitamin A, even 10,000 units daily, can lead to severe brain swelling. You actually need no vitamin A, but you do need the family of carotenoids, the best known being beta carotene. This family includes beta carotene, astaxanthin, and lycopene. All are precursors to vitamin A and are safe at very high doses. I prefer 25,000 units of beta carotene and 4 to 10 mg of astaxanthin daily. Lycopene and lutein are other members of the family and are, interestingly, increased in availability by cooking the most common source tomatoes.

CoQIO (Ubiquinone)—one of the major immune supporters. I prefer a minimum of 100 mg daily. Flavonoids—another fruit/vegetable family of antioxidants.

Polyphenols—the final fruit/vegetable antioxidants.

Essential Vitamins

Vitamin A see above.

The B Vitamins

B vitamins are essential for metabolism in general as well as production of energy and most importantly for brain and heart function. Despite the rather miniscule RDA's suggestion, in today's stressful environment, I think adults will be healthier if they take an average of 25 mg of the major ones

B1, Thiamine—deficiency of B1 leads to beriberi, Optic nerve damage, Korsakoff's syndrome, peripheral neuropathy, and heart failure. Up to 1000 mg daily is safe. Thiamine is absolutely required for metabolism of carbohydrates and alcohol, excess of which lead to beriberi. Up to 400 mg daily is safe.

B2, Riboflavin—B2 deficiency leads to inflammation of skin, mouth, tongue, and lips and anemia.

B3, Niacin—B3 deficiency leads to pellagra, which was rather common in the early twentieth century, again because of excess carbohydrate intake. This deficiency has a broader neurological/mental harm than virtually and other B vitamin. However, even 100 mg may cause significant flushing and a burning feeling in the skin. Another form of niacin, nicotinamide or niacinamide, is safe up to 1500 mg daily and may help arthritis symptoms and some schizophrenics.

B4—was once thought to be a vitamin, but it is "just" a critical component of DNA and RNA.

B5, Pantothenic acid—Pantothenic acid is primarily essential for energy, including proper metabolism of fat, carbohydrate, and protein. In general, it is quite safe up to 25 mg daily.

B6, Pyridoxine in one of the most commonly deficient B vitamins, even those who take the so-called RDA. Carpal tunnel syndrome, menstrual problems, and coronary artery disease are all major diseases of B6 deficiency. It is safe up to 100 mg daily.

B7, Biotin—B7 deficiency results from a really crummy diet and affects all aspects of mind and energy.

B8, Inositol in critical for function of brain, mind, and immune system. Up to 100 mg is safe.

B9, Folate (folic acid)—This is one of the most critical vitamins for function of mind, brain, and the integrity of the arteries. The RDA is ridiculously low, and it is safe up to 100 mg daily. Inadequate folic acid is a major contributor of homocysteine, a major cause of coronary disease, Alzheimer's disease, stroke, diabetes, and cancer, as well as malformations of babies. Blood levels above 7.5 are increasingly dangerous, and most labs ridiculously consider up to 14 "normal."

B10, PABA (Para amino benzoic acid) —B10 deficiency leads to many autoimmune diseases ranging from those affecting the skin, collagen system, and even the penis! It is safe up to 2000 mg twice a day and can help prevent sunburn.

B11, Salicylic acid—In general B11 can be manufactured by the body if you have adequate intake of phenylalanine, an essential amino acid. It is essential for the entire DNA system.

B12, Cobalamin (also Methylcobalamin)—B12 deficiency is best known as the cause of pernicious anemia, which leads not only to anemia but also to damage the spinal cord and brain. It is found only in animal protein! Vegans will inevitable develop B12 deficiency unless they take it as a supplement, and I like to remind them that it is still made by an animal—at the very least by yeast! Up to 5000 micrograms daily is quite safe.

Vitamin C (ascorbic acid)—Vitamin C is as critical as Vitamin D in supporting immune health.

The RDA of 60 mg is insanely low, and I believe adults with less than 1000 mg daily are at great risk.

Vitamin D3—80 percent of Americans are deficient in D3, largely because of the ridiculous advice of dermatologists to avoid sun and to use sun blocker. If you take at least 5000 units of D3 daily if you are an adult over 135 pounds.

Vitamin E, (Tocopherols and, more importantly, Tocotrienols)—One of the most basic antioxidant vitamins, working synergistically with A and C. 100 mg daily of gamma/delta Tocotrienols are essential for virtually every essential body function.

Carbohydrates

Carbohydrates are the broad field of sugars and starches. Essentially we do not need any carbs as we can make them out of fats or proteins. Naturally occurring carbohydrates, in general, are good, but "refined" and "enriched" carbohydrates are junk food! Table sugar, white flour, and fructose are plain rubbish, and they are major contributors to diabetes, heart disease, depression, ADHD, and cancer.

Honey is a blend of natural glucose and fructose and is much superior to sugar, since it is sweeter and contains some amino acids and vitamins. Used in moderation by all except diabetics, it is the only sweetener I recommend.

Fats

In general, naturally occurring fats in healthy meats, seeds, and nuts are good for you. Artificially hydrogenated or "hardened" fats are seriously dangerous, poisonous junk.

Omega-3—0mega-3s are alpha Linolenic acid (ALA), Eicosapentaenoic acid (EPA), and Docosahexaenoic acid (DHA). They are essential fats. Deficiencies lead to inflammation and every known disease! Best sources are wild salmon and grass fed beef and poultry.

Omega-6—The only healthy sources are nut oils, evening primrose, and black currant oils. Other vegetable sources such as corn oil, sunflower oil, safflower oil, cottonseed, peanut, and soy oil are to be avoided!!

Omega-9—These monounsaturated fats are not essential but in general are healthy, with the very best being from virgin olive oil and avocados.

Essential Amino Acids

There are nine really essential amino acids and on "conditionally" essential.

Histidine in needed to make histamine, as well as to stabilize hemoglobin and inhibit carbon monoxide. Those with allergies may be deficient.

Branched Chain Amino Acids: Isoleucine, Leucine, and Valine. These three are essential for building muscle and protecting cartilage, the "glue" substance that ties everything together, and for making and keeping cartilage healthy. Deficiencies weaken the immune system and increase risk of anxiety and depression.

Methionine is a sulfur-containing amino acid which can be widely used but with inadequate folic acid, B6, and B12 can lead to homocysteine, which is highly toxic.

Phenylalanine is essential for making the major stress essential triad: dopamine, norepinephrine, and epinephrine as well as for maintaining muscle.

Taurine is the most prevalent amino acid in the body CUT is deficient in 84 percent of depressed patients. It work synergistically with magnesium to stabilize cell membrane potential. It is especially helpful in depression, hyperextension, epilepsy, insomnia and anxiety. Up to 6000 mg daily may be tried.

Threonine is essential for making collagen, bones, teeth and preventing neurological spasticity. A major cause of deficiency is leaky gut!

Tryptophan is perhaps the best known amino acid and it is used to make serotonin, the most stabilizing mood neurochemical. Of course, you cannot make serotonin without B6, B3, and lithium.

Conditionally Essential Amino Acids...

Arginine is critical for maintaining muscle mass and for production of nitric oxide, a chemical essential to every cell function, including energy, immunity, and blood pressure.

After a certain age, arginine loses its significant contribution to nitric oxide (NO), because it is needed to maintain muscle mass.

Cysteine can usually be manufactured from methionine, if there are adequate amounts of B12, B6, and folate. It is a major contributor to energy.

Glutamine is made by healthy bacteria in the intestines and is also a "food" for growing more of the healthy probiotics which stabilize intestinal health.

Tyrosine is usually manufactured from the essential amino acid phenylalanine and would be deficient only in severe malnutrition.

Glycine is again a general malnutrition problem, as it is in all quality protein foods.

Ornithine deficiency is another general malnutrition problem. It works synergistically with arginine to assist in enhancing growth hormone release.

Proline is made in the body if there is not malnutrition. It is essential for maintaining cartilage.

Serine is manufactured from glycine and is deficient only in malnutrition.

There are a number of other amino acids which will be deficient only in general malnutrition—alanine, asparagine, aspartic acid, and glutamic acid.

Minerals

Calcium is one of the mega minerals and in adults requires an intake of about 1000 mg daily. However, if you take adequate vitamin D3 and eat a good diet, you do not need supplements.

Carbon is a building block for all organic matter.

Chlorine is ordinarily eaten as salt and very few people will be deficient if they eat a wide variety of foods. Excess salt can cause hypertension and related diseases.

Hydrogen is another building block of organic matter.

Magnesium is needed in over 350 enzymes and is second only to potassium and calcium in quantity. It is deficient in 80 percent of Americans because of high carbohydrate junk food and inadequate magnesium in the soil. It is far better absorbed through the skin than orally.

Phosphorus is prominent in all foods and would be deficient only in severe malnutrition.

Soda pop, a major junk food, is loaded with excess phosphorus.

Potassium is the third of the major minerals and comes mostly from fruits and vegetables.

Sodium deficiency would ordinarily occur only in malnutrition. Excess occurs because of overabundance of salt in many packaged foods.

Sulfur comes mainly from the sulfur containing amino acids and as methyl sulfonyl sulfate.

It is essential for supporting joints, cartilage, and making DHEA.

Trace Minerals

Boron is essential for preventing inflammation, for making testosterone, and for keeping bones strong. Most adults should take 9 mg.

Chromium is primarily necessary for production of insulin.

Cobalt is essential for making blood and balancing brain/mind.

Copper is mainly an anti-inflammatory and is a balancer with zinc.

Iodine is essential and for this is deficient in 80 percent of Americans. It is essential for thyroid function, energy, and immune strength.

Iron is best known for its role in hemoglobin.

Lithium is critical for making serotonin and stabilizing mood.

Manganese is critical for brain function.

Molybdenum is needed for many enzyme functions.

Selenium is needed for immune strength.

Silicon is important for strong bones.

Vanadium is critical to prevent diabetes and hypertension.

Zinc is essential for immune strength and general overall metabolic balance.

Toxic Minerals should be avoided! These include aluminum, arsenic, cadmium, fluoride, lead, mercury, and uranium.

Artificial & Processed Additives

The food industry has prostituted our food supply for the last century and created all these JUNK products: artificial flavors, aspartame, high fructose corn syrup, margarine, monosodium glutamate, Olestra, Splenda, and "American" or processed cheese. Avoid ALL!

The body is essentially alkaline—it has a pH that is above neutral. Blood and saliva should have a pH of 7.4. Urine, which gets rid of many waste products, should be acid at a pH 5.5 to a maximum of 6.5. Therefore, you should choose as least 80 percent of your foods from the alkaline producers!

Fruits: For anyone who is not overweight or diabetic, two to three servings of fruit daily are excellent. In general, a serving is 4 ounces of fruit or 6 ounces of juice. They are best raw, second best frozen, third best canned or dried. All fruits except cranberries, plums/prunes, and rhubarb are alkaline producing!

Vegetables: All are alkaline producing!

Grains: Acid Producing.

Legumes: Acid producing (except for string beans, snap beans, and snow peas.)

Eggs: Acid producing.

Dairy: Acid producing.

Meats: Acid producing.

Seafood: Acid producing.

Starchy Vegetables: Acid producing.

Spices: Neutral.

Now, with hundreds of different foods and scores of variety in preparation, you have no excuse for not having a minimum of 5 servings daily of fruits and vegetables, plus some quality protein!

The exciting variations in preparing this potpourri of excellent foods are virtually endless. In general, your major concerns should be excluding artificial foods discussed earlier and avoiding the seriously dangerous GMO foods. Ideally, it is best to obtain as much as possible from real farmers who use no poisonous chemical pesticides or herbicides good luck achieving this from prison.

However, there is another widely prevalent substance in food that is potentially a serious health threat—lectins. At least 30 percent of all natural foods contain lectins, with the highest concentrations being in whole grains, peanuts, kidney beans, and soybeans. Tomatoes, eggplant, peppers, and Irish potatoes are relatively high, and it appears that sensitivities to these nightshades is very much an individual reaction and not nearly as universal as the problems with wheat. In addition to gluten, the other widely produced lectins are prime contributors to autoimmune diseases, such as Hashimoto's thyroiditis, rheumatoid arthritis, multiple sclerosis, etc. If your intestines contain enough natural mucin, the lectins bind to it and may pass unnoticed. If you are low in mucin, lectins bind to the intestinal linings and create serious bowel problems. Lectins include:

- √ Grains (wheat, oats, buckwheat, rye, barley, millet, corn, and possibly rice, although most of the lectins in rice are not in the part that gets eaten)
- √ Legumes (any kind of bean plus peanuts, which have a particularly bad lectin)
- √ Soy

It's long been known that certain foods like kidney beans and castor beans contain especially toxic lectins. In fact, the lectin Ricin, which is found in castor beans, is so toxic that it's used as a weapon in biochemical warfare!

The most critical advice of all in relation to nutrition is that 80 percent of your food should come from the alkaline fruits and vegetables and only 20 percent from the acid producing foods.

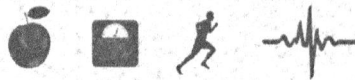

TOO MUCH SALT

HOW A DIET TOO HIGH IN SODIUM CAN AFFECT YOUR HEART, BRAIN, AND EVEN BONE HEALTH

Salt has always been of high importance to humanity. In ancient Egypt, salt was an integral part of religious ceremonies, and the Moors in Africa would trade salt pound for pound with gold. Part of our adoration for salt, however, lies in its main ingredient, sodium. (It's also composed of chloride and iodine sources.) According to the American Heart Association, about 75 percent of the sodium we consume comes not from the salt shaker, but rather in processed and restaurant food.

Our Love Affair With Salt

Sodium is essential to human health. The mineral helps to regulate fluids by letting the body know when it's time to replenish or dispose of water. Along with that, sodium also maintains nerve transmissions and muscle contractions—functions vital to our survival. As a result, our bodies evolved a desire for sodium akin to addiction to ensure that we never went without enough.

A 2011 Australian study found that the brain responds to sodium similar to how it does for substances such as heroin, cocaine, and nicotine, which may explain why so many of us tend to overindulge in high-sodium foods. Unfortunately, too much of a good thing can actually prove deadly.

Your Brain On Salt

A 2011 Canadian study on 1,200 older sedentary adults with normal brain function found that over the course of three years, high-sodium diets were linked to increased risk of cognitive decline. This result was "independent of hypertension and global diet quality" and "suggests that sodium intake alone may affect cognitive function in sedentary older adults above and beyond the effects of overall diet," the researchers wrote.

The reason why sodium is detrimental to the brain is not fully understood, but according to Dr. David L. Katz, a researcher involved in the study, physical exercise may be able to protect the brain from the effects of too much salt, Medscape reported.

Kidneys

Sodium plays a key role in balancing the levels of fluid in our bodies by signaling to the kidneys when to retain water and when to get rid of water. A high-sodium diet can interfere with this delicate process and reduce kidney function. The result is less water removed from the body, which may lead to higher blood pressure. As explained by The World Action on Salt and Health, this excess strain on the kidneys can lead to kidney disease or exacerbate kidney problems in those already with the condition.

High-sodium diets may also increase your risk of developing renal stones, also known as kidney stones. The main cause of kidney stones is urinary calcium, a mineral which is noted to increase in those with high-sodium intake.

Bones

Excessive calcium excretion in the urine is believed by some experts to increase the risk of bone thinning. According to WASH, over long periods of time, this excessive calcium loss is associated with osteoporosis, especially in postmenopausal women.

Heart

Due to salt's fluid retention effect, in some individuals excessive amounts of salt in their diet can lead to high blood pressure. High blood pressure is the force of blood pushing against the walls of the arteries as the heart pumps blood, and high blood pressure can lead to many serious conditions, such as stroke and heart failure. Although blood pressure increases naturally with age, according to the American Heart Association, reducing your salt intake can help prevent your blood pressure from increasing too much.

Skin

Excessive salt in the diet can cause a symptom known as edema. As reported by Medical News Today, edema is characterized by swelling, particularly in the hands, arms, ankles, legs, and feet, caused by fluid retention. Excessive salt consumption commonly causes edema; however, the symptom can be caused by a number of other health concerns ranging from menstruation to genetic disposition. Edema is non-life threatening and is a symptom of another underlying health condition, rather than a condition on its own.

While edema may be an extreme symptom of excessive salt consumption, even something as simple as having an extra-large popcorn the night before can leave your skin looking a bit puffier than usual. Dr. Neal B. Schultz, a dermatologist practicing in New York City, told Shape that susceptibility to swelling due to salt consumption increases with age.

Stomach

A 1996 study published in the International Journal of Epidemiology found that death from stomach cancer in both men and women was closely linked to salt consumption. High salt intake is also associated with stomach ulcers. The reason for this is not completely understood, but one study theorized that the salt may have an adverse effect on the mucous lining of the stomach and cause the stomach tissue to become abnormal and unhealthy, according to Livestrong.

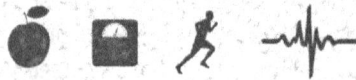

WHAT CHEMICAL COCKTAIL
IS IN YOUR FOOD

Story at-a-glance

- √ Since the 1950s, the number of food additives allowed in U.S. food has grown from about 800 to more than 10,000
- √ GRAS, or "generally recognized as safe," is a loophole created in 1958; food companies are tasked with determining such status for their own ingredients
- √ Once an additive is granted GRAS status by an industry-hired panel, the company doesn't need to inform the FDA that the ingredient is used, and no independent third-party objective evaluation is required

By Dr. Mercola

One of the simplest choices you can make in support of your health is to eat real food. Real food refers to vegetables, meats and wild-caught seafood, nuts, seeds, eggs, fruits and raw grass-fed dairy; foods that are in their whole, primarily unaltered form.

Such foods will not only hydrozincite you with rich concentrations of vitamins, minerals, fiber and antioxidants, but they're also beneficial for what they do not contain—food additives.

If you eat processed foods, you're consuming a chemical cocktail with each bite. Even seemingly simple foods like bread, processed cheese, salad dressing or pasta sauce are typically loaded with preservatives, emulsifiers, flavorings, colorings and other "enhancers."

9 TOP FOOD ADDITIVES TO AVOID

Since the 1950s, the number of food additives allowed in U.S. food has grown from about 800 to more than 10,000. We're not talking only about simple natural ingredients like vinegar and table salt anymore, but countless chemical concoctions that are putting Americans' health at risk.

What little risk assessment done on such chemicals is typically done on individual chemicals in isolation, but mounting research suggests that when you consume multiple additives in combination, the health effects may be more serious than previously imagined.

One assessment by the National Food Institute at the Technical University of Denmark found that even small amounts of chemicals can amplify each other's adverse effects when combined.

Really, the only way to avoid this chemical cocktail is to avoid processed foods. But at the very least, you'll want to read food labels carefully and avoid those that follow.

1.   High-Fructose Com Syrup (HFCS)

It's often claimed that HFCS is no worse for you than sugar, but this is not the case.

Because high-fructose com syrup contains free-form mono-saccharides of fructose and glucose, it cannot be considered biologically equivalent to sucrose (sugar), which has a glycosidic bond that links the fructose and glucose together, and which slows its breakdown in your body.

Fructose is primarily metabolized by your liver, because your liver is the only organ that has the transporter for it.

Since all fructose gets shuttled to your liver, and, if you eat a typical Western-style diet, you consume high amounts of it, fructose ends up taxing and damaging your liver in the same way alcohol and other toxins do.

And just like alcohol, fructose is metabolized directly into fat—it just gets stored in your fat cells, which leads to mitochondrial malfunction, obesity and obesity-related diseases.

The more fructose or HFCS a food contains, and the more total fructose you consume, the worse it is for your health.

For example, female mice fed a diet that contained 25 percent of calories from com syrup had nearly twice the death rate and 26 percent fewer offspring compared to those fed a diet in which 25 percent of calories came from table sugar.[2]

As a standard recommendation, I advise keeping your TOTAL fructose consumption below 25 grams per day, which is very difficult to do if you eat processed foods.

For most people it would also be wise to limit your fructose from fruit to 15 grams or less, as you're virtually guaranteed to consume "hidden" sources of fructose if you drink beverages other than water and eat processed food.

Fifteen grams of fructose is not much—it represents two bananas, one-third cup of raisins, or two Medjool dates. The average 12-ounce can of soda contains 40 grams of sugar, at least half of which is fructose, so one can of soda alone would exceed your daily allotment.

2.   Artificial Sweeteners

Experiments have found that sweet taste, regardless of its caloric content, enhances your appetite, and consuming artificial sweeteners has been shown to lead to even greater weight gain than consuming sugar.

Aspartame has been found to have the most pronounced effect, but the same applies for other artificial sweeteners, such as acesulfame potassium, sucralose and saccharin. Yet, weight gain is only the beginning of why artificial sweeteners should generally be avoided.

Aspartame, for instance, is a sweet-tasting neurotoxin. As a result of its unnatural structure, your body processes the amino acids found in aspartame very differently from a steak or a piece of fish.

The amino acids in aspartame literally attack your cells, even crossing the blood- brain barrier to attack your brain cells, creating a toxic cellular overstimulation, called excitotoxicity, similar to monosodium glutamate (MSG).

Further, inflammatory bowel disease may be caused or exacerbated by the regular consumption of the popular artificial sweetener Splenda (sucralose), as it inactivates digestive enzymes and alters gut barrier function.

Previous research also found that sucralose can destroy up to 50 percent of your beneficial gut flora. While you certainly don't want to overdo it on sugar, there's little doubt in my mind that artificial sweeteners can be even worse for your health than sugar and even fructose.

3.   Monosodium Glutamate (MSG)

This flavor enhancer is most often associated with Chinese food, but it's actually in countless processed food products ranging from frozen dinners and salad dressing to snack chips and meats.

MSG is an excitotoxin, which means it overexcites your cells to the point of damage or death, causing brain dysfunction and damage to varying degrees—and potentially even triggering or worsening learning disabilities, Alzheimer's disease, Parkinson's disease, Lou Gehrig's disease and more.

Part of the problem is that free glutamic acid (MSG is approximately 78 percent free glutamic acid) is the same neurotransmitter that your brain, nervous system, eyes, pancreas and other organs use to initiate certain processes in your body.

Although the U.S. Food and Drug Administration (FDA) continues to claim that consuming MSG in food does not cause these ill effects, many other experts say otherwise.

4.   Synthetic Trans Fats

Synthetic trans fats, found in margarine, vegetable shortening, and partially hydrogenated vegetable oils, are known to promote inflammation, which is a hallmark of most chronic and/or serious diseases.

These synthetic fats have been linked to stroke, cancer, diabetes, decreased immune function, reproductive problems, heart disease and more.

Fortunately, in June 2015 the FDA announced partially hydrogenated oils (a primary source of trans fat) will no longer be allowed in food due to their health risks, unless authorized by the agency.

According to the FDA, this change may help prevent around 20,000 heart attacks and 7,000 heart disease deaths each year.

The new regulation won't take effect until 2018. In the interim, food companies have to either reformulate their products to remove partially hydrogenated oils or file a limited use petition with the FDA to continue using them.

5.   Artificial Colors

Fifteen million pounds of artificial food dyes are added into U.S. foods every year—and that amount only factors in eight different varieties.3 As of July 2010, most foods in the European Union (EU) that contain artificial food dyes were labeled with warning labels stating the food "may have an adverse effect on activity and attention in children."

The British government also asked that food manufacturers remove most artificial colors from foods back in 2009 due to health concerns. Nine of the food dyes currently approved for use in the U.S. are linked to health issues ranging from cancer and hyperactivity to allergy-like reactions—and these results were from studies conducted by the chemical industry itself.

For instance, Red # 40, which is the most widely used dye, may accelerate the appearance of immune system tumors in mice, while also triggering hyperactivity in children. Blue # 2, used in candies, beverages, pet foods and more, was linked to brain tumors.

And Yellow 5, used in baked goods, candies, cereal and more, may not only be contaminated with several cancer-causing chemicals, but it's also linked to hyperactivity, hypersensitivity and other behavioral effects in children. Even the innocuous-sounding caramel color, which is widely used in brown soft drinks, may cause cancer due to 4-methylimidazole (4-Mel), a chemical byproduct formed when certain types of caramel coloring are manufactured.

Some U.S. companies are moving ahead of regulatory agencies to get these controversial additives out of their products. Mars, Inc., for instance, announced in February 2016 that it will be removing synthetic food dyes from its entire line of food products, including M&Ms candies.6

6.   Sodium Sulphite

This is a widely used food preservative. People who are sulfite sensitive can experience headaches, breathing problems and rashes. In severe cases, sulfites can actually cause death.

7.   Butylated Hydroxyanisole (BHA) and Butylated Hydroxytoluene (BHT)

Butylated Hydroxyanisole (BHA) 'is a preservative that affects the neurological system of your brain, alters behavior and has the potential to cause cancer. It can be found in breakfast cereal, nut mixes, chewing gum, butter spread, meat, dehydrated potatoes, popcorn, chips and beer, just to name a few.

BHA is known to cause cancer in rats, and may be a cancer-causing agent in humans as well. According to the U.S. Department of Health and Human Services National Toxicology Program's 2011 Report on Carcinogens, BHA "is reasonably anticipated to be a human carcinogen."

The international cancer agency categorizes it as a possible human carcinogen, and it's listed as a known carcinogen under California's Proposition 65.

BHA may also trigger allergic reactions and hyperactivity. BHA is banned from infant foods in the U.K. and is banned from use in all foods in certain parts of the EU and Japan. In the U.S., the FDA considers BHA to be a GRAS additive. BHT is chemically similar to BHA and the two preservatives are often used together. While BHT is not considered a carcinogen like BHA, it has been linked to tumor development in animals.

It's also been linked to developmental effects and thyroid changes in animal studies, which suggests it may be an endocrine-disrupting chemical. In the U.S., BHA is given GRAS (generally recognized as safe) status.

8.   Sulphur Dioxide

Sulphur additives are toxic, and in the U.S. they have been prohibited in raw fruit and vegetables. Adverse reactions include bronchial problems, low blood pressure and anaphylactic shock.

9.   Potassium Bromate

Nearly every time you eat bread in a restaurant or consume a hamburger or hotdog bun you are consuming bromide, an endocrine-disrupting chemical commonly used in flours. The use of potassium bromate as an additive in commercial breads and baked goods has been a huge contributor to bromide overload in Western cultures. Bromated flour is "enriched" with potassium bromate.

Commercial baking companies use it because it makes the dough more elastic and better able to stand up to bread hooks. However, Pepperidge Farm and other successful companies manage to use only unbromated flour without any of these so-called "structural problems."

Studies have linked potassium bromate to kidney and nervous system damage, thyroid problems, gastrointestinal discomfort, and cancer. The International Agency for Research on Cancer classifies potassium bromate as a possible carcinogen. Potassium bromate is banned for food use in Canada, China and the EU.

GRAS Loophole Makes Processed Foods a Chemical Minefield

GRAS, or generally recognized as safe, is a loophole created in 1958. At the time, the first law regulating food additives had just been put into place, which required food companies to submit new ingredients to the FDA for review.

Congress didn't want the FDA to waste time reviewing common staple ingredients like table salt and vinegar, so they added the loophole that companies could prove certain ingredients to be GRAS, with no FDA review required. One of the most alarming problems with the GRAS loophole is that food companies are tasked with determining such status for their own ingredients.

So a company can simply hire an industry insider to evaluate the chemical, and if that individual determines the chemical meets federal safety standards, it can be deemed GRAS. Once an additive is granted GRAS status by the hired panel, the company doesn't even need to inform the FDA that the ingredient is used, and no independent third-party objective evaluation is ever required.

According to the Center for Science in the Public Interest (CSPI), at least 1,000 ingredients are added to U.S. foods that the FDA has no knowledge of. Many of these additives may be imported from overseas, making their actual contents and safety profiles largely unknown. As reported by the Epoch Times.

"Many of the companies making the additives are headquartered overseas, like the China based Hanzhong TRG Biotech which makes at least 40 of the chemicals NRDC National Resources Defense Council says have undisclosed GRAS safety determinations.

Such imported additives are triply difficult for the FDA when the companies self- declare them as safe, said Erik Olsen, Ph.D. senior strategic director for health and food at the Natural Resources Defense Council. The FDA does not realize the additive is being used, has not evaluated the additive itself, and lacks a mechanism for assessing the safety of imported products. Buyer beware.

Chemical and Drug Companies Are Making Many Food Additives

You might expect that food additives are at least being made by food companies like Kraft. But some of the major players in the industry are not food companies at all but rather are more well-known as chemical and drug makers; Merck and BASF Cognis Nutrition and Health are among them.

The bottom line is that it's not safe to assume that anyone is looking out for the safety of additives in our food. Hundreds of food chemicals have been simply declared safe by their manufacturers, and in many instances the FDA doesn't even know they're added to your food, let along what their health effects may be and neither do you. NRDC published an eye-opening report on this subject in 2014, which revealed:

- √ "275 chemicals used by 56 companies appear to be marketed as GRAS and used in many food products based on companies' safety determinations that, pursuant to current regulations, did not need to be reported to the FDA or the public. This is probably just the tip of the iceberg."

- √ "Information obtained under the federal Freedom of Information Act shows that when FDA does learn of a chemical proposed to be used in food, the agency often asks tough questions, but because of the GRAS loophole a company is not bound to answer them and not prohibited from continuing to sell the chemical for use in food."

- √ "Based on information from notices submitted to the FDA, but later withdrawn, companies have sometimes certified their chemicals as safe for use in food despite potentially serious allergic reactions, or adverse reactions in combination with common drugs, or have proposed using amounts of the chemicals in food at much higher levels than company established safe levels."

√ "When companies seek FDA's voluntary review of their GRAS safety determination, the agency rejects or triggers withdrawal of that determination in one out of every 5 cases. At least in some instances, companies may have withdrawn their notices in order to avoid having an FDA rejection made public."

√ "The public and FDA are in the dark about hundreds of chemicals found in our food because companies aren't required to submit the safety determination to FDA for its review."

Are You Ready to Ditch Processed Foods?

Scottish author Joanna Blythman has written a behind-the-scenes book, *Swallow This: Serving Up the Food Industry's Darkest Secrets*, that delves into the details of what makes processed food the antithesis of a healthy diet. If you have any concerns about the food you're eating, this is a must-read book. It will radically increase your appreciation of just how processed your food really is and enlighten you to many of the deceptive tricks the industry uses to fool you.

Even aside from the additives, a processed food diet sets the stage for obesity and any number of chronic health issues. In fact, many of the top diseases plaguing the U.S. are diet-related, including heart disease, diabetes, and cancer. The answer to these health problems lies not in a pill but in the food choices you make each and every day.

When it comes to staying healthy, avoiding processed foods and replacing them with fresh, whole foods is the *secret* you've been looking for. This might sound daunting, but if you take it step-by-step as described in my nutrition plan it's quite possible, and manageable, to painlessly remove processed foods from your diet. Remember, people have thrived on vegetables, meats, eggs, fruits and other whole foods for centuries, while processed foods were only recently invented.

I believe you should spend 90 percent of your food budget on whole foods and only 10 percent on processed foods (unfortunately most Americans currently do the opposite). This requires that you plan your meals in advance. Ideally, this will involve scouting out your local farmer's markets for in-season produce that is priced to sell and planning your meals accordingly, but you can also use this same premise with supermarket sales.

Try to plan a week of meals at a time, make sure you have all ingredients necessary on hand, and then do any prep work you can ahead of time so that dinner is easy to prepare if you're short on time in the evenings (and you can use leftovers for lunches the next day). Processed foods are addictive, so if cravings are a problem for you please see my article on how to eliminate junk food cravings.

One of the most effective strategies to eliminate sugar cravings is intermittent fasting, along with diet modifications that effectively help reset your body's metabolism to burn fat instead of sugar as its primary fuel.

If your junk food cravings are linked to an emotional challenge, a psychological acupressure technique called the Emotional Freedom Techniques (EFT) can rapidly help you control your emotional food cravings. If you're currently sustaining yourself on fast food and processed foods, cutting them from your diet is one of the most positive life changes you could ever make.

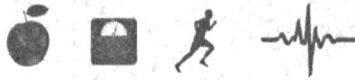

THE CASE FOR ESSENTIAL AMINO ACIDS
By Scott Robinson

If you're looking to build more muscle, why not supplement with the building block itself?

Let's face it: Deep down inside, every gym goer fantasizes about finding that magic bullet, the secret sauce that can build muscle, burn fat, and generally help you realize fitness goals faster and more efficiently. Thousands of exercise supplements promise just that, but let's face this: If we're honest with ourselves, we know that few are based on actual science and that the ones that do "work" owe their effectiveness to the magical ingredient known as placebo.

But there is one nutritional supplement that proponents say truly speeds the muscle-building process: amino acids.

A quick biology refresher: Muscle, we know, is tissue that's made up of protein. That tissue is composed of fibers—and those fibers comprise chains of amino-acid molecules.

All told, there are 20 amino acids that build protein. The body produces 11 of them on its own (the so-called nonessential acids); the remaining nine, the essential amino acids (eeas), come from food. So when you tuck into a T-bone steak (or some edamame pods), the digestive system breaks down the protein into amino acids, transporting the little guys via the bloodstream to the muscles so they can get to work on building new muscle fibers.

Now think about what happens at the gym. You're breaking down muscle fibers; muscle building is the healing process. More amino acids, more muscle, the thinking goes. But most guys rightfully don't want to gnaw on a steak between sets.

But it's not only brute strength. Some people who supplement their diets with amino acids say they have more energy to push through hard workouts and bounce back from bouts quicker.

The exercise community has, for decades, studied the effectiveness of amino acid supplements, branched-chain amino acids (BCAAs), in particular. They comprise leucine, isoleucine, and valine.

Still, there's little consensus in the scientific community of the supplement's effectiveness. A study out of the University of Charleston which appeared to show that BCAAs helped guys maintain muscle mass during periods of caloric restriction was criticized for drawing sunnier conclusions than the data would suggest. (The study authors would later revise their findings, acknowledging that more work needed to be done.)

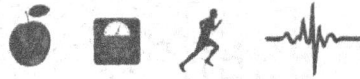

DIET—A PERSPECTIVE
By Bo Lozoff

Diet isn't a simple issue, as if we merely have to find out what's good for us and then "eat right." That's often a very uptight way to live. Of course, to eat whatever our crazed minds desire doesn't work too well, either. Neither extreme seems to produce happy, free, or powerful people.

On one hand, a great amount of dietary wisdom has influenced most of us during the past 20 years or so. The move away from junk food, away from fatty and heavy meat diets, the discoveries of the harmful effects of sugar and caffeine; the acceptance of various nutrition principles from other cultures—the effects of yogurt, the benefits or whole grains, balancing yin and yang in a macrobiotic diet, etc.

But on the other hand, food is still a prop, and so is the body. They both belong solely to the world of appearances. Time brings, time takes away. Good food or junk food—all end up in the same pile of bones eventually. Their only real meaning, their only lasting value, is to help us in our spiritual work, which involves a lot more than physical health.

In the past ten or fifteen years, our culture has made the healthy body into an object of worship and of obsessive focus. Diet and fitness are multi-billion-dollar industries in America. It's been easy to get sidetracked from the view of "honoring the body as a temple" into the view of worshipping the body as if it were the God inside the temple. It surely makes sense to stay in shape, but the intensity of our own concern is just another youth-oriented, death-denying trap in the world of illusion.

There's got to be a good balance, and though I hate to sound like a broken record, we each must find and honor our own unique balance within ourselves. The law of nutrition and chemistry would seem to treat us all equally, but actually any worldly laws are changeable depending on our states of mind and Spirit. A Big Mac can become manna, and brown rice become poison, depending on who's eating which, and how uptight they're feeling while they're doing it.

I studied Aikido for a short time in Colorado. My Sensei, or teacher, was a very gentle and powerful master from Japan. When we walked in the room, it was very easy to feel the "Ki" power that the martial arts are about. Everything about him felt natural and perfectly balanced; he seemed always at ease, yet it was obvious he couldn't be caught off-guard. He was certainly a living expression of the path he was teaching.

One day I walked by his office on my way out of the Dojo, and I saw him and his wife (also a black-belt) eating a lunch of all the worst junk food imaginable: Big Macs, Dunkin' donuts, cokes, fries, etc. After so many years of being careful about my diet, I couldn't help but be shocked that such "high beings" would treat their bodies so recklessly. I said, "Sensei, how can you put this food into your body?" He looked up at me, hardly missing a bite, and said, "Bo, whether food does you good or harm depends on your Ki, on your attitude! Have a good attitude, any food good; have bad attitude, any food bad." He smiled respectfully and went on with his meal.

Driving home, thinking it over, it all made perfect sense. And already the visions of Dairy Queen, Taco Bell, and M&M's were floating through my mind—all the stuff I used to love before becoming a strict yogi. I let go of the dietary controls I'd acquired over the years, and started eating anything and everything I wanted. The problem was—as I realized while groaning on the toilet one day—I wanted to believe as he did, but deep down, I still believed those foods were bad for me. The same food that nourished him was ruining me, because all I was doing was making excuses for a lot of food that I had repressed for years. This game is played far deeper than our conscious whims and passing fancies.

I still know he's right about attitudes. Mine have been steadily opening and changing (as well as my diet) since then. But it's a slower, more subtle process than I had realized; and we have to honestly live by whatever stage of it we're in at any given time.

The struggle to find our own best diet is rich with teachings about self-honesty, self-discipline self-righteousness, and wisdom. Any diet could benefit one person and harm another, so obviously our needs are unique—as are the lessons we need to learn.

Self-honesty comes up because God always finds a way to force us to look inward for answers rather than to any outside source no matter how popular or authoritative. Outside sources supply us with information (one expert usually contradicting another), and then we have to run it through our own minds and hearts to see what rings a bell or doesn't. It's more a process of recognizing, rather than "choosing," what we believe our bodies need.

What self-honesty shows us may be at odds with what our taste buds desire, and that's where self-discipline comes in. If my body seemed to be telling me something wrong, I'd have to pursue it and see where it leads—cutting out cigarettes or sugar or coffee or whatever I believed was being the problem. If I decided to follow a specific religion, I'd obey the dietary laws of that path in order to give the total system a fair chance. If I got heavily into Hatha Yoga, I'd be a stricter vegetarian and cut way down on spices and stimulants; again, because it's a total system. Self-discipline is what gives us the freedom to alter our diets to suit our needs.

But after gaining enough self-honesty and self-control to experiment with any diets we choose, most of us fall into the trap that what we believe about diet is absolute and final Truth. Now come the lessons of self-righteousness. If we allow them to happen, these lessons are more embarrassing than painful. We can laugh at the time we refused to eat turkey with our families on Thanksgiving, etc. But if we try to hold on tight to philosophies about food rather than opening up to higher teachings, we'll miss out on many experiences and a great deal of wisdom.

Diet takes on an even more confusing role in prison. On the streets, it's mostly a free-choice situation, and the struggle is usually one of self-discipline to clean up our diets without becoming neurotic about it. But in the joint, the struggle is often the opposite: most cons would love to get more wholesome foods—whole grains, fresh vegetables and fruit, "holistic" foods like! tofu, yogurt, nuts and so forth, but it's nearly impossible to do.

The self-discipline is often the opposite too, because in a no-choice situation, the spiritual warrior's way is to eat, with a happy mind, whatever food is available, and to let go of anxieties about cholesterol, fats, sugar, additives, etc. This is where my Sensei's advice about attitude becomes an important key for staying healthy. If you can't change your diet, change your attitude.

Another mystical secret: When choices are taken away, a perfect path remains.

"Bad" food can be transformed into Spirit-food. Remember, physical laws and "facts" don't always hold true. Reality isn't so unbending. Trust the magic!

All food; all drink—depending only on how we see it and deal with it. If there's any degree of choice, it's a good idea to eat fresh fruits and vegetables, less sugar and white flour, less coffee, more water, more whole grains like brown rice and buckwheat, fewer heavy meats like beef and pork, and maybe cut down a little bit on dairy products.

But the other stuff is still the body and blood of Christ.

As I learned from my own experience, a head-trip isn't the same as a genuine change of attitude. Genuine changes, deep changes, usually require conscious effort. It's spiritual work, just like yoga or meditation. The best time for this work is before and during each meal. Without drawing much attention to yourself, take a minute or so before eating to:

1. Get calm and centered.
2. Look at the food on your plate and realize that all of its energy came ultimately from the Sun; vegetables grow from sun-power, cows and hogs and chickens grow from eating sun-grown grasses and grains—all food-energy ultimately comes from sun energy, which is pure LIGHT.
3. Instruct your body to be receptive to this Light, and not worry about the rest.
4. Rather than feeling "resigned" about eating this food, give thanks instead, because dealing with this teaching is bound to increase your wisdom and power.
5. Pay attention as you eat, consciously consuming this food for perfect physical and spiritual health. If possible, eat alone for a while so you can concentrate better.

"This food is my body; this drink is my blood." —Jesus

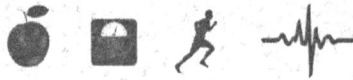

FOOD POINSONING

Food Poisoning Facts

- √ Food poisoning is a common infectious condition that affects millions of people in the United States each year.
- √ Most commonly, people complain of
    - √ vomiting
    - √ diarrhea and
    - √ cramping abdominal pain
- √ People should seek medical care if they have an associated fever, blood in their stool (rectal bleeding), signs and symptoms of dehydration, or if their symptoms do not resolve after a couple of days.
- √ Treatment for food poisoning focuses on keeping the affected person well hydrated.
- √ Prevention is key and depends upon keeping food preparation areas clean, proper hand washing, and cooking foods thoroughly.

What is food poisoning?

Food poisoning is a food borne disease. Ingestion of food that contains a toxin, chemical or infectious agent (like a bacterium, virus, parasite, or prion) may cause adverse symptoms in the body. Those symptoms may be related only to the gastrointestinal tract causing vomiting or diarrhea or they may involve other organs such as the kidney, brain, or muscle.

Typically most food borne diseases cause vomiting and diarrhea that tend to be short lived and resolve on their own, but dehydration and electrolyte abnormalities may develop. The Center for Disease Control and Prevention (CDC) estimates approximately 48 million people become ill from food- related diseases each year resulting in 128,000 hospitalizations, and 3,000 deaths.

According to the CDC, in 2011, the most common foodborne illnesses in the United States each year are caused by Norovirus, and the bacteria

Campylobacter, Clostridium perfringens, and Salmonella.

This article introduces the major causes of food poisoning and is not meant to be all-inclusive.

What are the signs and symptoms of food poisoning?

Food poisoning most commonly causes:

- √ abdominal cramps
- √ vomiting
- √ diarrhea

This can cause significant amounts of fluid loss and diarrhea along with nausea and vomiting may make it difficult to replace lost fluid, leading to dehydration d. In developing countries where infectious epidemics cause diarrheal illnesses, thousands of people die because of dehydration.

As noted in the section above, other organ systems may be infected and affected by food poisoning. Symptoms will depend upon what organ system is involved (for example, encephalopathy due to brain infection).

Are food poisoning and stomach flu the same thing?

Food poisoning and the stomach flu may or may not be the same thing, depending if the causative agent is transmitted by contaminated food, or if the agent is transmitted by non-food mechanisms such as body secretions. Most health-care professionals equate stomach flu to viral gastroenteritis.

Stomach flu is a non-specific term that describes an illness that usually resolves within 24 hours and is caused commonly by the adenovirus HI, Norwalk virus or rotavirus, (rotavirus is most commonly found in children).

If numerous cases of "stomach flu" occur in a situation where many people have been eating, it certainly may be considered food poisoning. Norwalk virus is responsible for many cases of food borne illness outbreaks on cruise ships.

How long does food poisoning last?

Most cases of food poisoning last about 1 to 2 days and symptoms resolve on their own. If symptoms persist longer than that, the affected person should contact their health-care professional.

Cyclospora infections may be difficult to detect and diarrhea may last for weeks, health-care professionals may consider this parasite as the potential cause of food poisoning in patients with prolonged symptoms.

What are the types of food poisoning?

Most frequently, food poisoning may be due to infection caused by bacteria, viruses, parasites, and infrequently, prions. More than 200 infectious causes exist. Sometimes it is not the bacteria that causes the problem, but rather the toxin that bacteria produce in the food before it is eaten. This is the case with Staphylococcal food poisoning and with botulism.

Other illnesses may involve chemical toxins that are produced in certain foods that are poorly cooked or stored. For example, scombroid poisoning occurs due to a large release of histamine chemical from the fish when it is eaten. It causes facial swelling, itching, and difficulty breathing and swallowing-just like an allergic reaction. Scombroid poisoning is sometimes confused with a shellfish allergy.

Some "food poisonings" may not be due to toxins or chemicals in food but to infectious agents that happen to contaminate the food. E. coli 0157:H7 (hemorrhagic E. coli) usually occurs when contaminated food is eaten, but it also can spread from contaminated drinking water, a contaminated swimming pool, or passed from child to child in a daycare center.

Listeria is a type of bacteria that has caused the two most deadly outbreaks of food poisoning in United States history. In 1985, an outbreak in California was traced to eating a type of fresh cheese, and in 2011, Listeria food poisoning was traced to a cantaloupe farm and processing operation in Colorado. It is most often associated with eating soft cheeses, raw milk, contaminated fruits, vegetables, poultry, and meats. Newborns, the elderly and others with compromised immune systems are at higher risk of becoming ill with Listeria infections. Pregnant women are also at higher risk of contracting Listeria infections and are recommended to avoid soft cheeses like brie, camembert, and blue (cream cheese is safe) to avoid infection and to prevent transmission to the fetus.

What are the causes of food poisoning?

There many causes of food poisoning. Sometimes they are classified by how quickly the symptoms begin after eating potentially contaminated food. Think of this as the incubation time from when food enters the body until symptoms begin. The following are examples of how this time classification can be arranged:

Short incubation of less than 16 to 24 hours

Chemical causes

- √ Scombroid poisoning usually is due to poorly cooked or stored fish. The affected person will experience flushing, shortness of breath, and difficulty swallowing within 1 to 2 hours of eating.

- √ Ciguatera poisoning is another fish toxin that occurs after eating fish such as grouper, snapper, and barracuda. Symptoms include vomiting and diarrhea, muscle aches, and neurologic complaints including headache, numbness and tingling, hallucinations, and difficulty with balance (ataxia).

- √ Mushroom ingestions can cause initial symptoms like vomiting and diarrhea. Eating Amanita mushrooms can cause liver and kidney failure leading to death.

- √ Bacterium Causes

- √ Staphylococcus aureus poisoning is due to a toxin that is performed in food before it is eaten. It causes vomiting within 1 to 6 hours after eating the contaminated food.

- √ Bacillus cereus is an infection that occurs after eating poorly cooked or raw rice.

- √ Clostridium perfringens produces a spore that may germinate in cooked meat that has been stored in an environment that was too warm. Within 8 to 12 hours, it may cause profuse diarrhea.

Intermediate incubation from about 1 to 3 days

Infections of the large intestine or colon can cause bloody, mucousy diarrhea associated with crampy abdominal pain.

- √ Campylobacter, according to CDC data, is the number one cause of food-borne disease in the United States.

- √ Shigella contaminate food and water and cause dysentery (severe diarrhea often containing mucus and blood).

- √ Salmonella infections often occur because of poorly or undercooked cooked, and poor handling of the chicken and eggs. In individuals with weakened immune systems, including the elderly, the infection can enter the bloodstream and cause potentially life-threatening infections.

- √ Vibrio parahaemolyticus can contaminate saltwater shellfish and cause a watery diarrhea.

Diarrhea due to small bowel infection tends not to be bloody, but infections may affect both the small and large intestine at the same time.

- √ E. coli (enterotoxigenic) is the most common cause of traveler's diarrhea. It lacks symptoms such as fever or bloody diarrhea.

√ Vibrio cholerae, often from contaminated drinking, water produces a voluminous watery diarrhea resembling rice-water.

√ Viruses such as Norwalk, rotavirus and adenovirus tend to have other symptoms associated with an infection including fever, chills, headaches. and vomiting.

√ Botulism is caused by Clostridium botulinum toxin and may present with fever, vomiting, mild diarrhea, numbness, and weakness leading to paralysis.

Long incubation of 3 to 5 days

√ Hemorrhagic £ coli (mainly £ coli 0157.H7) can cause inflammation of the colon leading to bloody stools. In some children, about a week after infection, it can progress to hemolytic uremic syndrome (HUS). Elderly individuals may contract thrombotic thrombocytopenic purpura (TTP). Toxins from the bacteria enter the blood stream and hemolyze or destroy red blood cells. In addition, the toxins cause kidney failure and uremia, where waste products build up in the body.

√ Yersinia enterocolitica may cause inflammation of lymph nodes in the lining of the abdomen and may mimic appendicitis.

Very long incubation of up to a month

Parasites

√ Giardiasis may occur after drinking water from lakes or rivers that have been contaminated by beavers, muskrats, or sheep that have been grazing. It also can be passed from person to person, for example in day care settings.

√ Amoebiasis is encountered in contaminated drinking water, usually in tropical or semitropical climates and can be passed person to person.

√ Trichinosis is due to an infection from eating undercooked pork or wild game such as bear meat. Aside from fever and gastrointestinal complaints, symptoms include muscle pain, facial swelling, and bleeding around the eyes and under the fingernails.

√ Cysticercosis is often seen in developing countries where water is contaminated with pork tapeworms and the person swallows the ova form the tapeworm. The infection can invade the brain (neurocysticercosis) causing seizures.

√ Cyclospora is a one celled parasite that infects the small intestine causing explosive, watery bowel movements. The infection is acquired from contaminated food or water and does not usually spread from person to person. Symptoms may also include headache, body aches, and malaise and can mimic a viral type infection. Without antibiotic treatment, Cyclospora infection will gradually resolve over the course of many weeks, but may come and go (relapse) over that time period.

Bacteria

√ Listeriosis usually occurs after foods contaminated with Listeria bacteria are ingested. These include unpasteurized, raw milk, soft cheeses, and processed meats and poultry. Vegetables and fruits may also become infected with Listeria. The bacteria may lay dormant in or on the surface of the food products for weeks.

√ Brucellosis occurs by ingesting raw or unpasteurized milk and cheese, especially goat's milk contaminated with Brucella.

√ **Virus**

√ Hepatitis A is spread by poor food handling, and not due to blood exposure such as in hepatitis B and C.

√ **Protozoans**

√ Toxoplasmosis is usually transmitted to humans from cat feces containing Toxoplasma parasites; most infections are

√ asymptomatic, but people who have diminished immune systems can develop systemic disease symptoms.

Prion

Bovine Spongiform encephalopathy (mad cow disease) is acquired by eating foods containing prions (transmissible agents that induce abnormal folding of brain protein) contaminating brain or spinal cord from infected cows.

When should the doctor be called for food poisoning?

With a clear fluid diet and rest, most infections resolve on their own within 24 hours. A health-care professional should be contacted if the vomiting and diarrhea are associated with one or more of the following symptoms:

√ fever

√ blood in the stools

√ signs of dehydration including lightheadedness when standing, weakness, decreased urination

√ diarrhea that lasts longer than 72 hours, and/or

√ repeated vomiting that prevents drinking and rehydrating (replacing the fluids lost due to fever, diarrhea, and vomiting).

How is food poisoning diagnosed?

Most times, the diagnosis of food poisoning is made by history and physical examination. Often, the patient volunteers the diagnosis when they come for medical care. For example, "I got sick after eating potato salad at a picnic," or, "I drank a raw egg protein shake."

The health-care professional may ask questions about the symptoms, when they started, and how long they have lasted. A review of systems may help give direction as to what type of infection is present. For example, a patient with numbness of their feet and weakness may be asked about whether they have opened any home canned food recently.

Travel history may be helpful to see if the patient had been camping near a stream or lake and the potential for drinking contaminated water, or if they have travelled out of the country recently and have eaten different foods than they normally do, such as raw eggs or wild game.

Physical examination begins with taking the vital signs of the patient (blood pressure, pulse rate, and temperature). Clinical signs of dehydration include dry, tenting skin, sunken eyes, dry mouth, and lack of sweat in the armpits and groin. In infants, in addition to the above, subtle signs of dehydration may include poor muscle tone, poor suckling, and sunken fontanelle.

Routine blood tests are not usually ordered unless there is concern about something more than the vomiting and diarrhea. In patients with significant dehydration, the health-care professional may want to check electrolyte levels in the blood as well as kidney function. If there is concern about hemolytic uremic syndrome, a complete blood count (hemogram, CBC) to check the red blood cells, white blood cells, and platelet count may be ordered. If there is concern about hepatitis, liver function tests may be ordered.

Stool samples may be useful especially if there is concern about infections caused by Salmonella, Shigella, and Campylobacter, the common non traveler's diarrhea. This is especially true when the patient presents with bloody diarrhea, thought to be due to infection. If there is concern about a parasite infection, stool samples can be examined also for the presence of parasites. Some parasites may be very difficult to see under the microscope, including Cyclospora, because it is so tiny.

Depending on the suspected cause of the food poisoning, there are some immunological tests (for example, detection of Shiga toxins) that the CDC recommends. Cyclospora DNA may be detected in the stool using molecular testing called polymerase chain reaction (PCR). Other methods may be used (for example, detection of prions in tissue samples).

What is the treatment for food poisoning?

Maintaining good hydration is the first priority when treating food poisoning. Hospitalization may be appropriate if the patient is dehydrated or if they have other underlying medical conditions that become unstable because of the fluid or electrolyte imbalance in their body.

Medications may be prescribed to help control nausea and vomiting.

Medications to decrease the frequency of diarrhea may be indicated, but if food poisoning is suspected, it is best to consult a health-care professional before taking OTC (over-the-counter) medications such as loperamide (Imodium), because it may cause increased problems for the patient.

Except for specific infections, antibiotics are not prescribed in the treatment of most food poisoning. Often, the health- care professional will decide upon their use based on multiple factors such as the intensity of the disease symptoms, the additional health factors of the patient, a serious response to infection (sepsis), and organ system compromise. For example, a pregnant woman suspected of having listeriosis will likely be treated with IV antibiotics because of the effect of the infection on the fetus.

Complications of certain types of food poisoning are best treated in consultation with infectious disease specialists (for example, HUS, TTP, bovine spongiform encephalopathy).

Are there any home remedies for food poisoning?

The key to home care is being able to keep the affected person hydrated. Oral rehydration therapy with water or a balanced electrolyte solution such as Gatorade or Pedialyte is usually adequate to replenish the body with fluids. A person can lose a significant amount of fluid with each diarrheal bowel movement, and that fluid has to be replaced to rehydrate. People who show any signs of dehydration such as decreased urination, dizziness, or dry mucous membranes, especially in the young or elderly, should see a health-care professional.

How can food poisoning be prevented?

Prevention of food borne illness begins at home with proper food preparation technique.

- √ Foods should be cooked thoroughly. This especially applies to eggs, poultry, and meat. A meat thermometer can be used to measure the internal temperature of a meat dish.

- √ Leftovers should be refrigerated immediately so bacteria and viruses do not have time to start growing.

- √ Wash fruits and vegetables well before eating. This removes dirt, pesticides, chemicals, or other infectious agents used on, or exposed to, the foods in the fields or storage facilities.

√ Wash hands routinely before and after handling food to help prevent the spread of infection.

√ Thoroughly clean counters and other areas that are used to clean, prepare, and assemble foods. Cross contamination of food is common and can cause food poisonings. For example, a cutting board and knife used to cut raw chicken should be washed thoroughly before cutting up fruit and vegetables to prevent the spread of Salmonella.

√ In restaurants, meals are prepared by others. Health inspectors check restaurants routinely and their reports on sanitary practices are usually available online. Make certain the food ordered is thoroughly cooked, especially meats such as hamburger.

√ Pregnant women and people who have compromised immune systems, such as those undergoing chemotherapy or who are taking medication such as prednisone, should avoid eating soft cheeses like camembert, brie, blue, and feta because of the risk of contracting Listeria. Be very sure all fruits and vegetables are cleaned thoroughly prior to eating, no matter the source.

What are the complications of food poisoning?

The first and most important complication of food poisoning is dehydration. Food poisoning can cause significant loss of body water and changes in the electrolyte levels in the blood.

If the affected individual has underlying medical conditions requiring medication, persistent vomiting may make it difficult to swallow and digest those medications.

Other complications of food poisoning are specific to the type of infection. Some are listed in the causes of food poisoning such as HUS, TTP, or encephalopathy.

What is the prognosis for someone with food poisoning?

Fortunately, most cases of food poisoning resolve within a few hours to days and the affected individual returns to normal function.

Depending upon the cause of the infection, and the patient's underlying medical condition, the infection may cause significant organ damage and even death.

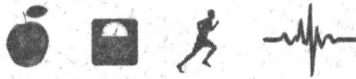

BRUSH YOUR TEETH

Taking good care of your mouth, teeth and gums is a worthy goal in and of itself. Good oral and dental hygiene can help prevent bad breath, tooth decay and gum disease—and can help you keep your teeth as you get older.

Researchers are also discovering new reasons to brush and floss. A healthy mouth may help you ward off medical disorders. The flip side? An unhealthy mouth, especially if you have gum disease, may increase your risk of serious health problems such as heart attack, stroke, poorly controlled diabetes and preterm labor.

The case for good oral hygiene keeps getting stronger. Understand the importance of oral health—and its connection to your overall health.

What's In Your Mouth Reveals Much About Your Health

What does the health of your mouth have to do with your overall health? In a word, plenty. A look inside or a swab of saliva can tell your doctor volumes about what's going on inside your body.

Many Conditions Cause Oral Signs & Symptoms

Your mouth is a window into what's going on in the rest of your body, often serving as a helpful vantage point for detecting the early signs and symptoms of systemic disease—a disease that affects or pertains to your entire body, not just one of its parts. Systemic conditions such as AIDS or diabetes, for example, often first become apparent as mouth lesions or other oral problems. In fact, according to the Academy of General Dentistry, more than 90 percent of all systemic diseases produce oral signs and symptoms.

Saliva: Helpful Diagnostic Tool

Your doctor can collect and test saliva to detect a variety of substances. For example, cortisol levels in saliva are used to test for stress responses in newborn children. And fragments of certain bone-specific proteins may be useful in monitoring bone loss in women and men prone to osteoporosis. Certain cancer markers are also detectable in saliva.

Routine saliva testing can also measure illegal drugs, environmental toxins, hormones and antibodies indicating hepatitis or HIV infection, among other things. In fact, the ability to detect HIV-specific antibodies had led to the production of commercial, easy-to-use saliva kits. In the future, saliva testing may replace blood testing as a means of diagnosing and monitoring diseases such as diabetes, Parkinson's disease, cirrhosis of the liver and many infectious diseases.

Protection Against Harmful Invaders: How Saliva Disables Bacteria & Viruses

Saliva is also one of your body's main defenses against disease-causing organisms, such as bacteria and viruses. It contains antibodies that attack viral pathogens, such as the common cold and HIV. And it contains proteins called histatins, which inhibit the growth of a naturally occurring fungus called Candida albicans. When these proteins are weakened by HIV infection or other illness, Candida can grow out of control, resulting in a fungal infection called oral thrush.

Saliva also protects you against disease causing bacteria. It contains enzymes that destroy bacteria in different ways, by degrading bacterial membranes, inhibiting the growth and metabolism or certain bacteria, and disrupting vital bacterial enzyme systems.

The Problem with Dental Plaque: Link To Infections & Diseases

Though your saliva helps protect you against some invaders, it can't always do the job. More than 500 species of bacteria thrive in your mouth at any given time. These bacteria constantly form dental plaque—a sticky, colorless film that can cling to your teeth and cause health problems.

Your Mouth As Infection Source

If you don't brush and floss regularly to keep your teeth clean, plaque can build up along your gum line, creating an environment for additional bacteria to accumulate in the space between your gums and your teeth. This gum infection is known as gingivitis. Left unchecked, gingivitis can lead to a more serious gum infection called periodontitis. The most severe form of gum infection is called acute necrotizing ulcerative gingivitis, also known as trench mouth.

Bacteria from your mouth normally don't enter your bloodstream. However, invasive dental treatments—sometimes even just routine brushing and flossing if you have gum disease—can provide a port of entry for these microbes. Medications or treatments that reduce saliva flow and antibiotics that disrupt the normal balance of bacteria in your mouth can also compromise your mouth's normal defenses, allowing these bacteria to enter your bloodstream.

If you have a healthy immune system, the presence of oral bacteria in your bloodstream causes no problems. Your immune system quickly dispenses with them, preventing infection. However, if your immune system is weakened, for example because of a disease or cancer treatment, oral bacteria in your bloodstream may cause you to develop an infection in another part of your body. Infective endocarditis, in which oral bacteria enter your bloodstream and stick to the lining of diseased heart valves, is an example of this phenomenon.

Plaque As Cause Of Common Conditions?

Long-term gum infection can eventually result in the loss of your teeth. But the consequences may not end there. Recent research suggests that there may be an association between oral infections—primarily gum infections—and poorly controlled diabetes, cardiovascular disease and preterm birth. More research is needed to determine whether oral infections actually cause these conditions.

A Compelling Case For Good Habits

If you didn't already have enough reasons to take good care of your mouth, teeth and gums, the relationship between your oral health and your overall health provides even more. Resolve to practice good oral hygiene every day. You're making an investment in your overall health, not just for now, but the future, too.

Great Dental Hygiene Tips

1. Proper Brushing : One of the easiest steps to do to help your teeth keep clean. When brushing your teeth, position the bristles at an angle of 45 degrees near the gum line. Both the gum line and the tooth surface should be in contact with the bristles. Brush the outer surfaces of the teeth using a back-and-forth, up-and-down motion, making sure to be done

gently in order to avoid bleeding. To clean the inside surfaces of the teeth and gums, place the bristles at a 45-degree angle again and repeat the back-and-forth, up-and-down motion. Lastly, brush the surfaces of your tongue and the roof of your mouth to remove bacteria, which might cause bad breath.

2. Flossing: we know, it's a chore and a lot of times easy to forget after brushing if heading to bed or rushing out the door. However, flossing can help remove food particles and other detrimental substances that brushing regularly cannot. Flossing allows you to reach deep between your teeth where the toothbrush bristles cannot reach or even mouthwash cannot wash away. We recommend flossing at least once a day.

3. Avoid Tobacco: This will be a big favor to your teeth. One, it will save you from Oral cancer and periodontal complications. Two, it will save you from the countless ill effects caused by the agents used to mask the smell of tobacco. For example, if you smoke a cigarette, you may use candies, tea or coffee to mask the smoky breath and odor. This doubles the amount of damage caused.

4. Limit Sodas, Coffee, And Alcohol: Although these beverages contain a high level of phosphorous, which is a necessary mineral for a healthy mouth, too much phosphorous can deplete the body's level of calcium. This causes dental hygiene problems such as tooth decay and gum disease. Beverages containing additives such as corn syrup and food dye can make pearly white teeth appear dull and discolored. Therefore, it is best to choose beverages like milk, which helps strengthen teeth and build stronger enamel, giving you a healthy smile and water which hydrates your body longer than sugary drinks. You should drink tap water when possible, too, so you can reap the rewards of the decay-preventive benefits of fluoride.

5. Consume Calcium & Other Vitamins That Are Good For The Body: You need plenty of calcium for your teeth. It is essential for the teeth as well as your bones. It is better to drink milk, fortified orange juice and to eat yogurt, broccoli, cheese, and other dairy products. You can also take a calcium supplement, taking different doses according to your age and necessity as per prescription. Calcium and Vitamin D are necessary for maintaining the health of gums and teeth. Vitamin B complex is also essential for the protection of gums and teeth from cracking and bleeding. Copper, zinc, iodine, iron and potassium are also required for maintaining healthy dental hygiene.

6. Visit Your Dentist: You should visit your dentist at least twice a year to have a full hygiene treatment performed, though most prisons that I've been to will only do one.

7. Use Mouthwash Along Side of Brushing & Flossing: Mouthwash is not particularly necessary and not all mouthwashes are useful. Mouthwashes containing Listerine or chloride dioxide are very helpful because they help to kill and maintain the bacteria in your mouth. It can maintain good breath as well as help maintain strong teeth. Mouthwash cannot do all the work, but if you're already brushing, flossing, visiting the dentist and eating well –following a proper nutritious diet not only helps keep your body healthy, but your mouth as well! Mouthwash is the cherry on top that will make your dental health great.

8. Monitor Your Low-Carb Lifestyle: Despite their popularity, low-carb diets can cause bad breath. A balanced, dental-healthy diet can help prevent tooth decay.

9. Having a Toothache Or Noticing Other Dental Symptoms: If you are having tooth and jaw pain, make an appointment as soon as possible. Your dentist needs to diagnose the underlying cause and correct it before it becomes a bigger problem.

10. Clean Your Tongue: Clean the surface of your tongue daily. By using a professional tongue cleaner (many toothbrushes now come with them on the flipside of the bristles) your remove countless bacteria that otherwise live, particularly on the rougher top surface of your tongue. These can contribute to bad breath (halitosis) and negatively affect your dental health.

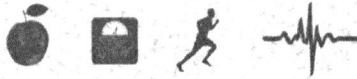

TIPS FOR HEALTHY SKIN

With new research, new products and new skin protection advice popping up all the time, it is hard to find out the best things to do to improve and protect your skin.

A skin care program is the combination of skin care products and a routine that will be most beneficial to the skin. You will first need to consider yourdiet and type of lifestyle since these two factors play an important role in the health of a person's skin.

These days we seem to be living in the fast-food age and the condition of your skin is often neglected. Prison food isn't going to be any better for your skin than fast food. You still can't beat the old fruit and vegetable diet when it comes to good health and a good complexion. Remember to feed and nourish your skin by eating the proper foods if you can. Give your skin a drink, too. Those eight glasses of water a day your Mom always told you to be sure to drink are essential to maintaining your skin's elasticity and suppleness, say experts. And don't count coffee (a staple in the inmate diet) or caffeinated sodas as part of the eight glasses because caffeine is dehydrating. It may be wise to keep a water bottle close at hand, or simple drink a glass or two with your meals, and a few in between.

Help keep environmental pollutants from being absorbed into the skin with a good moisturizer that also acts as a skin barrier, check the labels for those with added vitamin A, and E, which help block the penetration of pollutants. And wear sunscreen! Not only can the sun cause you skin cancer, it will age you. Too many prisoners go out into the sun all day, burning their skin in the process.

A good exercise program such as calisthenics can active and rejuvenate the skin and improve circulation and blood flow. Also, body sweat triggers production of sebum, which is the skin's own natural moisturizer.

Get serious about stress reduction. Skin conditions such as acne appear on many people who get stressed out, and chronic skin conditions tend to get worse. Set aside quiet time to meditate or reflect (see a connection/pattern in all of these health care tips?). Be sure to get enough sleep. To avoid morning eye or facial puffiness, sleep on your back so fluid doesn't collect there. And, you should try to keep your hair out of your face, so the oils from your hair don't transfer. Don't forget: too much stress can affect your overall health as well as your complexion

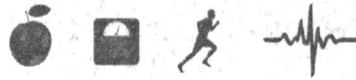

THINK BEFORE YOU INK
By Dr. Mercola

Tattoos Last, and So Does the Pain for 1 in 10

About one in five US adults, or 21 percent, has at least one tattoo. This is up from 14 percent in 2008, according to a Harris poll. Tattoos have been around for more than 5,000 years. They were used in ancient Egypt as a way to identify peasants and slaves.

They were discovered on a 5,000-year-old mummy identified as the "Iceman," and it's thought his tattoos may have been placed as a therapeutic tool on areas prone to joint pain and degeneration.

In Samoa, extensive tattoos were given as a show of courage, endurance, and dedication to cultural traditions, while around the word different cultures valued the designs as status symbols, signs of religious beliefs, declarations of love, beautifications, or as a form of punishment. Obviously, some people get tattoos to represent gangs.

In the US, tattoos, once thought of as more of a fringe or alternative practice, are becoming practically mainstream and are often used as a form of self-expression. There are still some stereotypes remaining, however.

While 73 percent of voters said they would hire someone with a visible tattoo, 27 percent of respondents to a Harris poll believed people with tattoos are less intelligent and 50 percent believed they were more rebellious.

Most people getting a tattoo are not doing so to appease the views of others, of course, but there is one consideration you might not have considered: your health. If you've ever gotten a tattoo, or thought about it, chances are high that you weighed the artistic and social aspects of it far more than the health aspects.

But, unbeknownst to many, a significant number of people with tattoos have experienced lasting health issues as a result.

10 Percent of People with Tattoos Experienced Abnormal Reactions

Researchers from the NYU Langone Medical Center surveyed 300 people in New York's Central Park. Of those who had a tattoo, more than 10 percent said they developed abnormal reactions as a result, including pain, itching, and infection that sometimes required antibiotics.

In 4 percent of the cases, the symptoms went away within four months, but for 6 percent, symptoms such as itching, scaling skin, and swelling lasted much longer. Chronic reaction occurred more often in people with more colors in their tattoo, particularly shades of red.

Past research has also found "red pigments are the commonest cause of delayed tattoo reactions. One study conducted actual skin biopsies from red tattoo reactions and determined interface dermatitis was the primary problem, in many cases due to an allergic response.

In many cases, however, "overlapping patterns were identified," which suggests the red pigment was irritating the skin and body via multiple mechanisms. In addition to red, pink and purple colors were commonly involved in reactions.

The featured study's lead author was actually motivated to conduct the study after seeing a patient who seemed to develop an intolerance to red tattoo dye after receiving her multiple tattoos. She told CNN:

"Dr. Marie C. Leger, assistant professor of dermatology at NYU Langone Medical Center... got motivated to study tattoo complications after treating a patient who developed itching and raised, scaly skin around only the red parts of a tattoo on her arm.

She had the first tattoo for years but the symptoms started after getting a more recent tattoo on her foot. In addition to the problems at the tattoo site, she developed a rash over her whole body.

'It was like her body decided after being exposed to red dye more than once, that it just didn't like it,' Leger said. There are many questions over what is causing these undesirable side effects. Leger said she suspects that allergic reactions to the dyes, especially red dye, are responsible for some of the chronic reactions lasting more than four months."

Tattoo Ink Is Unregulated

While tattoo parlors are often inspected to ensure safe practices such as the use of single-use needles), however tattoo inks typically fly under the radar. Inks and ink colorings (pigments) used for tattoos are technically subject to regulation by the US Food and Drug Administration (FDA) as cosmetics and color additives.

However, the Agency states that because of other public health priorities and a "previous lack of evidence of safety concerns," they have NOT traditionally regulated such products.

It has been said that "tattoo ink is remarkably nonreactive histologically, despite the frequent use of different pigments of unknown purity and identity by tattoo artists."

However, University of Bradford researchers using an atomic force microscope (AFM) that allows them to examine skin with tattoos at the nano-level have found evidence that suggests otherwise. In preliminary study (the first to use AFM to examine tattoos), the researchers found that the tattoo process remodels collagen (your body's main connective tissue).

Carcinogenic Nanoparticles Found in Tattoo Ink

In 2011, a study in The British Journal of Dermatology revealed that nanoparticles are indeed found in tattoo ink, with black pigments containing the smallest particles (white pigments had the largest particles and colored pigments were in between).

Nanoparticles are ultra-microscopic in size, making them able to readily penetrate your skin and travel to underlying blood vessels and your bloodstream. Evidence suggests that some nanoparticles may induce toxic effects in your brain and cause nerve damage, and some may be carcinogenic.

Further, nanoparticles from tattoo ink were found to exist in both the collagenous network of the skin as well as around blood vessels, according to the University of Bradford researchers.

This suggests the ink particles are leaving the surface of your skin and traveling elsewhere in your body, where they could potentially enter organs and other tissues. This is particularly worrisome because tattoo inks are known to contain cancer-causing compounds. And this is the "good," "professional" ink we're talking about here. The stuff used in real shops. Can you imagine what could be found in burned plastic or handballs or whatever else inmates use?

(Note: I have many tattoos. I've used many things over the years. The best I've found to burn is Baby Oil or even cooking oil. And though I can't be sure, I'd think that would be healthier than burning a handball.)

Black Tattoo Ink May Also Carry Unique Risks

While red ink appears to be associated with chronic skin reactions and those that are allergic in nature, black ink is also implicated in health problems. This might be, in part, because of its high concentration of nanoparticles.

"The black pigments were almost pure NPs nanoparticles], i.e. particles with at least one dimension <100 nm," researchers said in the British Journal of Dermatology. Writing in Experimental Dermatology, researchers highlighted the dangerous potential of tattoo inks (particularly black) even beyond nanoparticles:

"Black tattoo inks are usually based on soot, are not regulated and may contain hazardous polycyclic aromatic hydrocarbons (PAHs). Part of PAHs possibly stay lifelong in skin, absorb UV radiation and generate singlet oxygen which may affect skin integrity.

"...Tattooing with black inks entails an injection of substantial amounts of phenol and PAHs into the skin. Most of these PAHs are carcinogenic and may additionally generate deleterious singlet oxygen inside the dermis when skin is exposed to UVA (e.g. solar radiation)."

That being said, all tattoo inks have toxic potential. Some tattoo pigment may migrate from your skin into your body1s lymph nodes, for instance. Other potential health effects include:

- √ Potentially carcinogenic
- √ May cause inflammation and DNA damage
- √ May contain carcinogenic Polycyclic Aromatic Hydrocarbons (PAHs) like benzo(a)pyrene (a Class 1 carcinogen according to the International Agency for Research on Cancer)

Think Before You Ink

While I certainly value artistic and self-expression, I do urge you to "think before you ink" for the sake of your health. No systematic studies have been performed on the safety of tattoo inks, and many of those used are industrial grade colors suitable for printers' ink or automobile paint.

And this is just the dangers of the inks—even the professionally made inks. There are obviously other dangers from dirty equipment. NEVER use anyone else's needle or barrel, and make sure you at least know what your ink is and where it comes from to avoid things like HIV and Hep C.

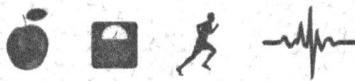

SCABIES

Overview

Scabies is an itchy skin condition caused by a tiny burrowing mite called Sarcoptes scabiei. The presence of the mite leads to intense itching in the area of its burrows. The urge to scratch may be especially strong at night.

Scabies is contagious and can spread quickly through close physical contact in a family, child care group, school class, nursing home or prison. Because of the contagious nature of scabies, doctors often recommend treatment for entire families or contact groups.

Scabies is readily treated. Medications applied to your skin kill the mites that cause scabies and their eggs, although you may still experience some itching for several weeks.

Symptoms

Scabies signs and symptoms include:

- √ Itching, often severe and usually worse at night
- √ Thin, irregular burrow tracks made up of tiny blisters or bumps on your skin
- √ The burrows or tracks typically appear in folds of your skin. Though almost any part of your body may be involved, in adults and older children scabies is most often found:
- √ Between fingers
- √ In armpits
- √ Around your waist
- √ Along the insides of wrists
- √ On your inner elbow
- √ On the soles of your feet
- √ Around breasts
- √ Around the male genital area
- √ On buttocks
- √ On knees
- √ On shoulder blades

In infants and young children, common sites of infestation include the:

- √ Scalp
- √ Face
- √ Neck

√ Palms of the hands

√ Soles of the feet

If you've had scabies before, signs and symptoms may develop within a few days of exposure. However, if you've never had scabies, it could take as long as six weeks for signs and symptoms to begin. It's important to remember that you can still spread scabies even if you don't have any signs or symptoms yet.

When to see a doctor

Talk to your doctor if you have signs and symptoms that may indicate scabies.

Many skin conditions, such as dermatitis or eczema, are associated with itching and small bumps on the skin. Your doctor can help determine the exact cause and ensure that you receive proper treatment. Bathing and over-the-counter preparations won't eliminate scabies.

Causes

The eight-legged mite that causes scabies in humans is microscopic. The female mite burrows just beneath your skin and produces a tunnel in which it deposits eggs. The eggs hatch, and the mite larvae work their way to the surface of your skin, where they mature and can spread to other areas of your skin or to the skin of other people. The itching of scabies results from your body's allergic reaction to the mites, their eggs and their waste.

Close physical contact and, less often, sharing clothing or bedding with an infected person can spread the mites.

Dogs, cats and humans all are affected by their own distinct species of mite. Each species of mite prefers one specific type of host and doesn't live long away from that preferred host. So humans may have a temporary skin reaction from contact with the animal scabies mite. But people are unlikely to develop full-blown scabies from this source, as they might from contact with the human scabies mite.

Complications

Vigorous scratching can break your skin and allow a secondary bacterial infection, such as impetigo, to occur. Impetigo is a superficial infection of the skin that's caused most often by staph (staphylococci) bacteria or occasionally by strep (streptococci) bacteria.

A more severe form of scabies, called crusted scabies, may affect certain high-risk groups, including:

People with chronic health conditions that weaken the immune system, such as HIV or chronic leukemia

People who are very ill, such as people in hospitals or nursing facilities

Older people in nursing homes

Crusted scabies, also called Norwegian scabies, tends to be crusty and scaly, and to cover large areas of the body. It's very contagious and can be hard to treat.

Prevention

To prevent re-infestation and to prevent the mites from spreading to other people, take these steps:

Clean all clothes and linen. Use hot, soapy water to wash all clothing, towels and bedding used within three days before beginning treatment. Dry with high heat. Dry clean items you can't wash at home.

Starve the mites. Consider placing items you can't wash in a sealed plastic bag and leaving it in a place, such as in your garage, for a couple of weeks. Mites die after a few days without food.

Diagnosis

To diagnose scabies, your doctor examines your skin, looking for signs of mites, including the characteristic burrows. When your doctor locates a mite burrow, he or she may take a scraping from that area of your skin to examine under a microscope. The microscopic examination can determine the presence of mites or their eggs.

Treatment

Scabies treatment involves eliminating the infestation with medications. Several creams and lotions are available with a doctor's prescription. You usually apply the medication over all your body, from your neck down, and leave the medication on for at least eight hours. A second treatment is needed if new burrows and rash appear.

Because scabies spreads so easily, your doctor will likely recommend treatment for all household members and other close contacts, even if they show no signs of scabies infestation.

Medications commonly prescribed for scabies include:

√ Permethrin cream, 5 percent (Elimite). Permethrin is a topical cream that contains chemicals that kill scabies mites and their eggs. It is generally considered safe for adults, pregnant women, and children ages 2 months and older. This medicine is not recommended for nursing mothers.

√ Lindane lotion. This medication—also a chemical treatment—is recommended only for people who can't tolerate other approved treatments, or for whom other treatments didn't work. This medication isn't safe for children younger than age 2 years, women who are pregnant or nursing, the elderly, or anyone who weighs less than 110 pounds (50 kilograms).

√ Crotamiton (Eurax). This medication is available as a cream or a lotion. It's applied once a day for two days. This medication isn't recommended for children or for women who are pregnant or nursing. Frequent treatment failure has been reported with crotamiton.

√ Ivermectin (Stromectol). Doctors may prescribe this oral medication for people with altered immune systems, for people who have crusted scabies, or for people who don't respond to the prescription lotions and creams. Ivermectin isn't recommended for women who are pregnant or nursing, or for children who weigh less than 33 pounds (15 kg).

Although these medications kill the mites promptly, you may find that the itching doesn't stop entirely for several weeks.

Doctors may prescribe other topical medications, such as sulfur compounded in petrolatum, for people who don't respond to or can't use these medications.

Lifestyle and home remedies

Itching may persist for some time after you apply medication to kill the mites. These steps may help you find relief from itching:

√ Cool and soak your skin. Soaking in cool water or applying a cool, wet washcloth to irritated areas of your skin may minimize itching.

√ Apply soothing lotion. Calamine lotion, available without a prescription, can effectively relieve the pain and itching of minor skin irritations.

√ Take antihistamines. At your doctor's suggestion, you may find that over-the-counter antihistamines relieve the allergic symptoms caused by scabies.

Preparing for your appointment

Make an appointment with your family doctor or pediatrician if you or your child has signs and symptoms common to scabies.

Here's some information to help you get ready for your appointment and know what to expect from your doctor.

Information to gather in advance

√ List any signs or symptoms you or your child has had, and for how long.

√ List any possible sources of infection, such as other family members who have had a rash.

√ Write down key medical information, including any other health problems and the names of any medications you or your child is taking.

√ Write down questions you want to be sure to ask your doctor.

Below are some basic questions to ask your doctor about scabies.

√ What is the most likely cause of these signs and symptoms?

√ Are there any other possible causes?

√ What treatment approach do you recommend?

√ How soon do you expect symptoms to improve with treatment?

√ Whenwill you see me or my child to determine whether the treatment you've recommended is working?

√ Are there any home remedies or self-care steps that could help relieve symptoms?

√ Am I or is my child contagious? For how long?

√ What steps should be taken to reduce the risk of infecting others?

What to expect from your doctor

Your doctor is likely to ask you a number of questions. Being ready to answer them may reserve time to go over any points you want to talk about in-depth. Your doctor may ask:

√ What signs and symptoms have you noticed?

√ When did you first notice these signs and symptoms?

√ Have these signs and symptoms gotten worse over time?

√ If you or your child has rash, what parts of the body are affected?

√ Has anyone else with whom you have frequent, close contact had a rash, an itch or both within the past several weeks?

√ Are you currently pregnant or nursing?

√ Are you or is your child currently being treated or have you or your child recently been treated for any other medical conditions?

√ What medications are you or your child currently taking, including prescription and over-the-counter drugs, vitamins and supplements?

√ Is your child in child care?

What you can do in the meantime

In the time leading up to your appointment, try at-home and over-the-counter (OTC) remedies to help reduce itching. Cool water, antihistamines and calamine lotion may provide some relief. Ask your doctor what OTC medications and lotions are safe for your child.

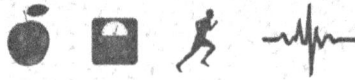

STAPH INFECTIONS

OVERVIEW

Staph infections are caused by staphylococcus bacteria, types of germs commonly found on the skin or in the nose of even healthy individuals. Most of the time, these bacteria cause no problems or result in relatively minor skin infections.

But staph infections can turn deadly if the bacteria invade deeper into your body, entering your bloodstream, joints, bones, lungs or heart. A growing number of otherwise healthy people are developing life-threatening staph infections.

Treatment usually involves antibiotics and drainage of the infected area. However, some staph infections no longer respond to common antibiotics.

SYMPTOMS

Staph infections can range from minor skin problems to endocarditis, a life-threatening infection of the inner lining of your heart (endocardium). As a result, signs and symptoms of staph infections vary widely, depending on the location and severity of the infection.

Skin infections

Skin infections caused by staph bacteria include:

- √ Boils. The most common type of staph infection is the boil, a pocket of pus that develops in a hair follicle or oil gland. The skin over the infected area usually becomes red and swollen.

- √ If a boil breaks open, it will probably drain pus. Boils occur most often under the arms or around the groin or buttocks.

- √ Impetigo. This contagious, often painful rash can be caused by staph bacteria. Impetigo usually features large blisters that may ooze fluid and develop a honey-colored crust.

- √ Cellulitis. Cellulitis—an infection of the deeper layers of skin—causes skin redness and swelling on the surface of your skin. Sores (ulcers) or areas of oozing discharge may develop, too.

- √ Staphylococcal scalded skin syndrome. Toxins produced as a result of a staph infection may lead to staphylococcal scalded skin syndrome. Affecting mostly babies and children, this condition features fever, a rash and sometimes blisters. When the blisters break, the top layer of skin comes off—leaving a red, raw surface that looks like a burn.

Food poisoning

Staph bacteria are one of the most common causes of food poisoning. Symptoms come on quickly, usually within hours of eating a contaminated food. Symptoms usually disappear quickly, too, often lasting just half a day.

A staph infection in food usually doesn't cause a fever. Signs and symptoms you can expect with this type of staph infection include:

- √ Nausea and vomiting
- √ Diarrhea
- √ Dehydration
- √ Low blood pressure

Septicemia

Also known as blood poisoning, septicemia occurs when staph bacteria enter a person's bloodstream. A fever and low blood pressure are signs of septicemia. The bacteria can travel to locations deep within your body, to produce infections affecting:

- √ Internal organs, such as your brain, heart or lungs
- √ Bones and muscles
- √ Surgically implanted devices, such as artificial joints or cardiac pacemakers Toxic shock syndrome

Toxic Shock Syndrome

This life-threatening condition results from toxins produced by some strains of staph bacteria and has been linked to certain types of tampons, skin wounds and surgery. It usually develops suddenly with:

- √ A high fever
- √ Nausea and vomiting
- √ A rash on your palms and soles that resembles sunburn
- √ Confusion
- √ Muscle aches
- √ Diarrhea
- √ Abdominal pain

Septic arthritis

Septic arthritis is often caused by a staph infection. The bacteria often target the knees, shoulders, hips, and fingers or toes. Signs and symptoms may include:

- √ Joint swelling
- √ Severe pain in the affected joint
- √ Fever

When to see a doctor

Go to the doctor if you or your child has:

- √ An area of red, irritated or painful skin
- √ Pus-filled blisters
- √ Fever
- √ You may also want to consult your doctor if:
- √ Skin infections are being passed from one family member to another

√ Two or more family members have skin infections at the same time

CAUSES

Many people carry staph bacteria and never develop staph infections. However, if you develop a staph infection, there's a good chance that it's from bacteria you've been carrying around for some time.

These bacteria can also be transmitted from person to person. Because staph bacteria are so hardy, they can live on inanimate objects such as pillowcases or towels long enough to transfer to the next person who touches them.

Staph bacteria are able to survive:

√ Drying
√ Extremes of temperature
√ Stomach acid
√ High levels of salt

RISK FACTORS

A variety of factors—including the status of your immune system to the types of sports you play—can increase your risk of developing staph infections.

Underlying health conditions

Certain disorders or the medications used to treat them can make you more susceptible to staph infections. People who may be more likely to get a staph infection include those with:

√ Diabetes who use insulin
√ HIV/AIDS
√ Kidney failure requiring dialysis
√ Weakened immune systems—either from a disease or medications that suppress the immune system
√ Cancer, especially those who are undergoing chemotherapy or radiation
√ Skin damage from conditions such as eczema, insect bites or minor trauma that opens the skin
√ Respiratory illness, such as cystic fibrosis or emphysema

Current or recent hospitalization

Despite vigorous attempts to eradicate them, staph bacteria remain present in hospitals, where they attack the most vulnerable, including people with:

√ Weakened immune systems
√ Burns
√ Surgical wounds

Invasive devices

Staph bacteria can travel along the medical tubing that connects the outside world with your internal organs. Examples include:

√ Dialysis tubing
√ Urinary catheters

√ Feeding tubes

√ Breathing tubes

√ Intravascular catheters

Contact sports

Staph bacteria can spread easily through cuts, abrasions and skin-to-skin contact. Staph infections may also spread in the locker room through shared razors, towels, uniforms or equipment.

Unsanitary food preparation

Food handlers who don't properly wash their hands can transfer staph from their skin to the food they're preparing. Foods that are contaminated with staph look and taste normal.

COMPLICATIONS

If staph bacteria invade your bloodstream, you may develop a type of infection that affects your entire body. Called sepsis, this infection can lead to septic shock—a life-threatening episode with extremely low blood pressure.

PREVENTION

These commonsense precautions can help lower your risk of developing staph infections:

√ Wash your hands. Careful hand-washing is your best defense against germs. Wash your hands briskly for at least 20 seconds, then dry them with a disposable towel and use another towel to turn off the faucet. If your hands aren't visibly dirty, you can use a hand sanitizer containing at least 60 percent alcohol.

√ Keep wounds covered. Keep cuts and abrasions clean and covered with sterile, dry bandages until they heal. The pus from infected sores often contains staph bacteria, and keeping wounds covered will help keep the bacteria from spreading.

√ Reduce tampon risks. Toxic shock syndrome is caused by staph bacteria. Since tampons left in for long periods can be a breeding ground for staph bacteria, you can reduce your chances of getting toxic shock syndrome by changing your tampon frequently, at least every four to eight hours. Use the lowest absorbency tampon you can, and try to alternate tampons with sanitary napkins whenever possible;

√ Keep personal items personal. Avoid sharing personal items such as towels, sheets, razors, clothing and athletic equipment. Staph infections can spread on objects, as well as from person to person.

√ Wash clothing and bedding in hot water. Staph bacteria can survive on clothing and bedding that isn't properly washed. To get bacteria off clothing and sheets, wash them in hot water whenever possible.

√ Also, use bleach on any bleach-safe materials. Drying in the dryer is better than air-drying, but staph bacteria may survive the clothes dryer.

√ Take food safety precautions. Wash your hands before handling food. If food will be out for a while, make sure that hot foods stay hot—above 140 F (60 C)—and that cold foods stay at 40 F (4.4 C) or below. Refrigerate leftovers as soon as possible.

DIAGNOSIS

To diagnose a staph infection, your doctor will:

✓ Perform a physical exam. During the exam, your doctor will closely examine any skin lesions you may have.

✓ Collect a sample for testing. Most often, doctors diagnose staph infections by checking a tissue sample or nasal secretions for signs of the bacteria.

TREATMENT

Treatment of a staph infection may include:

✓ Antibiotics. Your doctor may perform tests to identify of the staph bacteria behind your infection, and to help choose the antibiotic that will work best. Antibiotics commonly prescribed to treat staph infections include certain cephalosporins, nafcillin or related antibiotics, sulfa drugs, or vancomycin.

✓ Vancomycin increasingly is required to treat serious staph infections because so many strains of staph bacteria have become resistant to other traditional medicines. But vancomycin and some other antibiotics have to be given intravenously.

✓ If you're given an oral antibiotic, be sure to take it as directed, and to finish all of the medication prescribed by your doctor. Ask your doctor what signs and symptoms you should watch for that might indicate your infection is worsening.

✓ Wound drainage. If you have a skin infection, your doctor will likely make an incision into the sore to drain fluid that has collected there.

✓ Device removal. If your infection involves a device or prosthetic, prompt removal of the device is needed. For some devices, removal might require surgery.

Antibiotic Resistance

Staph bacteria are very adaptable, and many varieties have become resistant to one or more antibiotics. For example, only about 10 percent of today's staph infections can be cured with penicillin.

The emergence of antibiotic-resistant strains of staph bacteria—often described as methicillin-resistant Staphylococcus aureus (MRSA) strains—has led to the use of IV antibiotics, such as vancomycin, with the potential for more side effects, such as vancomycin.

Preparing for your appointment

While you may initially consult your family physician, he or she may refer you to a specialist, depending on which of your organ systems is affected by the infection. For example, a dermatologist specializes in skin conditions, while a cardiologist treats heart disorders. Or you may be referred to a doctor who specializes in infectious diseases.

What you can do

You may want to write a list that includes:

✓ Detailed descriptions of your symptoms

✓ Information about medical problems you've had

✓ Information about the medical problems of your parents or siblings

✓ All the medications and dietary supplements you take

✓ Questions you want to ask the doctor

✓ For staph infection, some basic questions to ask your doctor include:

✓ What's the most likely cause of my symptoms?

√ What kind of tests do I need?

√ What's the best treatment for a staph infection?

√ Am I contagious?

√ How can I tell if my infection is getting better or worse?

√ Are there any activity restrictions that I need to follow?

√ I have other health conditions. How can I best manage these conditions together?

√ Do you have any brochures or other printed material that I can take home with me? What websites do you recommend?

What to expect from your doctor

Your doctor will likely ask you a number of questions, such as:

√ When did you first notice your symptoms? Could you describe them to me?

√ How severe are your symptoms?

√ Have you been around anyone with a staph infection?

√ Do you have any implanted medical devices, such as an artificial joint or a pacemaker?

√ Do you have any ongoing medical conditions, including an impaired immune system?

√ Have you recently been in the hospital?

√ Do you play contact sports?

What you can do in the meantime

If you suspect you have a staph infection on your skin, keep the area clean and covered until you see your doctor so that you don't spread the bacteria. And, until you know whether or not you have staph, don't prepare food.

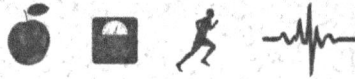

UPPER RESPIRATORY INFECTION

Most upper respiratory infections (URIs) are cause by a virus. A URI affects the nose, throat, and upper air passage. The most common type of URI is often called "the common cold."

Home Care

- √ Take medications only as told by your doctor.
- √ Gargle warm saltwater or take cough drops to comfort to throat as told by your doctor.
- √ Use a warm mist humidifier or inhale steam from a shower (or hotpot) to increase air moisture. This may make it easier to breathe.
- √ Drink enough fluid to keep your urine clear or pale yellow.
- √ Eat soup and other clear broths.
- √ Have a healthy diet.
- √ Rest as needed.
- √ You may want to wear a face mask and wash your hands often to avoid spread of the virus.
- √ Use your inhaler more if you have asthma.
- √ Do NOT use any tobacco products, including cigarettes, chewing tobacco, or e-cigarettes. If you need help quitting, ask your doctor.

Get Help If

- √ You are getting worse, not better.
- √ Your symptoms are not helped by medicine.
- √ You have chills.
- √ You are getting more short of breath.
- √ You have brown or red mucus.
- √ You have yellow or brown discharge from your nose.
- √ You have pain in your face, especially when you bend forward.
- √ You have a fever.
- √ You have swollen neck glands.
- √ You have pain while swallowing.
- √ You have white areas in the back of your throat.

Get Help Right Away If

- √ You have a very bad or constant:

- √ Headache.
- √ Ear Pain.
- √ Pain in your forehead, behind your eyes, and over your cheekbones.
- √ You have chronic lung disease and any of the following:
  - √ Wheezing.
  - √ Long-lasting cough.
  - √ Coughing up blood.
  - √ A change in your usual mucus.
- √ You have a stiff neck.
- √ You have changes in your:
  - √ Vision.
  - √ Hearing.
  - √ Thinking.
  - √ Mood.

Make Sure You

- √ Understand these instructions.
- √ Will watch your condition.
- √ Will get help right away if you are not doing well or get worse.

ACUTE BRONCHITIS

Bronchitis is inflammation of the airways that extend from the windpipe into the lungs. The inflammation often causes mucus to develop. This leads to a cough, which is the most common symptom of bronchitis.

In acute Bronchitis, the condition usually develops suddenly and goes away over time, usually in a couple weeks. Smoking, allergies, and asthma can make bronchitis worse. Repeated episodes of bronchitis may cause further lung problems.

Causes

Acute bronchitis is most often caused by the same virus that causes a cold. The virus can spread from person to person through coughing, sneezing, and touching contaminated objects.

Signs & Symptoms

- √ Cough.
- √ Fever.
- √ Coughing up mucus.
- √ Body aches.
- √ Chest congestion.
- √ Chills.
- √ Shortness of breath.
- √ Sore throat.

Diagnosis

Acute bronchitis is usually diagnosed through a physical exam. Your health care provider will also ask you questions about your medical history. Tests, such as chest X-rays, are sometimes done to rule out other conditions.

Treatment

Acute bronchitis usually goes away in a couple weeks. Oftentimes, no medical treatment is necessary. Medicines are sometimes given for relief of fever or cough. Antibiotic medicines are usually not needed but may be prescribed in certain situation. In some cases, an inhaler may be recommended to help reduce shortness of breath and control and cough. A cool mist vaporizer may also be used to help thin bronchial secretions and make it easier to clear the chest.

Home Care Instructions

√ Get plenty of rest.

√ Drink enough fluids to keep your urine clear or pale yellow (unless you have a medical condition that requires fluid restriction). Increasing fluids may help thin your respiratory secretions and reduce chest congestion, and it will help prevent dehydration.

√ Take medicines only as directed by your health care provider.

√ If you were prescribed an antibiotic medicine, finish it all even if you start to feel better.

√ Avoid smoking and secondhand smoke. Exposure to cigarette smoke or irritating chemicals will make bronchitis worse. If you are a smoker, consider using nicotine gum or skin patches to help control withdrawal symptoms. Quitting smoking will help your lungs heal faster.

√ Reduce the chances of another bout of acute bronchitis by washing your hands frequently, avoiding people with cold symptoms, and trying not to touch your hands to your mouth, nose or eyes.

√ Keep all follow-up visits as directed by your health care provider.

Seek Medical Care If

√ Your symptoms do not improve after one week of treatment.

Seek Immediate Medical Care If

√ You develop an increased fever of chills.

√ You have chest pain.

√ You have severe shortness of breath.

√ You have bloody sputum.

√ You develop dehydration.

√ You faint or repeatedly feel like you are going to pass out.

√ You develop repeated vomiting.

√ You develop a severe headache.

Make Sure You

√ Understand these instructions.

√ Will watch your condition.

√ Will get help right away if you are not doing well or get worse.

PHARYNGITIS

Pharyngitis is redness, pain, and swelling of your pharynx.

Causes

Pharyngitis is usually caused by infection. Most of the time, these infections are from viruses and are part of a cold. However, sometimes pharyngitis is caused by bacteria. Pharyngitis can also be caused by allergies. Viral pharyngitis may be spread from person to person by coughing, sneezing, and personal items or utensils (cups, forks, spoons). Bacterial pharyngitis may be spread from person to person by more intimate contact, such as kissing.

Signs & Symptoms

√ Symptoms of pharyngitis include:

√ Sore throat.

√ Tiredness.

√ Low-grade fever.

√ Headache.

√ Joint pain and muscle aches.

√ Skin rushes.

√ Swollen lymph nodes.

√ Plaque-like film on throat or tonsils.

Diagnosis

Your health care provider will ask you questions about your illness and your symptoms. Your medical history, along with a physical exam, is often all that is needed to diagnose pharyngitis. Sometimes, a rapid strep test is done. Other lab tests may also be done, depending on the suspected cause.

Treatment

Viral pharyngitis will usually get better in 3-4 days without the use of medicine. Bacterial pharyngitis is treated with medicines that kill germs (antibiotics).

Home Care Instructions

√ Drink enough water and fluids to keep your urine clear or pale yellow.

√ Only take over-the-counter or prescription medicines as directed by your health care provider:

√ If you are prescribed antibiotics, make sure you finish them even if you start to feel better.

√ DO NOT take aspirin.

√ Get lots of rest.

√ Gargle with 8 oz of salt water (1/2 tsp of salt per 1 qt or water) as often as every 1-2 hours to soothe your throat.

√ Throat lozenges (if you are not at risk for choking) or sprays may be used to soothe your throat.

Seek Medical Care If

√   You have large, tender lumps in your neck.

√   You have a rash.

√   You cough up green, yellow-brown, or bloody spit.

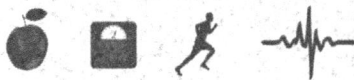

AVOID CANCER

Take Control of Your Health and Reduce Your Cancer Risk!

There are choices you can make that can help reduce your risk of getting cancer. Many of the things you can do to help prevent cancer help fight heart disease, stroke, and diabetes, too. The changes you can make may be easier than you think.

Stay Away from Tobacco

There is not safe form of tobacco. If you smoke (or chew), stop! Encourage the people around you to quit. Smoking increases cancer risk for smokers and everyone around them.

Get to And Stay at a Healthy Weight

Aim to be as lean as possible without being underweight. If you are overweight or obese, losing even a few pounds will improve your health and is a good place to start. The best way to do this is to combine a healthy diet with plenty of physical activity.

Being overweight or obese is linked with and increased risk of developing several types of cancer (and other serious health problems). Overweight and obese people can lower their risk for health problems by losing weight.

What is the "right" weight? Knowing your body mass index (BMI) can tell you if your weight is right for someone your height. You can learn your BMI by asking your doctor. Watching what and how much you eat and being more active are keys to weight control.

Get Moving

Physical activity can lower the risk of several types of cancer by helping you get and stay as a healthy weight. Physical activity also affects the levels of some hormones that contribute to cancer formation.

How much activity do you need? As an adult, get at least 150 minutes of moderate or 75 minutes of vigorous activity each week, or an equivalent combination. Spreading this activity throughout the week is better than trying to do it all in 1 or 2 days. And remember, anything is better than nothing! Doing any intentional physical activity above your usual activities can have many health benefits. Don't be a "couch" (or bunk) potato! Spend less time sitting or lying down and less time watching TV.

Have fun and be fit. The more movement you do, the better. Your daily amount of activity doesn't need to be continuous, but is most valuable if done at least 20 minutes at a time.

Eat A Variety of Healthy Foods, with More from Plant Sources

This may be a bit more difficult in prison than the outside, but still do what you can.

Choose foods and beverages in amounts that help you get to and stay at a healthy weight.

Do you best to be aware of portion sized and calories consumed. Remember: low-fat or non-fat does not always mean low-calorie some of these foods have lots of calories from added sugar. With canteen and package items, check the labels and learn which are the better foods for your diet.

Eat smaller portions of high-calorie foods. Eat vegetables, whole fruit, and other low-calorie foods instead of high-calorie foods such as chips, ice cream, doughnuts, and other sweets. Limit the number of sugar-sweetened beverages you drink, such as soft drinks, sports drinks, and fruit drinks.

Limit the amount of processed meat and red meat you eat! This is difficult in prison, because almost every meat they give us is processed. Sometimes they even give us meat not for human consumption. But if you're fortunate enough to be able to choose, eat less processed meats such as bacon, sausage, luncheon meats, and hot dogs. Try to eat fish, poultry, or beans instead of red meat. If you eat red meat, eat smaller portions.

Try to eat 2.5 cups of more of vegetables and fruits each day even if you have to trade your processed meat to the someone next to you, for his veggies and fruit. A lot of folks don't eat the veggies on their tray. Take advantage of this. Prison veggies may not be the best (try to get them raw if possible), but they're better than the processed meat, for sure!

Eat whole grains if possible, rather than refined grain products. If you buy cereal, buy whole grain cereal, such as barley and oats. Brown rice over white rice.

Limit how much you eat of refined carbohydrate foods, such as pastries, candy, sweetened breakfast cereals, and other high-sugar foods.

Drinking alcohol can increase your cancer risk. Alcohol increases your risk for developing several types of cancer (including breast, mouth, throat, larynx, esophagus, liver, colon, and rectum cancers) and several other health problems.

Protect Your Skin

About 90 percent of skin cancers diagnosed each year could be prevented with proper sun protection! Try to avoid the direct sun between 10am and 4pm. Instead, stay inside or seek the shade. When you are in the sun, cover up with protective clothing. Use sunscreen with an SPF of 30 or higher, even on hazy or overcast days.

Cover your head with a wide-brimmed hat that shades your face, ears, and neck. If you choose a baseball hat, remember to protect your ears and neck with sunscreen. Some guys like to wear a bandanna on their head, under their hat, and let it hang down. Wear sunglasses with 99 percent to 100 percent UV absorption to protect your eyes and the surrounding skin.

And know your skin. Be aware of all moles and spots on your skin, and report any changes to your doctor right away.

Know Yourself and Your Risks

Your parents and ancestors help determine some of who you are. Your tobacco use, eating and exercise habits, and lifestyle also help define your health and your risk for some diseases, such as cancer. You may be at increased risk for cancer because of the choices you make and your family history. Know yourself and your family history, and talk about these things with your doctor or nurse.

Get Regular Check-Ups

Many cancers can start to grow and spread without causing and symptoms. Regular screening tests can find some cancers in their early stages when they are small, have not spread, and are easier to treat. Be aware of any changes in your body, do regular self-exams, and visit your doctor regularly for cancer screenings.

The cancers that most often affect men are prostate, colon, lung, and skin cancers. Knowing about these cancers and what you can do to help prevent them or find them early (when they are small and easy to treat) may help save your life!

Prostate Cancer

The chance of getting prostate cancer goes up as a man gets older. Most prostate cancers are found in men over the age of 65. For reasons that are still unknown, African American men are more likely to develop prostate cancer than men of any other races. Having one or more close relatives with prostate cancer also increases a man's risk of having prostate cancer.

What you can do:

The American Cancer Society recommends that men make an informed decision with their health care provider about whether to be tested for prostate cancer. Research has not yet proven that the benefits outweigh the harms of testing and treatment. The ACS believes that men should not be tested without learning about what they know and don't know about the risks and possible benefits of testing and treatment.

Starting at age 50, talk to your provider about the pros and cons of testing so you can decide if getting tested is the right choice for you. If you are African American or have a father or brother who had prostate cancer before age 65, you should have this talk with your provider starting at age 45. If you decide to be tested, you should have the PSA blood test with or without a rectal exam. How often you are tested will depend on your PSA level.

Colon Cancer

Most colon cancers (cancers of the colon and rectum) are found in people age 50 or older. People with a personal or family history of this cancer, or who have polyps in their colon or rectum, or those with inflammatory bowel disease are more likely to have colon cancer. Also, being overweight, eating a diet mostly of high-fat foods (especially from animal sources), smoking, and being inactive can make a person more likely to have this cancer.

What you can do:

Colon cancer almost always starts with a polyp—a small growth on the lining of the colon or rectum. Testing can save lives by finding polyps before they become cancer. If pre-cancerous polyps are removed, colon cancer can be prevented.

For people of average risk, the American Cancer Society recommends getting tested, starting at age 50. The tests that are designed to find both early cancer and polyps should be your first choice if these tests are available to you and you're willing to have one of them. Talk to a health care provider about which test is best for you.

If you are at high risk of colon cancer based on family history or other factors, you may need to be tested at a younger age with colonoscopy. Talk to your yard doctor about your risk for colon cancer to know when you should start testing.

Lung Cancer

About 8 out of 10 lung cancer deaths are thought to result from smoking. People who don't smoke can also have lung cancer.

What you can do:

Lung cancer is one of the few cancers that can often be prevented simply by not smoking. If you are a smoker, quit. If you don't smoke, don't start, and avoid breathing in other people's smoke. If your friends and loved ones are smokers, help them quit. For help quitting, have them call the American Cancer Society as 1-800-227-2345 to find out how they can help improve your chances of quitting for good.

Certain men at high risk for lung cancer may want to talk to their doctor about getting yearly low-does CT scans to test for early lung cancer. Testing may benefit adults who are current or former smokers between the ages of 55 and 74 who are in good health and have a 30 pack-year smoking history.

Skin Cancer

Anyone who spends time in the sun can have skin cancer. People with fair skin, especially those with blond or red hair, are more likely to get skin cancer than people with darker coloring. People who have had a close family member with melanoma and those who had severe sunburns as children are more likely to get skin cancer.

What you can do:

Most skin cancers can be prevented by limiting exposure to ultraviolet (UV) rays from the sun. When outside, try to stay in the shade, especially during the middle of the day. If you're going to be in the sun, wear hats with brims, long-sleeve shirts, sunglasses, and use broad-spectrum sunscreen with an SPF of 30 or higher on all exposed skin. Be aware of all moles and spots on your skin, and report any changes to your health care provider right away.

The best defense against cancer is doing what you can to prevent getting it in the first place. Knowing about cancer and what you can do to help reduce your risk of it can save your life. The next key is early detection. Finding cancer early, before it has spread, gives you the best chance to do something about it.

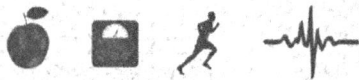

KNOW THY NUTS

Testicular cancer only occurs in 1% of the male population, but it is the most common type of cancer in young males, ages 15 to 35. Although it is alarming to be diagnosed with any form of cancer, the good news is that when caught in the early stages, testicular cancer is highly treatable. According to the American Cancer Society, there is a 99% survival rate in cases that are treated prior to the spread of the disease beyond the testicles.

Regular self-exams to look and feel for any lumps or abnormalities is extremely important for young males in order to catch the disease before it progresses.

HERE ARE THE 10 MOST COMMON EARLY WARNING SIGNS OF TESTICULAR CANCER THAT YOU NEED TO READ.

1. Small Lump or Hardened Area

The most common sign of testicular cancer is a small lump—usually pea-sized— or a hardened area found on one of the testicles. It is important to understand that a healthy testicle will feel bumpy, because it houses numerous blood vessels, sperm tubes, and reproductive tissue. However, if the lump you feel is hard like a bean or feels different from tissue on the other testicle, it is important to follow up with a physician for a more thorough examination. Just because you find a lump, does not necessarily mean that you have testicular cancer; it could be symptomatic of a less serious disorder, including varicocele (an enlargement of blood vessels), a small cyst called a spermatocele, or an inguinal hernia. Since early diagnosis is the best predictor of a successful recovery, it is important not to put off a trip to the doctor. No matter what the cause, it will require some form of treatment.

2. Change in Size of Testicles

It is completely normal for one testicle to be larger than the other, or hang down further. However, if there is a noticeable change in the size of one of your testicles that is not due to temperature change or sexual activity, either enlargement or significant shrinkage, this could be cause for concern. Other possible causes for an enlargement of the testes may include inflammation, hydrocele (a buildup of fluid in the membrane surrounding the testicles), or an infection. While testicular cancer does not cause pain in the early stages, these other disorders may also be accompanied by pain and discharge.

3. Pain or Tenderness

Frequently testicular cancer is characterized by a painless lump or enlargement of one of the testicles. However, pain or tenderness of the testicles, either with or without a lump, could also be a sign of cancer. Any type of pain is never normal, so it is important to find out the root cause and treat it accordingly. The pain may just be from an infection of the testicle (orchitis) or the epididymis that is found behind the testis, but both would require antibiotics. Infection may sometimes be accompanied by fever and discharge. An inguinal hernia could also be the source of your pain and may require surgery. Torsion of the testis, which occurs when a testicle rotates, and therefore, cuts off blood supply can also be extremely painful and cause swelling. This is a surgical emergency and requires immediate medical intervention to save the affected area.

4. Feeling of Heaviness in the Scrotum

If you notice a change in the way that your testicle feels—one testicle feels firmer, fuller, or heavier than before--this could be a sign of a serious problem. A sudden collection of fluid in the scrotum could be the culprit. This is never normal and may be an indicator of testicular cancer.

5. Dull Ache in the Lower Abdomen

In cases of testicular cancer where the symptoms include some type of discomfort, it is generally characterized as more of a dull ache than a sharp pain. The ongoing ache is commonly felt in the groin area, but may also be felt in the lower abdominal region. This type of discomfort is also common with inguinal hernia.

6. Developing a Blood Clot

In some instances, there may not be any early warning signs or symptoms of testicular cancer. In middle-age men, the development of deep vein thrombosis (DVT), or what is more commonly referred to as a blood clot, may be the first symptom that there is something wrong. A DVT occurs in the large veins and is usually characterized by pain and swelling in the affected leg. If the blood clot moves to the lungs, it could cause shortness of breath and can be extremely serious.

7. Tenderness of Breast Tissue

Although it is uncommon, in some instances, the tumor may produce the female hormone, estrogen. The imbalance of the female hormone estrogen and the male hormone testosterone may lead to a condition known as gynecomastia, where the male breast tissue becomes tender and swells like that of a woman. Gynecomastia may also be caused by certain drugs or malnutrition, but it is always symptomatic of another problem.

8. Early Signs of Puberty

Some tumors may also produce male sex hormones. While testicular cancer is highly uncommon in pre-pubescent boys, if your son is suddenly showing signs of puberty at an early age, this could be a symptom of a developing tumor. Puberty in males usually occurs gradually. If you notice your child is quickly changing at an abnormal age, such as the growth of facial and body hair and deepening of his voice, it is a good idea to take him to the physician for further examination.

9. Lower Back Pain

Cancer typically spreads to the lymph nodes first, which can be found in the back of abdominal region. The onset of chronic lower back pain without excessive physical strain or injury may be indicative of metastasis of testicular cancer. There are some instances where there are no noticeable symptoms until the cancer progresses, so any unusual warning signs in males 15-35 should be evaluated further.

10. Shortness of Breath

Testicular cancer may also spread to the lungs, liver, or brain. Chest pain, a chronic cough that may or may not expel bloody sputum, and a shortness of breath may all be symptoms of cancer that has metastasized to the lungs. Abdominal pain and bloating could indicate that the cancer has spread to the lymph nodes and liver. Severe headaches and confusion may occur if the cancer has spread to the brain. While these may all be symptoms of other conditions as well, it is important to seek further medical advice to diagnose and treat the problem quickly and accurately.

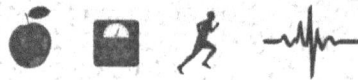

COLON CANCER FACTS

Colon cancer facts

√ Colorectal cancer is a malignant tumor arising from the inner wall of the large intestine (colon) or rectum.

√ Colorectal cancer is the third leading cause of cancer in both men and women in the U.S.

√ Common risk factors for colorectal cancer include increasing age, African-American race, a family history of colorectal cancer, colon polyps, and long-standing ulcerative colitis.

√ Most colorectal cancers develop from polyps. Removal of colon polyps can aid in the prevention of colorectal cancer.

√ Colon polyps and early cancer may have no cancer-specific early signs or symptoms. Therefore, regular colorectal cancer screening is important.

√ Diagnosis of colorectal cancer can be made by sigmoidoscopy or by colonoscopy with biopsy confirmation of cancerous tissue.

√ Treatment of colorectal cancer depends on the location, size, and extent of cancer spread, as well as the health of the patient.

√ Surgery is the most common medical treatment for colorectal cancer.

√ Early-stage colorectal cancers are typically treatable by surgery alone.

√ Chemotherapycan extend life and improve quality of life for those who have had or are living with metastatic colorectal cancer. It can also reduce the risk of recurrence in patients found to have high-risk colon cancer findings at surgery.

What is cancer?

Every day within our bodies, a massive process of destruction and repair occurs. The human body is comprised of about 15 trillion cells, and every day billions of cells wear out or are destroyed. In most cases, each time a cell is destroyed the body makes a new cell to replace it, trying to make a cell that is a perfect copy of the cell that was destroyed because the replacement cell must be capable of performing the same function as the destroyed cell. During the complex process of replacing cells, many errors occur. Despite remarkably elegant systems in place to prevent errors, the body still makes tens of thousands of mistakes daily while replacing cells either because of random errors or because there are outside pressures placed on the replacement process that promote errors. Most of these mistakes are corrected by additional elegant systems or the mistake leads to the death of the newly made cell, and another normal new cell is produced. Sometimes a mistake is made, however, and is not corrected.

Many of the uncorrected mistakes have little effect on health, but if the mistake allows the newly made cell to divide independent of the checks and balances that control normal cell growth, that cell can begin to multiply in an uncontrolled manner. When this happens, a tumor (essentially a mass of abnormal cells) can develop.

Tumors fall into two categories: there are benign (noncancerous) tumors and malignant (cancerous) tumors. So what is the difference? The answer is that a benign tumor grows only in the tissue from which it arises. Benign tumors sometimes can grow quite large or rapidly and cause severe symptoms, even death, although most do not. For example, a fibroid tumor in a woman's uterus is a type of benign tumor. It can cause bleeding or pain, but it will never travel outside the uterus and grow as a new tumor elsewhere. Fibroids, like all benign tumors, lack the capacity to shed cells into the blood and lymphatic system, so they are unable to travel to other places in the body and grow. A cancer, on the other hand, can shed cells that can travel through the blood or lymphatic system, landing in tissues distant from the primary tumor and growing into new tumors in these distant tissues. This process of spreading to distant tissues, called metastasis, is the defining characteristic of a cancerous or malignant tumor.

Benign tumor cells often look relatively normal in appearance when examined under the microscope. Malignant or cancerous cells usually look more abnormal in appearance when similarly viewed under the microscope.

Cancer is a group of more than 100 different diseases, much like infectious diseases. Cancers are named by the tissues from which the first tumor arises. Hence, a lung cancer that travels to the liver is not a liver cancer but is described as lung cancer metastatic to the liver, and a breast cancer that spreads to the brain is not described as a brain tumor but rather as breast cancer metastatic to the brain. Each cancer is a different disease with different treatment options and varying prognoses (likely outcomes or life expectancy). In fact, each individual with cancer has a unique disease, and the relative success or lack thereof of treatment among patients with the same diagnosis may be very different. As a result, it is important to treat each person with a diagnosis of cancer as an individual regardless of the type of cancer.

What is the colon, and what does it do?

The colon and the rectum are the final portions of the tube that extends from the mouth to the anus. Food enters the mouth where it is chewed and then swallowed. It then travels through the esophagus and into the stomach. In the stomach, the food is ground into smaller particles and then enters the small intestine in a carefully controlled manner. In the small intestine, final digestion of food and absorption of the nutrients contained in the food occurs. The food that is not digested and absorbed enters the large intestine (colon) and finally the rectum. The large intestine acts primarily as a storage facility for waste; however, additional water, salts, and some vitamins are further removed. In addition, some of the undigested food, for example, fiber, is digested by colonic bacteria and some of the products of digestion are absorbed from the colon and into the body. (It is estimated that 10% of the energy derived from food comes from these products of bacterial digestion in the colon.) The remaining undigested food, dying cells from the lining of the intestines, and large numbers of bacteria are stored in the colon and then periodically passed into the rectum. Their arrival into the rectum initiates a bowel movement that empties the colonic contents from the body as stool.

Although the large intestine is a tube, it is structurally a complicated tube, more like a steel belted radial tire than a garden hose. The tube is comprised of four layers. The first is an inner layer of cells that line the cavity through which the undigested and digesting food travels, called the mucosa. The mucosa is attached to a thin second layer, the submucosa, that is attached itself to a layer of muscle, the muscularis. The entire tube is surrounded by fibrous (scar-like) tissue called the serosa. The most common cancers of the large intestine (the type called adenocarcinoma) arise from the mucosa, the inner layer of cells. These cells are exposed to toxins from food and bacteria as well as mechanical wear and tear, and they are relatively turning over rapidly (dying off and being replaced). Mistakes (usually a series of mistakes involving genes within the replacement cells) lead to abnormal cells and uncontrolled proliferation of the abnormal cells that give rise to cancer. The rapid turnover allows for more mistakes to occur as compared with tissues that do not turn over so rapidly (for example, liver tissue).

Where is the colon located?

Most of the large intestine rests inside a cavity in the abdomen called the peritoneal cavity. Parts of the colon are able to move quite freely within the peritoneal cavity as the undigested food is passing through it. As the colon heads towards the rectum, it becomes fixed to the tissues behind the peritoneal cavity, an area called the retroperitoneum. The end portion of the large intestine, the part that resides in the retroperitoneum, is the rectum. Unlike much of the rest of the colon, the rectum is fixed in place by the tissues that surround it. Because of its location, treatment for rectal cancer often is different than treatment for cancer of the rest of the colon.

How long is the human colon?

The human large intestine (colon) is about 6 feet long.

What is colorectal cancer?

Cancers of the colon and rectum (colorectal cancer) start when the process of the normal replacement of colon lining cells goes awry. Mistakes in cell division occur frequently. For reasons that are poorly understood, sometimes mistakes occur that escape our editing systems. When this occurs, these cells begin to divide independently of the normal checks and balances that control growth. As these abnormal cells grow and divide, they can lead to growths within the colon called polyps. Polyps vary in type, but many are precancerous tumors that grow slowly over the course of years and do not spread. As polyps grow, additional genetic mutations further destabilize the cells. When these precancerous tumors change direction (growing into the wall of the tube rather than into the space in the middle of it) and invade other layers of the large intestine (such as the submucosa or muscular layer), the precancerous polyp has become cancerous. In most cases this process is slow, taking at least eight to 10 years to develop from those early aberrant cells to a frank cancer. Colorectal cancer is typically an adenocarcinoma, a term that refers to a cancer that has formed in certain types of lining tissues in the body.

Once a colorectal cancer forms, it begins to grow in two ways. First, the cancer can grow locally and extend through the wall of the intestine and invade adjacent structures, making the mass (called the primary tumor) more of a problem and harder to remove. Local extension can cause additional symptoms such as pain or fullness, perforation of the colon, or blockages of the colon or nearby structures. Second, as the cancer grows it begins the process of metastasis, shedding thousands of cells a day into the blood and lymphatic system that can cause cancers to form in distant locations. Colorectal cancers most commonly spread first to local lymph nodes before traveling to distant organs. Once local lymph nodes are involved, spread to the liver, the abdominal cavity, and the lung are the next most common destinations of metastatic spread.

Colorectal cancer is the third most common cause of cancer in the U.S. in both men and women. It affects over 135,000 people annually, representing 8% of all cancers. About 4.3% of people will be diagnosed with colon or rectum cancer at some point in their lives.

What are the causes and risk factors of colon cancer?

Health care professionals are certain that colorectal cancer is not contagious (a person cannot catch the disease from a cancer patient). Some people are more likely to develop colorectal cancer than others. Factors that increase a person's risk of colorectal cancer include increasing age, African-American race, high fat intake, a family history of colorectal cancer and polyps, the presence of polyps in the large intestine, and inflammatory bowel diseases, primarily chronic ulcerative colitis.

Age

Increasing age is the main risk factor for colorectal cancer. Around 90% of colorectal cancers are diagnosed after age 50.

Race

African Americans have a higher incidence of colorectal cancer than people of other races.

Diet and colorectal cancer

Diets high in fat have been shown in numerous research studies to predispose people to colorectal cancer. In countries with high colorectal cancer rates, the fat intake by the population is much higher than in countries with low cancer rates. It is believed that the digestion of fat that occurs in the small intestine and the colon leads to the formation of cancer-causing chemicals (carcinogens). Likewise, research studies also reveal that diets high in vegetables and high-fiber foods such as whole-grain breads and cereals contain less fat that produces these carcinogens and may counter the effects of the carcinogens. Both effects would help reduce the risk of cancer.

Colon polyps and colorectal cancer

Research has shown that most colorectal cancers develop in colorectal polyps. Therefore, removing benign (but precancerous) colorectal polyps can prevent colorectal cancer. Precancerous colorectal polyps are most commonly called adenomatous polyps. They develop when chromosomal damage occurs in cells of the inner lining of the colon. The damage produces abnormal cells, but the cells have not yet developed the ability to spread, the hallmark of cancer. Instead, the growing tissue remains localized within the polyp. When chromosomal damage increases further within the polyp, cell growth becomes uncontrolled, and the cells begin to spread, that is, they become cancer. Thus, colon polyps which are initially benign acquire additional chromosome damage to become cancerous.

Ulcerative colitis and colorectal cancer

Chronic ulcerative colitis causes inflammation of the inner lining of the colon. Colon cancer is a recognized complication of chronic ulcerative colitis. The risk for cancer begins to increase after eight to 10 years of colitis. The risk of developing colon cancer in a patient with ulcerative colitis also is related to the location and the extent of his or her disease.

Patients at higher risk of cancer are those with a family history of colon cancer, a long duration of ulcerative colitis, extensive colon involvement with ulcerative colitis, and those with ulcerative colitis-associated liver disease, sclerosing cholangitis.

Since the cancers associated with ulcerative colitis have a more favorable outcome when caught at an earlier stage, yearly examinations of the colon often are recommended after eight years of known extensive disease. During these examinations, samples of tissue (biopsies) are taken to search for precancerous changes in the cells lining the colon. When precancerous changes are found, removal of the entire colon may be necessary to prevent colon cancer.

Genetics and colorectal cancer

A person's genetic background is an important factor in colon cancer risk. Having a first-degree relative with colorectal cancer, especially if the cancer was diagnosed before the age of 55 years, roughly doubles the risk of developing the condition.

Even though a family history of colon cancer is an important risk factor, a majority (80%) of colon cancers occur sporadically in patients with no family history of colon cancer. Approximately 20% of cancers are associated with a family history of colon cancer.

Chromosomes contain genetic information, and chromosomal damage causes genetic defects that lead to the formation of colon polyps and later colon cancer. In sporadic polyps and cancers (polyps and cancers that develop in the absence of family history), the chromosome damages are acquired (develop in a cell during adult life). The damaged chromosomes can only be found in the polyps and the cancers that develop from that cell. But in hereditary colon cancer syndromes, the chromosomal defects are inherited at birth and are present in every cell in the body. Patients who have inherited the hereditary colon cancer syndrome genes are at risk of developing colon polyps, usually at young ages, and are at very high risk of developing colon cancer early in life; they also are at risk of developing cancers in other organs.

Familial adenomatous polyposis (FAP) is one hereditary colorectal cancer syndrome where the affected family members will develop countless numbers (hundreds, sometimes thousands) of colon polyps starting during their teens. Unless the condition is detected and treated early (treatment involves removal of the colon), a person affected by FAP is almost sure to develop colon cancer from these polyps. Cancers almost certainly develop by the time a person is in their 40s. These patients are also at risk of developing other cancers such as cancers in the thyroid gland, stomach, and the ampulla (part of the bile duct where it drains into the small intestine from the liver) as well as benign tumors called desmoid tumors. FAP arises from a mutation in a specific gene called the APC gene. The specific mutation can be identified in most people with appropriate testing, and such testing is recommended for individuals diagnosed with FAP as well as their family members.

Attenuated familial adenomatous polyposis (AFAP) is a milder version of FAP. Affected members develop fewer than 100 colon polyps. Nevertheless, they are still at very high risk of developing colon cancers at a young age. They are also at risk of having gastric polyps and duodenal polyps.

Hereditary nonpolyposis colon cancer (also known as Lynch Syndrome or HNPCC) is a hereditary colorectal cancer syndrome where affected family members can develop colon polyps and cancers, usually in the right colon, in their 30s to 40s. Patients with HNPCC are also at risk of developing uterine cancer, stomach cancer, ovarian cancer, and cancers of the ureters (the tubes that connect the kidneys to the bladder), and the bile ducts. Ironically, it appears that while colon cancer occurs more frequently in patients with HNPCC, these cancers may be more easily cured than "sporadic" colon cancers. The specific genetic abnormalities associated with HNPCC have been identified, and patients and family members can be tested to determine if HNPCC is present and if family members carry the abnormality and are likely to develop cancer.

MYH polyposis syndrome is a recently discovered hereditary colorectal cancer syndrome. Affected members typically develop 10 to 100 polyps at around 40 years of age and are at high risk of developing colon cancer. Here, too, the genetic abnormality has been identified.

It is important to remember that the overwhelming majority of colorectal cancers do not have a single, identifiable chromosomal abnormality that can be looked for in relatives in order to identify individuals at risk for colorectal cancer.

What are the signs and symptoms of colon cancer?

Symptoms of colorectal cancer are numerous and nonspecific. They include fatigue, weakness, shortness of breath, change in bowel habits, narrow stools, diarrhea or constipation, red or dark blood in stool, weight loss, abdominal pain, cramps, or bloating. Other conditions such as irritable bowel syndrome (spastic colon), ulcerative colitis, Crohn's disease, diverticulosis, and peptic ulcer disease can have symptoms that mimic colorectal cancer.

Colorectal cancer can be present for several years before symptoms develop. Symptoms vary according to where in the large intestine the tumor is located. The right colon is wider and more flexible. It can even be called relatively spacious as compared to the rest of the colon. Cancers of the right colon can grow to large sizes before they cause any abdominal symptoms. Typically, right-sided cancers cause iron deficiency anemia due to the slow loss of blood over a long period of time. Iron deficiency anemia causes fatigue, weakness, and shortness of breath. The left colon is narrower than the right colon. Therefore, cancers of the left colon are more likely to cause partial or complete bowel obstruction. Cancers causing partial bowel obstruction can cause symptoms of constipation, narrowed stool, diarrhea, abdominal pains, cramps, and bloating. Bright red blood in the stool may also indicate a growth near the end of the left colon or rectum.

What tests can be done to detect and diagnose colon cancer?

When colon cancer is suspected, a colonoscopy is typically performed to confirm the diagnosis and locate the tumor.

Colonoscopy is a procedure whereby a health care professional inserts a long, flexible viewing tube into the rectum for the purpose of inspecting the inside of the entire colon. Colonoscopy is generally considered more accurate than barium enema X-rays, especially in detecting small polyps. If colon polyps are found, they usually are removed through the colonoscope and sent to the pathologist. The pathologist examines the polyps under the microscope to check for cancer. Colonoscopy is the best procedure to use when cancer of the colon is suspected. While the majority of the polyps removed through colonoscopes are benign, many are precancerous. Removal of precancerous polyps prevents the future development of colon cancer from these polyps.

Sigmoidoscopy is a procedure performed using a shorter flexible scope to examine just the left colon and rectum. It is more easily prepared for and performed than a complete colonoscopy but has obvious limitations in terms of not being long enough to assess both the right and transverse colons. Polyp removal and cancer biopsy can be performed through the sigmoidoscope.

If cancerous growths are found during colonoscopy, small tissue samples (biopsies) can be obtained and examined under the microscope to determine if the polyp is cancerous. If colon cancer is confirmed by a biopsy, staging examinations are performed to determine whether the cancer has already spread to other organs. Since colorectal cancer tends to spread to the lungs and the liver, staging tests usually include CT scans of the lungs, liver, and abdomen. Positron emission tomography (PET) scans, a newer test which looks for the increased metabolic activity that is common in cancerous tissue, also are employed frequently to look for the spread of colon cancer to lymph nodes or other organs.

Sometimes, the health care professional may obtain a "tumor marker" blood test called a carcinoembryonic antigen (CEA) if there is a suspicion of cancer. CEA is a substance produced by some colon and rectal cancer cells as well as by some other types of cancers. It is sometimes found in high levels in patients with colorectal cancer, especially when the disease has spread. It can serve as a useful test to follow if it is found to be elevated before the cancer is removed. However, not all patients with colorectal cancer will have an elevated CEA even if their cancer has spread. (Some colorectal cancers don't produce it.) Additionally, some patients without cancer can have an elevated CEA blood test. About 15% of smokers, for example, will have an elevated CEA without colon cancer. So the CEA is not used to diagnose colorectal cancer but rather to follow the effects of treatment of colorectal cancer in someone with a known history of the disease because, again, in some patients the amount of cancerous tissue correlates with the level of CEA.

What are the stages of colon cancer?

When a colorectal cancer is diagnosed, additional tests are performed to determine the extent of the disease. This process is called staging. Staging determines how advanced a colorectal cancer has become. The staging for colorectal cancer ranges from stage I, the least advanced cancer, to stage IV, the most advanced cancer. Stage I colorectal cancers involve only the innermost layers of the colon or rectum. The likelihood of cure (excellent prognosis) for stage I colorectal cancer is over 90%. Stage II cancers exhibit greater growth and extension of tumor through the wall of the colon or rectum into adjacent structures. Stage III colorectal cancers manifest spread of the cancer to local lymph nodes. Stage IV (metastatic) colorectal cancers have spread, or metastasized, to distant organs or lymph nodes far from the original tumor.

With each subsequent stage of colon cancer, the risk for recurrent cancer and death due to spread of the cancer (metastasis) rises. As noted, earlier cancers have lower risks of recurrence and death. By the time an individual has stage IV colorectal cancer, the prognosis is poor. However, even in stage IV colorectal cancer (depending on where the cancer has spread) the opportunity for cure exists.

What are the treatments for colon cancer?

Surgery is the most common initial medical treatment for colorectal cancer. During surgery, the tumor, a small margin of the surrounding healthy intestine, and adjacent lymph nodes are removed. The surgeon then reconnects the healthy sections of the bowel. In patients with rectal cancer, the rectum sometimes is permanently removed if the cancer arises too low in the rectum. The surgeon then creates an opening (colostomy) on the abdominal wall through which solid waste from the colon is excreted. Specially trained nurses (enterostomal therapists) can help patients adjust to colostomies, and most patients with colostomies return to a normal lifestyle.

For early colon cancers, the recommended treatment is surgical removal. For most people with early stage colon cancer (stage I and most stage II), surgery alone is the only treatment required. Chemotherapy may be offered to some people with stage II cancers who have factors suggesting that their tumor may be at higher risk of recurrence. However, once a colon cancer has spread to local lymph nodes (stage III), the risk of the cancer returning remains high even if all visible evidence of the cancer has been removed by the surgeon. This is due to an increased likelihood that tiny cancer cells may have escaped prior to surgery and are too small to detect at that time by blood tests, scans or even direct examination. Their presence is deduced from higher risk of recurrence of the colon cancer at a later date (relapse). Medical cancer doctors (medical oncologists) recommend additional treatments with chemotherapy in this setting to lower the risk of the cancer's return. Drugs used for chemotherapy enter the bloodstream and attack any colon cancer cells that were shed into the blood or lymphatic systems prior to the operation, attempting to kill them before they set up shop in other organs.

This strategy, called adjuvant chemotherapy, has been proven to lower the risk of cancer recurrence and is recommended for all patients with stage III colon cancer who are healthy enough to undergo it, as well as for some higher risk stage II patients whose tumor may have been found to have obstructed or perforated the bowel wall prior to surgery.

There are several different options for adjuvant chemotherapy for the treatment of colon cancer. The treatments involve a combination of chemotherapy drugs given orally or into the veins. The treatments typically are given for a total of six months. It is important to meet with an oncologist who can explain adjuvant chemotherapy options as well as side effects to watch out for so that the right choice can be made for a patient as an individual.

Chemotherapy usually is given in a health care professional's clinic, in the hospital as an outpatient, or at home. Chemotherapy usually is given in cycles of treatment followed by recovery periods without treatment. Side effects of chemotherapy vary from person to person and also depend on the agents given. Modern chemotherapy agents are usually well tolerated, and side effects for most people are manageable. In general, anticancer medications destroy cells that are rapidly growing and dividing. Therefore, normal red blood cells, platelets, and white blood cells that also are growing rapidly can be affected by chemotherapy. As a result, common side effects include anemia, loss of energy, and a low resistance to infections. Cells in the hair roots and intestines also divide rapidly. Therefore, chemotherapy can cause hair loss, mouth sores, nausea, vomiting, and diarrhea, but these effects are transient.

Treatment of stage IV colorectal cancer

Once colorectal cancer has spread distant from the primary tumor site, it is described as stage IV disease. These distant tumor deposits, shed from the primary tumor, have traveled through the blood or lymphatic system, forming new tumors in other organs. At that point, colorectal cancer is no longer a local problem but is instead a systemic problem with cancer cells both visible on scan and undetectable, but likely present elsewhere throughout the body. As a result, in most cases the best treatment is chemotherapy, which is a systemic therapy. Chemotherapy in metastatic colorectal cancer has been proven to extend life and improve the quality of life. If managed well, the side effects of chemotherapy are typically far less than the side effects of uncontrolled cancer. Chemotherapy alone cannot cure metastatic colon cancer, but it can more than double life expectancy and allow for good quality of life during the time of treatment.

Chemotherapy options for colorectal cancer treatment vary depending on other health issues that an individual faces. For fitter individuals, combinations of several chemotherapeutic drugs usually are recommended, whereas for sicker people, simpler treatments may be best. Different multidrug regimens combine agents with proven activity in colorectal cancer such as 5-fluorouracil (5-FU), which is often given with the drug leucovorin (also called folinic acid) or a similar drug called levoleucovorin, which helps it work better.

Capecitabine (Xeloda), is a chemotherapy drug given in pill form. Once in the body, it is changed to 5-FU when it gets to the tumor site. Other chemotherapy drugs for colorectal cancer are irinotecan (Camptosar), oxaliplatin (Elozatin), and trifluridine and tipiracil (Lonsurf), a combination drug in pill form. Chemotherapy regimens often have acronyms to simplify their nomenclature (such as FOLFOX, FOLFIRI, and FLOX).

Targeted therapies are newer treatments that target specific aspects of the cancer cell, which may be more important to the tumor than the surrounding tissues, offering potentially effective treatments with fewer side effects than traditional chemotherapy. Bevacizumab (Avastin), cetuximab (Erbitux), panitumumab (Vectibix), ramucirumab (Cyramza), regorafenib (Stivarga), and ziv-aflibercept (Zaltrap) are targeted therapies that have been used in the management of advanced colorectal cancer. These newer chemotherapeutic agents most often are combined with standard chemotherapy to enhance their effectiveness.

If the first treatment is not effective, second and third line options are available that can confer benefit to people living with colorectal cancer.

Radiation therapy in the primary treatment of colorectal cancer has been limited to treating cancer of the rectum. As noted earlier, whereas parts of the colon move freely within the abdominal cavity, the rectum is fixed in place within the pelvis. It is in intimate relationship to many other structures and the pelvis is a more confined space. For these reasons, a tumor in the rectum often is harder to remove surgically because the space is smaller and other structures can be involved with cancer. As a result, for all but the earliest rectal cancers, initial chemotherapy and radiation treatments (a local treatment to a defined area) are recommended to try and shrink the cancer, allowing for easier removal and lowering the risk of the cancer returning locally. Radiation therapy is typically given under the guidance of a radiation specialist called a radiation oncologist. Initially, individuals undergo a planning session, a complicated visit as the doctors and technicians determine exactly where to give the radiation and which structures to avoid. Chemotherapy usually is administered daily while the radiation is delivered. Side effects of radiation treatment include fatigue, temporary or permanent pelvic hair loss, and skin irritation in the treated areas.

Radiation therapy will occasionally be used as a palliative treatment to reduce pain from recurrent or metastatic colon or rectal cancer.

What is the follow-up care for colon cancer?

Follow-up exams are important for people with colorectal cancer. The cancer can come back near the original site, although this is unusual. If the cancer returns, it typically does so in a distant location such as the lymph nodes, liver, or lungs. Individuals diagnosed with colorectal cancer remain at risk of their cancer returning for up to 10 years after their original diagnosis and treatment, although the risk of recurrence is much higher in the first few years. Medical providers in the United States follow patients with physical examinations and blood tests including the CEA (if it was elevated before surgery) tumor marker every three months for the first two years and then with decreasing frequency thereafter. Patients are also followed with colonoscopies (starting one year after their diagnosis) and with CT scans (typically performed at least once yearly for the first two to five years).

If a recurrence is noted either locally or with metastatic spread, individuals may still be treated with the intention of cure. For example, if a new tumor were to recur in the liver, individuals can be treated with a combination of chemotherapy and surgery (or sophisticated radiation techniques) in hopes of eradicating the cancer completely. Evaluation in hospitals of excellence that specialize in liver surgery can help guide these complicated treatment decisions and increase the chances of cure even in the setting of metastatic disease.

In addition to checking for cancer recurrence, patients who have had colon cancer may have an increased risk of cancer of the prostate, breast, and ovary. Therefore, follow-up examinations in the clinic should include screening for these disease, as well.

What is the prognosis for patients with colorectal cancer?

Colorectal cancers are typically slow-growing cancers that take years to develop. Because they grow most often in a step-wise manner, screening can greatly reduce the likelihood of death associated with the disease. Whether with virtual colonoscopy or newer screening techniques, the future must focus first and foremost on better, more comprehensive screening programs that find polyps and early cancers before they become life-threatening. The public also must be educated on the value of screening programs.

For those living with cancer, intensive research is ongoing to better understand cancer biology and genetics so that specific approaches can be developed to attack specific types of cancers and, more importantly, specific individuals' cancers. Each person living with cancer has a disease with a unique biology and genetic code and the secret to better treatments involves unlocking that code. Cancer is very complex and scientists are just beginning to unravel its secrets. Progress is frustratingly slow for those battling the disease. With each passing year, however, our understanding increases and treatments become more refined. If you or your family member is living with colorectal cancer, speak with your doctor about ways you can participate in research through clinical trials to help increase our knowledge and improve our therapies for this difficult disease.

What are colon cancer survival rates?

Survival rates for any cancer are often reported by stage, the extent of spread when the cancer is identified. For colon and rectum cancer, around 39% are diagnosed at the local stage, before the cancer has spread outside the local area. The five-year survival for these patients with localized colon and rectum cancer is around 90%.

When the cancer has spread to the regional lymph nodes near the site of origin, the five-year survival rate is about 71%. When the cancer has metastasized to distant sites in the body (stage IV cancer), the five-year survival rate lowers to about 14%.

Is it possible to prevent colon cancer?

The most effective prevention for colorectal cancer is early detection and removal of precancerous colorectal polyps before they turn cancerous. Even in cases where cancer has already developed, early detection still significantly improves the chances of a cure by surgically removing the cancer before the disease spreads to other organs.

Regular physical activity is associated with lower risk of colon cancer. Aspirin use also appears to lower the risk of colon cancer. The use of combined estrogen and progestin in hormone replacement therapy lowers the risk of colon cancer in postmenopausal women. Hormone replacement therapy has risks which must be weighed against this effect, and should be discussed with a doctor.

Genetic counseling and testing

Blood tests are now available to test for hereditary colon cancer syndromes. Families with multiple members having colon cancers, multiple colon polyps, cancers at young ages, and other cancers such as cancers of the ureters, uterus, duodenum, and more, may take advantage of resources such as genetic counseling, followed possibly by genetic testing. Genetic testing without prior counseling is discouraged because of the extensive family education that is involved and the complicated nature of interpreting the test results.

The advantages of genetic counseling followed by genetic testing include: (1) identifying family members at high risk of developing colon cancer to begin colonoscopies early; (2) identifying high-risk members so that screening may begin to prevent other cancers such as ultrasound tests for uterine cancer, urine examinations for ureter cancer, and upper endoscopies for stomach and duodenal cancers; and (3) alleviating concern for members who test negative for the hereditary genetic defects.

Diet to prevent colon cancer

People can change their eating habits by reducing fat intake and increasing fiber (roughage) in their diet. Major sources of fat are meat, eggs, dairy products, salad dressings, and oils used in cooking. Fiber is the insoluble, non-digestible part of plant material present in fruits, vegetables, and whole-grain breads and cereals. It is postulated that high fiber in the diet leads to the creation of bulky stools which can rid the intestines of potential carcinogens. In addition, fiber leads to the more rapid transit of fecal material through the intestine, thus allowing less time for a potential carcinogen to react with the intestinal lining.

Screening for colorectal cancer

The term "screening" is properly applied only to the use of testing to look for evidence of cancer or pre-cancerous polyps in individuals who are asymptomatic and at only average risk for a type of cancer. Those patients who, for example, have a positive family history of colon cancer, or are symptomatic for a colon abnormality, undergo diagnostic testing rather than screening tests.

There are different types of screening tests for colorectal cancer: fecal (stool) occult blood testing, sigmoidoscopy, colonoscopy, digital colonoscopy, and DNA testing of the stool. The US Preventive Services Task Force (USPSTF) recommends strongly that screening begin at age 50 years for average-risk adults, but there is no specific recommendation for one screening test or strategy over another. The USPSTF advises that patients be offered a choice of screening options, using shared decision-making with the patient and physician to arrive at the best choice of screening programs for each individual.

Stool or fecal occult blood testing (FOBT)

Tumors of the colon and rectum tend to bleed slowly into the stool. The small amount of blood mixed into the stool usually is not visible to the naked eye. The commonly used stool occult blood tests rely on chemical color conversions to detect microscopic amounts of blood. These tests are both convenient and inexpensive. There are two kinds of fecal occult blood tests. The first is known as a guaiac FOBT. In this test, a small amount of stool is smeared on a special card for occult blood testing when a chemical is added to the card. Usually, three consecutive stool cards are collected. The other type of FOBT is an immunochemical test in which a special solution is added to the stool sample and analyzed in the laboratory using antibodies that can detect blood in a stool sample. The immunochemical test is a quantitative test that is more sensitive and specific for the diagnosis of polyps and cancer. It is preferred over the guaiac test.

A person who tests positive for stool occult blood has a 30%-45% chance of having a colon polyp and a 3%-5% chance of having a colon cancer. Colon cancers found under these circumstances tend to be small and not to have spread and have a better long-term prognosis.

It is important to remember that having stool tested positive for occult blood does not necessarily mean a person has colon cancer. Many other conditions can cause occult blood in the stool. However, patients with a positive stool occult blood test should undergo further evaluations to exclude colon cancer and to explain the source of the bleeding. It is also important to realize that stool that has tested negative for occult blood does not mean that colorectal cancer or polyps do not exist. Even under ideal testing conditions, a significant percentage of colon cancers can be missed by stool occult blood screening. Many patients with colon polyps do not have positive stool occult blood. In patients suspected of having colorectal polyps and in those at higher risk for developing colorectal polyps and cancer, screening flexible sigmoidoscopies or colonoscopies are performed even if the FOBT is negative.

Flexible sigmoidoscopy and colonoscopy

Flexible sigmoidoscopy is an exam of the rectum and the lower colon (60 cm or about 2 feet in from the outside) using a viewing tube (a short version of colonoscopy). Research studies have shown that the use of screening flexible sigmoidoscopy can reduce mortality from colon cancer. This is a result of the detection of polyps or early cancers in people with no symptoms. If a polyp or cancer is found, a complete colonoscopy is recommended. The majority of colon polyps can be completely removed at the time of colonoscopy without surgery; however, polyps in the proximal colon that cannot be reached by the sigmoidoscope will be missed. Flexible sigmoidoscopy is often combined with fecal occult blood testing for colorectal cancer screening.

Colonoscopy uses a long (120 cm-150 cm) flexible tube, which can examine the entire length of the colon. Through this tube, the doctor (typically a gastroenterologist) can both view and take pictures of the entire colon and also can take biopsies of colon masses and remove polyps.

Patients with a high risk of developing colorectal cancer may undergo screening colonoscopies starting at earlier ages than 50. For example, patients with a family history of colon cancer are recommended to start screening colonoscopies at an age 10 years before the earliest colon cancer diagnosed in a first-degree relative or five years earlier than the earliest precancerous colon polyp discovered in a first-degree relative. Patients with hereditary colon cancer syndromes such as FAP, AFAP, HNPCC, and MYH are recommended to begin colonoscopies early. The recommendations differ depending on the genetic defect. For example, in people with FAP, colonoscopies may begin during teenage years to look for the development of colon polyps. Patients with a prior history of polyps or colon cancer may also undergo colonoscopies to exclude recurrence. Patients with a long history (greater than 10 years) of chronic ulcerative colitis have an increased risk of colon cancer and should have regular colonoscopies to look for precancerous changes in the colon lining.

Virtual colonoscopy

Virtual colonoscopy (computerized tomographic or CT colonography) has been utilized in the clinic as a screening technique for colorectal cancer. Virtual colonoscopy employs a CT scan using low doses of radiation with special software to visualize the inside of the colon and look for polyps or masses. The procedure typically involves a bowel preparation with laxatives and/or enemas (although not always) followed by a CT scan after air is introduced into the colon. Because no sedation is necessary, individuals can return to work or other activities upon completion of the test. Virtual colonoscopies appear to be equally able to detect larger polyps (over 1 centimeter in size) as regular colonoscopies. The virtual colonoscopy cannot be used to biopsy or remove tissue from the colon. A follow-up sigmoidoscopy or colonoscopy must be done to accomplish that.

Stool DNA testing

The Cologuard test is available in the U.S. for in-home sample collection for adults over 50 at average risk for colon cancer. The sample is sent to a laboratory for analysis of DNA changes in DNA from cells shed by the intestinal lining into the stool or hemoglobin in the sample. In a research study, the test was able to find 92% of colon cancers and 69% of precancers of the colon. False-negative and false-positive results are also possible.

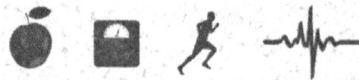

COLORECTAL CANCER

Doctor's know how to prevent colon or rectal cancer—and you can, too!

Colorectal cancer: Should you be concerned?

If you're 50 or older, the answer is yes. If you're 50 or older, you need to think about colorectal cancer. Most colon or rectal cancers occur in men and women who are 50 or older.

But no one in your family has had colorectal cancer?

Most people who get colorectal cancer have no family history of the disease. And you can have colorectal cancer and not even know it. If you have a parent, brother, sister, or child

who has had colon or rectal cancer, then testing is even more important for you. In fact, you may need to start testing before you're 50.

Get tested

You have the power to help stop colorectal cancer before it starts. Colorectal cancer begins with a growth called a polyp that's not yet cancer. Testing can help your health care provider tell whether there's a problem, andsome tests can find polyps before they become cancer.

Most people who have polyps removed never get colorectal cancer. If colorectal cancer is found, you have a good chance of beating it with treatment if it's found early (when it's small and has not spread). And testing can help find it early.

The ACS believes the preventing colorectal cancer (and not just finding it early) should be a major reason for getting tested. When polyps are found and removed, it can keep some people from getting colorectal cancer. Tests that have the best chance of finding both polyps and cancer should be your first choice if these tests are available and you're willing to have them.

Ask for the test

As you get older, you have more health concerns. Your health care provider has a lot to talk to you about. If your provider doesn't mention getting tested for colorectal cancer, don't be afraid to ask about it! There's more than one way to get tested, so you and your provider should choose the test that's best for you. You owe it to yourself and the people who love you to take care of yourself!

What is colorectal cancer?

Cancer of the colon or rectum is called colorectal cancer.

What do the colon and rectum do?

The colon and rectum help the body digest food. They hold waste until it passes out of the body.

If you're 50 or older, or have a family history of colorectal cancer, go to the clinic today and talk to your doctor about it!

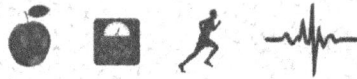

12 SIGNS OF SKIN CANCER

Cancer is the second leading cause of death in the U.S. and while it is a highly common condition that affects adults and children, there is no cure. Skin cancer is one of the most common forms of cancer and there are various forms the skin cancer can present with. While some parts of the body is affected more than other, skin cancer predominantly affects and harms the skin, with the potential for it to spread to other areas. Given that your skin is by far the largest organ of your human body, it is only reasonable to understand some of the warning signs and symptoms of skin cancer. Listed below are 12 important signs of skin cancer you need to know, especially if you live in an area that is at increased risk.

1. Moles.

Some people may consider these to be beauty marks of some sort, but moles are simply a cluster of melanocytes that reside on an area of your skin. While they may appear harmful when they are on the skin, many moles remain dormant and actually are harmless. However, some moles can develop into a cancerous form and begin to cause problems with your health. If you notice that a mole on your skin changes its shape, size, or even its color, then you should have your doctor or dermatologist check out your mole. A comprehensive skin exam may be useful, especially if you notice that you have multiple moles throughout your body.

2. Know the ABCDEs.

You learned this when you were much younger, but your ABCDEs are an important way to assess certain marks on your skin. To start off the acronym, A means asymmetry. This is meant to explain that any marking or skin mole that has an asymmetrical shape is a possible sign of skin cancer. The B stands for borders, implying that any irregularly shaped borders on a skin marking demonstrates possible skin cancer. The C represents a color change in the mole or marking. The D stands for diameter and any mole or skin lesion that is larger than a standard pencil eraser indicates possible skin cancer. Lastly, the E is the evolution of the mole and it can range from anything from where the mole starts from. Use these ABCDEs to help assess your skin informally and report it to your doctor for further evaluation.

3. Abnormal, Unusual, or Suspicious Growth.

Let's face it you look at your skin quite often. You view yourself in the mirror when you brush your teeth, dry off after a shower, or when you are doing your hair. While many of the looks you take during this time are to assess your looks, it subconsciously is a way for you to perform an informal assessment on your skin. During this assessment, you should be able to point out any new growths and unusual looking marks that have popped up on your skin. If you notice anything unusual, it is best to make note of it, observe it, and report it to your doctor.

4. Skin that Resembles a Scar.

When it comes to skin cancer, you now understand the ABCDEs of what to help look for. If you have an area on your skin that looks like a scar and maybe even feels like a scar, but you did not cut yourself recently, then this could be alarming. Sometimes, these areas could appear white or yellow and they may resemble wax on your skin. In addition, the borders of this "scar" looking piece of skin could have undefined borders, which fall right into the ABCDEs assessment. If you notice any part of your skin that has this appearance, you should contact your doctor or dermatologist for a full evaluation of your skin.

5. Genetic History.

This is not an exact, but one sign that you could end up or have skin cancer is if your parents of siblings have skin cancer. While there are environmental variables in play with this condition, the chances are higher if you have a parent or close relative that has skin cancer. Add any of the already mentioned signs of skin cancer to this and your risk is more than likely higher. Consider talking with your close relatives to see if they have any skin cancer signs on their skin and if so, make sure to report this to your doctor.

6. Severe Sunburns.

This is quite possibly the most risky thing you can do for your skin. A sunburn means you have been outdoors without proper UV protection and if your burn is severe, this could cause permanent damage to your skin. Some people who experience a severe sunburn report that a mole or dark mark appeared on the skin following the burn. If you notice that you develop a new mole on a spot where you recently had a sunburn then it is important to have your doctor look at this mole. This underscores the importance of wearing sunblock with proper UV protection anytime that you are outdoors.

7. Large Moles.

It is a fairly commonality to have a mole on your skin and as reported above, a mole is not always something to worry about. However, in the event the mole is cancerous, it is best to take a close watch as to how it grew. Is the mole bigger than a standard pencil eraser? If yes, then this could be an issue. Is it much bigger than a pencil eraser? If yes, then this is definitely something you should show your doctor. It is important to notice any and all marks that appear on your skin and visually follow them over time.

8. Asymmetric Cell Shape.

This is the first letter in the ABCDEs. Any large and darkened marks on your skin that have an asymmetrical shape, this could be an indicator of skin cancer. The asymmetry will mostly likely have some jagged edges or non-rounded corners, which is your clue that this is not a normal skin cell. If you notice a darkened cell on your skin with asymmetric borders then you should show this to your doctor as soon as possible. Time is important with the treatment of your skin cancer and if you notice any signs that are on this list, you should talk with your doctor for appropriate treatment if it is skin cancer.

9. Coloring.

There is no surprise that your skin is a particular color. Some people have more melanin than others, which can affect skin color. Regardless of the color of your skin; however, a major warning sign of skin cancer is when you have a skin cell that changes color. It could start out as a mole or cell that looks like a mole and progress to any color (mostly changes to pink, red, blue, or even white). If you notice any mole or skin cell that changes to any of these abnormal colors then this should be a sign to visit your doctor soon to have a check-up.

10. Bleeding.

There are many cells that appear on your skin throughout your life and chances are you are no stranger to something on your skin that has bled in the past. However, if you have a mole or skin cell that is crusty or bleeds then this should be alarming to you. Also, if this cell type is located on your nose or head area and even your lips then you especially want to be checked out by your doctor. This could be a sign of skin cancer that is possibly a carcinoma cancer cell and it can be treated if it is detected early in the growth phase.

11. Red Patchy Skin.

A skin rash is actually more common than skin cancer, but the two of these closely are related. A skin rash, or redness on your skin, can be present when a certain type of cancer appears on your skin. With this type of skin cancer, a rash or redness appears, and it may be hidden as eczema or even psoriasis. If you notice a small area on your skin and you think it is a rash, you should have your doctor evaluate your skin to see what exactly the condition may be. If caught early, the potential skin cancer can be treated effectively.

12. Fair Skin.

Fair skin people are the most at risk for skin cancer and this is mainly due to the reason that there are no melanocytes in this skin type. So when melanocyte cells appear on the skin this is a sign that skin cancer is affecting you. This is not to say that individuals who are not fair skinned have no risk to the condition, but it certainly increases your risk when you are lighter skinned. The best thing to do to avoid skin cancer is to follow the directions of your doctor (if you are under the care of a doctor) or make sure to take the necessary precautionary measures. Proper UV block is the first solution to blocking harmful sun rays and it can help to prolong your exposure outdoors without harmful effects.

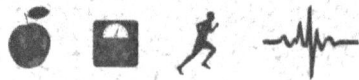

AN INTRODUCTION TO LIVER CARE

Why is the liver important?

The liver is the second largest organ in your body and is located under your rib cage on the right side. It weighs about three pounds and is shaped like a football that is flat on one side.

The liver performs many jobs in your body. It processes what you eat and drink into energy and nutrients your body can use. The liver also removes harmful substances from your blood.

What are the ways to take care of a liver?

Have a healthy lifestyle. Eating a healthy diet and exercising regularly help the liver to work well. Eat foods from all the food groups: grains, fruits, vegetables, meats and beans, milk, and oil. Maintain a healthy weight.

Limit the amount of alcohol you drink.

Alcohol can damage or destroy liver cells.

Manage you medications. When medicines are taken incorrectly—by taking too much or the wrong type of mixing—the liver can be harmed. Learn about medicines and how they can affect the liver. Follow dosing instruction. Talk to a doctor or nurse about the medications you are taking. And remember, mixing alcohol and medicines can harm you liver, even if they are not taken at the same time.

Avoid breathing in or touching toxins. Toxins can injure liver cells. Limit direct contact with toxins from cleaning and aerosol products, chemicals, etc.

Common liver diseases and prevention

One out of every 10 Americans is affected by liver disease. Liver disease is one of the top 10 causes of death in the United States. There are more than 100 liver diseases. Below are some of the most common liver diseases, and ways you can help prevent them and keep your liver healthy.

Hepatitis A: Hepatitis A is a liver disease caused by the hepatitis A virus (HAV). HAV can cause the liver to swell and not work well.

Prevention: Hepatitis A vaccination is the best way to prevent HAV. Other ways to stop the spread of HAV are:

- Always washing your hands with soap and warm water immediately after using the bathroom
- Always washing your hands with soap and warm water before preparing or eating food

Hepatitis B: Hepatitis B is a liver disease cause by the hepatitis B virus (HBV). HBV can cause the liver to swell and lead to cirrhosis and liver cancer.

Prevention: Hepatitis B vaccination is the best way to prevent HPV. Other ways to stop the spread of HBV are:

- ✓ Not sharing needles
- ✓ Practicing safe sex
- ✓ Not sharing razors, tooth brushes, or other personal items
- ✓ Using only clean needles for tattoos and body piercing

Hepatitis C: Hepatitis C is a liver disease caused by the hepatitis C virus (HCV). HCV can cause the liver to swell and lead to cirrhosis and liver cancer.

Prevention: There is NO vaccine to prevent HCV. The only way to prevent HCV is to avoid direct contact with infected blood. Other ways to stop the spread of HCV are:

Not sharing needles!

- ✓ Practicing safe sex
- ✓ Not sharing razors, toothbrushes, or other personal items
- ✓ Using only clean needles for tattoos and body piercings
- ✓ Getting medical care if you are exposed to blood or needle sticks

Fatty Liver Disease: Fatty liver disease is the buildup of fat in liver cells. It can cause the liver to swell and can lead to cirrhosis.

Prevention: Ways to prevent fatty liver disease are:

- ✓ Eating a healthy diet
- ✓ Maintaining a healthy weight
- ✓ Exercising regularly
- ✓ Limiting the amount of alcohol you drink
- ✓ Maintaining a normal cholesterol level

NASH (Nonalcoholic Steatohepatitis): NASH is a type of fatty liver disease. NASH causes the liver to swell and become damaged due to reasons unrelated to alcohol.

Prevention: Ways to prevent NASH are:

- ✓ Eating a healthy diet
- ✓ Maintaining a healthy weight
- ✓ Exercising regularly
- ✓ Limiting the amount of alcohol you drink
- ✓ Maintaining a normal cholesterol level

Alcohol-Related Liver Disease: Alcohol-related liver disease is caused by drinking too much alcohol. It can cause the liver to swell and can lead to cirrhosis.

Prevention: The best way to prevent alcohol-related liver disease is to not drink more alcohol than what your doctor recommends.

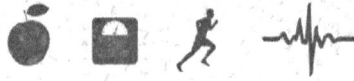

HEPATITIS C

For some reason, A LOT of prisoners share needles. This is something I never understood.

Many think it's OK if they just rinse them out with warm water. This is crazy to me. This is probably the major reason why so many prisoners have Hep C. For this reason I'm going to delve deeper into the disease.

What is hepatitis C? Hep C is a disease caused by a virus that infects the liver. The virus, also called HCV, is just one of the hep viruses, as you by now know. The others, hep A and hep B, differ somewhat from hep C in the way they are spread and treated.

How does hep C affect the liver? Hepatitis means inflammation, or swelling, of the liver. When the liver is inflamed, it has a harder time doing its job—processing everything you eat, drink, breathe, and absorb through your skin; turning nutrients into energy your body can use; and removing harmful substances from your blood.

Some people who get Hep C have it for a short time—up to six months—and then get better on their own. This is called acute hepatitis C. But most people, about 75-80 percent, will go on to develop long-term or chronic hep C, meaning it doesn't go away.

Anything that damages the liver over many years can lead the liver to form scar tissue. Fibrosis is the first stage of liver scarring. When scar tissue builds up and takes over most the liver, this is a more serious problem called cirrhosis. Unless successfully treated with medication, chronic hep C can eventually lead to cirrhosis, liver cancer and liver failure.

Who is at risk of having hep C?

You have a greater risk of infection with hep C if you:

- √ Shared needles to inject drugs (the most common way HCV is spread in prison, and the US in general) or straws to inhale them, even once many years ago
- √ Were born between 1945 and 1965 (baby boomers)
- √ Received a blood transfusion before July 1992
- √ Received a blood product for clotting problems made before 1987
- √ Had tattoos or body piercings using non-sterile equipment
- √ Needed to have your blood filtered by a machine (hemodialysis) for a long period of time because your kidneys weren't working
- √ Have HIV
- √ Less common risks include:
- √ Being born to a mother with HCV (about 4 of every 100 infants born to mothers with HCV become infected)

√ Having sexual contact with a HCV-infected partner

√ Sharing personal care items, such as toothbrushes or razors, that came in contact with the blood of a HCV-infected person

It should be noted that recent studies have shown an increased incidence of acute hep C in young people (under 30 years old) due to an increase of injection use among that age group!

What are the symptoms of hep C? Most people with acute or chronic hep C have no symptoms. When symptoms do occur, they may include:

√ jaundice (a yellowing of the skin and whites of the eyes)

√ itchy skin

√ tiredness

√ dark urine

√ muscle soreness

√ nausea

√ loss of appetite

√ stomach pain

Someone can have HCV for years or even decades without experiencing symptoms.

How is hepatitis C diagnosed?

There are two main blood tests used to diagnose Hep C. The Hep C Antibody Test looks for antibodies (proteins made by your body's immune system to fight infection) to the Hep C virus; it shows if you've ever been exposed to the virus. If the antibody test is positive, another blood test will be performed to determine if you're currently infected with hep C.

This test, called an RNA Test, looks for the generic material (RNA) of the Hep C virus.

If the RNA test is positive, it means you currently have Hep C and should talk to a doctor experienced in diagnosing the treating the disease.

If you think you may have Hep C, get tested today so you can get the proper treatment. If you are found negative for the virus, great! Make the necessary moves to ENSURE you never get it. In the unfortunate event you are found positive for the virus, here are some questions you should ask your health care provider:

√ What is my HCV genotype?

√ How much Hep C virus do I have in my body?

√ Has the virus damaged my liver?

√ What are the benefits and risks of treatment?

√ What treatment options are available to me?

√ Which option do you think is best for me and why?

√ How long will treatment last?

√ What side effects will I have, and how can I manage them?

√ How likely is it that I will develop cirrhosis or liver cancer?

√ What prescription or over-the-counter medications should I avoid?

√ Should I be vaccinated for Hep A and hep B?

√ What is the next step?

Fortunately, this is a hopeful time for people with hep C as treatment is rapidly changing for the better. With higher cure rates, shorter treatment times, and all-oral treatment regimens for most people with hep c, everyone should consider getting treated. Discuss the risk and benefits of pursuing treatment with your healthcare provider.

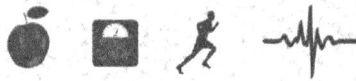

HCV/HIV COINFECTION

By now you have a basic understanding of HCV (hep C) and the horrible damage it can cause to your liver and overall health. But worse yet is an HCV/HIV coinfection.

What is the human immunodeficiency virus (HIV)? HIV is a virus that attacks the immune system. HIV is the virus that causes acquired immunodeficiency syndrome (AIDS).

What is HCV/HIC coinfection? A person with hepatitis C and HIV has HCV/HIV coinfection (having two or more viruses). One out of every four people with HIV also have HCV. (CDC 2015)

What is the relationship between HCV and HIV? HCV and HIV are viruses that are transmitted blood-to-blood. People with HCV or HIV often have no symptoms. Since HCV and HIV can be transmitted through SHARING INFECTED NEEDLES. MANY DRUG USERS ARE COINFECTED! Between 50 percent and 90 percent of HIV-infected injection drug users are also infected with HCV. (CDC 2015)

Can HIV make HCV worse? Yes. HCV/HIV coinfection can cause faster progression of liver deterioration and an increased risk for life threatening scarring of the liver (cirrhosis).

What are the difference in HCV therapy and HIV therapy? There is cure for HCV, but NOT for HIV. The goal of HCV medication is to remove the virus from someone's body. The goal of HIV medication is to suppress the virus so that it is not multiplying fast enough to enter the blood stream.

What are the treatment options for people who have HCV/HIV coinfection? There are many new medications to cure the hepatitis C infection. These medications are very effective in co-infected individuals and have almost no serious side effect. People with HCV and HIV need to talk to their doctors to determine their treatment options. Treatment options vary by person, and are determined by:

- √ Subtype of HCV virus patient has.
- √ How advanced the patient's liver disease is.
- √ Patient's got prior treatment history.
- √ Other treatment related steps people with HCV and HIV can take:
- √ Avoid alcohol.
- √ Talk to your doctor before taking any new medicines, including OTC, alternative, or herbal medicines, vitamins, and supplements that may harm your liver.
- √ Be vaccinated for Hep A and Hep B.
- √ What is the best way to stop the spread of HCV and HIV? There are no vaccines to prevent HCV or HIV. The only way to stop the spread of HCV and HIV is to avoid direct contact with infected blood.

√ Do not share needles.

√ Use clean needles and equipment for tattoos or body piercings.

√ Do not share toothbrushes, razors, and other personal items with others.

√ Wear gloves if you have to touch blood.

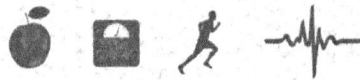

DIET AND YOUR LIVER

How does a healthy diet help the liver? Eating a healthy diet helps the liver to do its functions well and do them for a long time. Eating an unhealthy diet can lead to liver disease. For example, a person who eats a lot of fatty foods is at higher risk of being overweight and having non-alcoholic fatty liver disease.

For people who have liver disease, eating a healthy diet makes it easier to do its jobs and can help repair some liver damage. An healthy diet can make the liver work very hard and can cause more damage to it.

What does a healthy diet include?

- √ Eating foods from all the food groups: grains, proteins, dairy, fruits, vegetables, and fats.
- √ Eating food that have a lot of fiber such as fresh fruits and vegetables, whole grain breads, rice and cereals.

Are there diet changes for those with liver disease? It is important for people with liver disease to maintain a healthy weight by eating a balanced diet with foods from all food groups. Also,

- √ Do not eat uncooked shellfish such as oysters and clams.
- √ Limit eating foods that have a lot of sugar or salt.
- √ Limit eating fatty foods.

LIVER DISEASES AND DIET

Some liver diseases have specific diet recommendations.

Bile Duct Diseases: Bile is a liquid made in the liver that helps break down fats in the small intestine. Bile duct disease keeps bile from flowing to the small intestine.

Diet Recommendations:

- √ Use fat substitutes.
- √ Use kernel oil (i.e. canola, olive, corn, sunflower, peanut, flax seed oils) because it needs less bile to break down.

Cirrhosis: Cirrhosis is the scarring and hardening of the liver.

Diet Recommendations:

- √ Limit salt and foods that contain a lot of salt.
- √ Talk to your doctor about how much protein to have in your diet.

Hemochromatosis: Hemochromatosis is the buildup of iron in the liver.

Diet Recommendations:

- √ Do not eat foods that have iron.

✓ Do not use iron pots and pans.

✓ Do not take pills with iron.

✓ Do not eat uncooked shellfish.

Hepatitis C: Hepatitis c is a disease of the liver caused by the hepatitis C virus.

Diet Recommendations:

✓ Limit foods that have a lot of iron.

✓ Do not use iron pots and pans.

✓ Limit salt and foods that contain a lot of salt.

Wilson Disease: Wilson disease is the buildup of copper in the body.

Diet Recommendations:

✓ Limit foods that have copper such as chocolate, nuts, shellfish and mushrooms.

✓ Do not use copper pots.

How can alcohol and medicine affect the liver?

Alcohol can damage or destroy liver cells. Liver damage can lead to the buildup of fat in your liver, inflammation or swelling or your liver (alcoholic hepatitis), and/or scarring of your liver (cirrhosis). For people with liver disease, even a small amount of alcohol can make the disease worse. Talk to your doctor about alcohol and your liver health.

Different types of medicines are taken every day, including prescription medicines, vitamins dietary Supplements, and alternative medicines. Medicines can help you feel better. However when medicines are taken incorrectly—by taking too much or the wrong type or by mixing-your liver can be harmed.

✓ Learn about medicines and how they can affect your liver.

✓ Follow dosing instructions.

✓ Talk to your doctor often about all the medicines you are taking.

✓ Mixing alcohol and medicines can be harmful even if they are not taken at the same time.

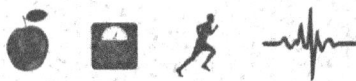

DIABETES

What is Diabetes?

Diabetes is a problem with your body that causes blood glucose (sugar) levels to rise higher than normal. This is also called hyperglycemia.

When you eat your body breaks food down into glucose and sends it into the blood. Insulin then helps move the glucose from the blood into your cells. When glucose enters your cells, it is either used as fuel for energy right away or stored for later use. In a person with diabetes, there is a problem with insulin. But, not all people with diabetes have the same problem.

The types of diabetes are type 1, type 2, and a condition called gestational diabetes, which happens when pregnant. If you have diabetes, your body either doesn't make enough insulin or can't use the insulin it does make very well.

What is Type 2 Diabetes?

In type 2 diabetes, your body does not make insulin properly. This is called insulin resistance. At first, the pancreas makes extra insulin to make up for it. But, over time your pancreas isn't able to keep up and can't make enough insulin to keep your blood glucose levels normal. Type 2 is treated with lifestyle changes, oral medications (pills), and insulin.

Some people with type 2 can control their blood glucose with healthy eating and being active. But, your doctor may need to also prescribe oral medications or insulin to help you meet your target blood glucose levels. Type 2 usually gets worse over time—even if you don't need medications at first, you may need them later on.

How is Type 2 Different From Type 1?

In type 1, your body treats the cells that make the insulin as invaders and destroys them. This can happen over a few weeks, months, or years. When enough of the cells are gone, your pancreas stops making insulin, or makes too little insulin.

Without insulin, your blood glucose rises higher than normal, so the insulin needs to be replaced.

What Causes Type 2 Diabetes?

Scientists do not know the exact cause of type 2 diabetes. However, development of type 2 diabetes has been associated with several risk factors. These risk factors include:

- √ history of hyperglycemia, prediabetes, and/or gestational diabetes (GDM)
- √ overweight and obesity
- √ physical inactivity
- √ genetics
- √ family history

√ race and ethnicity

√ age

√ high blood pressure

√ abnormal cholesterol

What Treatments Are Used For Type 2 Diabetes?

The two goals of diabetes treatment are to make sure you feel well day-to-day and to prevent or delay long-term health problems. The best way to reach those goals are by:

√ taking medications, if your doctor prescribes them

√ planning your meals—choosing what, how much, and when to eat

√ being physically active

What To Know About Diabetic Ketoacidosis (DKA)

DKA is a serious condition that can result from untreated or undiagnosed diabetes or from too little insulin. It can lead to a diabetic coma or even death.

Early Signs of DKA:

√ Feeling very thirsty

√ Urinating often

√ High blood glucose levels

√ High ketone levels in urine

√ Later, Extreme Signs:

√ Feeling weak or constantly sleepy

√ Dry/flushed skin

√ Nausea, vomiting, pain in abdomen

√ Difficulty breathing, fruity-smelling breath

If you think you may have diabetes, put in a sick call slip immediately, discuss it with your doctor and ask to be tested. If you have diabetes and want to learn more about it, there is a fantastic book you can get FREE by writing to Prison Legal News and requesting a copy. The book is titled *Prisoner Diabetes Handbook: A Guide to Managing Diabetes—for Prisoners, by Prisoners*. Order from :

Prison Legal News
POB 1151
Lake Worth, FL 33460

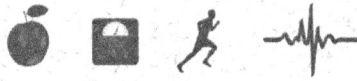

ULCERS ARE NO LAUGHING MATTER

Peptic ulcers, which are in the stomach and the duodenum (the first part of the intestine leading from the stomach) can occur at any age and affect both men and women. Untreated, sufferers can look forward to a long siege with them. But today's peptic ulcer sufferers have a brighter prospect for relief than did those even a single generation ago. There is now less than 1 chance in 18 that surgery will even be necessary and new medications act faster and better and offer more relief than ever before.

The warning sign of active ulcers you will most likely experience (if you get any warning at all) is a gnawing discomfort in the middle of the upper abdomen that typically comes between meals or in the middle of the night. Food or liquids, including antacids and milk, can provide some temporary relief, but milk might not be all that good a remedy since it stimulates production of hydrochloric acid and other digestive juices which further aggravates the pain.

Antacids blended from aluminum, calcium or magnesium salts, have long been the non-prescription drugs most people quickly reach for to get relief from their stomach pains. But, because antacids interfere with absorption of some medications, be sure to go over this with your doctor and get his approval.

You should never ignore any warning signs of ulcers. Ulcer complications are serious and in some cases can be life-threatening. If pain from ulcers persists after more than 10 to 14 days of self-treatment or comes back when treatment ends, you should see your doctor. The passing of blood through the bowels may be caused by some other problem, but it can also be an urgent warning of a bleeding ulcer.

Bleeding ulcers can cause anemia or, if the ulcer gets larger it may expand into a major blood vessel, a leak can turn into a hemorrhage, with only minutes available for life-saving treatment. Ulcers can also perforate and may erode completely through the wall of the stomach or duodenum. If this happens and the stomach's contents flow into the abdominal cavity, severe infection can result. A perforated ulcer is an emergency that requires immediate surgery.

It has been determined that smoking doubles a person's risk for the ulcer disease.

Physicians and researchers have found that ulcer heal a lot slower for smokers, and smokers also have a higher relapse rate.

And you're definitely at a risk for ulcers if you take aspirin and any of the other products containing aspirin. High-dose aspirin, Ibuprofen, Naproxen and Piroxicam are in wide use today for many conditions, especially to relieve pain and swelling among the millions of people who have arthritis. These medications can irritate the stomach's lining and cause gastrointestinal bleeding.

Ulcers have frequently been that target for humor in describing the stereotypical aggressive, pressured, goal-or-career oriented person. But for those who have them, ulcers are certainly no laughing matter. Peptic ulcers strike 1 out of every 50 Americans each year.

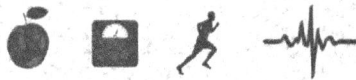

ARTHRITIS: SYMPTOMS, TREATMENT PREVENTION & RISKS

Is it Arthritis?

Chances are you or someone you know has arthritis. Arthritis is a general term for more than 100 types of arthritis and related conditions. More than 52 million adults and 300,000 children in the United States have some type of arthritis.

The word "arthritis" literally means joint inflammation. Arthritis can cause pain, stiffness and swelling in or around joints. Joints are where bones meet, such as your knee. The ends of the bones are covered by cartilage, a spongy material that keeps bones from rubbing together. The joint is enclosed in a capsule and lined with tissue called the synovium. This lining releases a slippery fluid that helps the joint move smoothly and easily. Muscles and tendons support the joint and help you move.

Different types of arthritis can affect one or more parts of the joint to produce pain and swelling, which can limit use of the joint. Certain types of arthritis can also affect other parts of the body, such as the skin, eyes, mouth and internal organs (e.g., the heart, lungs or kidneys).

Arthritis is usually chronic, meaning that it lasts a long time. For many people, it does not go away. Pain and stiffness usually will be worse in the morning after periods of inactivity.

In some types of arthritis, the skin over the joint may appear swollen and red and feel warm to the touch.

With some types of arthritis, you may have fatigue, a poor appetite or fever. If you have any of these signs for more than 2 weeks, see your doctor. These symptoms can develop suddenly or slowly. But there are many things you can do now to avoid arthritis or to reduce pain and keep moving and prevent joint and organ damage.

What Causes Arthritis?

The cause of most types of arthritis is unknown. Scientists are studying several major factors that are thought to be important in arthritis. These factors include: genes; the role of inflammation and the immune system in causing joint damage; and lifestyle factors, including injury to joints. The importance of these factors varies, depending on the type of arthritis.

How Is Arthritis Diagnosed?

It's important to find out what type of arthritis you have because treatments are different for the various types of arthritis. Early diagnosis and treatment are important to help slow or prevent damage to joints that can occur during the first few years with certain types of arthritis.

Your primary-care doctor is your best first stop for getting a: diagnosis. For some types of arthritis, this doctor may be the only one you need to see to manage your arthritis. But for others, you may need to see a rheumatologist, a physician who specializes in diagnosis and treatment of arthritis and related conditions.

When you see your doctor for the first time about your joint pain, expect at least three things to happen before you get an arthritis diagnosis.

- √ First, your doctor will talk to you about your symptoms and medical history.
- √ Next, your doctor will conduct a physical examination.
- √ Finally, your doctor may order x-rays and laboratory tests.

Your doctor will examine your joints to check for swelling and tender points, to see what movements cause pain, and to see if your joints move through their normal range of motion.

Your doctor will also check for other signs that may be found in some forms of arthritis, including Skin rashes, mouth sores, muscle weakness, eye problems of involvement or internal organs, such as the heart or lungs.

The results from your medical history, physical exam and tests help your doctor match your symptoms to the pattern of a specific disease or rule out other diseases.

Symptoms for some types of arthritis develop slowly and may appear similar to other types in its early stages. It may take several visits before your doctor can tell what type of arthritis you have.

Can Arthritis Be Prevented?

There are steps you can take to reduce your risk for getting certain types of arthritis or to reduce disability if you already have arthritis.

Doctors believe some people can reduce their risk of developing some types of arthritis or delay its onset by following these guidelines:

- √ Maintain a healthy weight or lose extra weight.
- √ Stay physically active.
- √ Avoid joint injury.
- √ Adjust jobs that require repetitive joint movement.
- √ Don't smoke.

What Type Of Arthritis Do I Have?

With more than 100 types of arthritis and related conditions, it is important to know which type you have so it can be treated properly. If you don't know which type you have, put in a request slip to see your doctor or ask at your next visit.

The most common types of arthritis and related conditions are described here:

Osteoarthritis: The most common type of arthritis is osteoarthritis, or OA. OA affects about 27 million Americans. OA is sometimes called degenerative arthritis or degenerative joint disease because it causes the breakdown of cartilage and bones over time, causing pain and stiffness. OA usually affects the fingers and weight-bearing joints, including the knees, hips, back and neck, but it can affect other joints and the hands. It affects both men and women and usually occurs after age 44.

Rheumatoid Arthritis: Rheumatoid arthritis, or RA, is an autoimmune disease. In autoimmune diseases, the body's immune system mistakenly attacks healthy tissue, causing inflammation of the joints. The exact cause of the disease is unknown. Inflammation begins in the joint lining and, over time, leads to damage of both cartilage and bone. RA often affects the same joints on both sides of the body. Hands, wrists, feet, knees, ankles, shoulders, neck, jaw and elbows can all have RA. RA affects about 1.5 million Americans and is more common in women than in men.

Psoriatic Arthritis: You may know psoriasis as a disease affecting the skin. But did you know about 30 percent of people with psoriasis also have inflammatory form of arthritis called psoriatic arthritis? Psoriasis usually shows up first. The disease usually appears between the ages of 30 and 55 in people who have psoriasis, but it can be diagnosed during childhood. Unlike many autoimmune diseases, men and women are equally at risk for developing this condition.

Lupus: Lupus is another autoimmune disease that affects the skin and joints. In some people, lupus also affects the internal organs such as the kidneys, lungs or heart. Lupus affects women about eight to 10 times more than men. Symptoms often first appear in women between ages 18 and 45. Some of the common symptoms include a rash over the cheeks and across the bridge of the nose, sun sensitivity and joint pain. Lupus occurs more often in African Americans than in Caucasians and also more frequently in Asian and Latino populations.

Gout: Gout occurs when the body produces too much of a substance called uric acid. Gout also happens when your body can't get rid of uric acid, leading to high levels of uric acid in the blood. This may lead to the formation of uric acid crystals in a joint, which causes severe pain and swelling. Gout most commonly affects the big toes, ankles and knees. More men than women have gout. Certain foods (such as sardines, anchovies and organ meats) and alcohol, especially beer, can raise the body's uric acid level.

Fibromyalgia: In contrast to arthritis, which is a disease of the joints, fibromyalgia does not affect joints but instead is a condition that involves widespread pain in the muscles and soft tissues. People with fibromyalgia often have fatigue, disturbed sleep, low mood and stiffness. Fibromyalgia is a common condition that usually affect women, but it can affect men. It does not cause muscle or joint damage.

Other Common Arthritis-Related Conditions

Low back pain can be caused by a back strain or injury, or by certain types of arthritis, such as osteoarthritis and ankylosing spondylitis.

Bursitis and tendinitis may be caused by irritation from injuring or overusing a joint, but in many cases occurs without a known cause. Bursitis affects a small sac called the bursa that helps cushion the muscles and tendons surrounding a joint. Tendinitis affects the tendons that attach muscle to bone.

Osteoporosis causes bone to lose mass and become thin and brittle. This can lead to painful fractures, rounded shoulders and loss of height. It does not directly affect the joints as arthritis does. Osteoporosis affects more than 40 million Americans, most of whom are women.

It is the major cause of bone fractures in postmenopausal women and senior citizens, including men. People with some forms of arthritis (such as RA or lupus) or who medications, such as corticosteroids are at risk for developing osteoporosis.

How Is Arthritis Treated?

Once you have a diagnosis, your doctor can work with you to develop a treatment plan. Your treatment plan likely will include multiple approaches to reducing your pain and stiffness, fighting inflammation and keeping you moving. These approaches may include medications and medical treatments as well as self-management approaches, such as diet and exercises.

Finding the right treatment plan may take time. Be sure to let your doctor know if your treatment is not working. Your treatment may change as your arthritis changes. Treatments for arthritis can be divided into several categories, some of which I'll now explain.

Medication

Many different drugs are used to treat arthritis and related diseases. The ones you should take will depend on the type of arthritis you have. Most arthritis medications are designed to relieve pain and/or reduce inflammation. Some arthritis medications are available without a prescription, or over-the-counter (OTC). They typically come in pill form, however, there are some topical creams and gels, too. Other medications require a prescription from your doctor. These medications may come in pill or gel form, or your doctor may inject them.

It is very important that your doctors are aware of all the medications you are taking, both prescription and OTC. Be sure to also tell your doctor about any supplements you are taking.

Physical Activity

Being physically active every day can keep you moving and independent. It lessens pain, increases range of motion, reduces fatigue, prevents weight gain and helps you look and feel better. People with arthritis should try to be active or exercise at least 30 minutes five days a week in addition to their everyday activities. Physical therapists and exercise physiologists can assist in designing exercises that minimize joint injury.

Pacing Your Activities

Pacing yourself saves energy by switching between periods of activity and periods of rest. Pacing helps protect your joints from the stress of repeated tasks and helps reduce fatigue. Alternate heavy or repeated tasks with easy ones. Changing tasks often so that you don't hold joints in one position for a long time. Plan rest breaks during your daily activities.

Joint Protection

You can learn to protect your joints by using them in ways that avoid excess stress. Protecting your joints makes it easier to do daily tasks. An occupational therapist can help you learn to use your joints in the best way to avoid excess stress on them. Use larger or stronger joints to carry things.

Weight Control

Weight control means staying close to your recommended weight or losing weight if you are overweight now. Weight control can reduce your risk for developing osteoarthritis in the knees. And if you already have knee OA, losing weight may lessen pain by reducing stress on your joints. Exercising and reducing calories will help you lose weight. If you need to lose a lot of Weight, work with your doctor or the prison's dietitian to find the best weight loss program for you.

Surgery

Most people with arthritis will never need surgery. Your prison probably won't give it to you anyway.

Self-Management Skills

You are the best manager of your arthritis. Being a good arthritis manager means understanding your disease and knowing what to expect. It also means planning your activities for when you feel best and learning to work with your doctor as a team. You can help yourself feel better by learning to manage your symptoms and how they affect your daily activities.

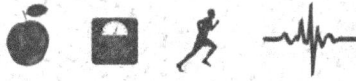

GIVE YOUR JOINTS A POUNDING

High-impact movements are the enemy of healthy knees, right? Dead wrong, says Paul Ochoa, a physical therapist in New York City. In fact, it's what keeps them going strong.

Popular opinion says that as we age, we need to give our joints a break. Box jumps and basketball are a younger man's game. Over time, too much pounding degrades cartilage, puts excess pressure on tendons, and causes arthritis. Or we simply creak when ascending a flight of stairs.

But that's just not how the body works. The way to keep your joints functioning properly is to work them out.

Think about the way you build and maintain muscle. When you lift weights and increase the load over time, your muscles adapt by getting stronger. Now take jumping and all the other moves that force you to get some air. When you land, you're placing a bigger-than-body-weight force on the bones. It puts stress—in a good way—on your limbs, helping to preserve bone density. You're also taxing the tendons that connect the muscles to those bones, forcing the tendons to get stronger, which is the best way to bolster strength and mobility.

If you haven't done sets of box jumps in a while, go easy to avoid ankle sprains. Try jumping jacks and high knees. Or choose a lower "box" for box jumps. But do something. If you don't use it, you'll lose it.

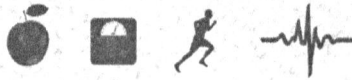

PAIN MANAGEMENT TIPS

Pain Has A Purpose

Pain is your body's alarm system—it tells you something is wrong. When your body is injured or battling diseases, nerves in the affected area release chemical signals. Other nerves send these signals to your brain, where they are recognized as pain.

How The Body Controls Pain

Pain signals travel through a system of nerves located in your extremities, spinal cord and brain. When you experience pain, your body may stop or limit pain be creating chemicals that help block pain signals traveling through your nerves. Different factors, such as your own thoughts and emotions, cause the body to produce pain-relieving substances called endorphins. For example, a father hurt in a car accident may not feel the pain of a broken arm if he's intensely worried about his child's well-being. That's because concern for his child causes the natural release of endorphins, which block the pain signal and prevent him from noticing his own pain.

Changing Your Reaction To Pain

You can learn to manage your pain by thinking of pain as a signal that may be changed by taking positive actions. Here are some examples:

Your mind plays an important role in how you feel about pain and how you respond to illness. Use these tips to build a sense of personal control by adjusting your thoughts and actions.

Keep a positive attitude. One way to rescue your pain is to build your life around wellness, not pain or sickness. This means thinking positive thoughts, having a sense of humor, eating a balanced diet, exercising regularly, surrounding yourself with positive people and enjoying activities with friends and family. It also means following your treatment plan, taking your medication properly and practicing relaxation.

Don't dwell. How often do you think about your pain? The amount of time you spend thinking about pain has a lot to do with how much discomfort you feel. People who dwell on their pain usually say it's worse than those who don't dwell on it.

Shift your focus. One way to take your mind off pain is to focus your mind on something else, like an enjoyable activity. The more you think about something outside of your body, such as a hobby or other activity, the less you'll think about physical discomfort.

Think about pain differently. Think of pain as your body's message to do something different. For example, if your pain is worse after sitting for a period of time, your body may be telling you to get up and move around.

Practice positive self-talk. What we say to ourselves often determines what we do and how we look at life. This is called self-talk. For example, you may say to yourself, "I don't think I want to exercise today. It's cloudy outside, there's no one to exercise with, and besides, I've already exercised twice this week." Approach the situation from a positive perspective instead: "I don't feel like exercising today, but I know I'll feel better afterward and have an easier time falling asleep." Practice turning your negative statements around.

Change your habits. It's easy to slip into the habit of taking more medicine or relying on unhealthy practices, such as drinking alcohol, to escape your pain. Try doing something

Create a pain management plan. Make a chart of your own pain-management methods to help track methods used and which ones work best for you. Work with your health care team to create a pain management plan.

Engage In Physical Activity

Regular physical activity can help you effectively manage pain. Through exercise, you can improve your overall health and fitness as well as your pain. Exercise can:

- ✓ Keep joints moving.
- ✓ Strengthen the muscles around joints.
- ✓ Maintain bone strength and health.
- ✓ Help you do daily activities more easily.
- ✓ Improve your overall health and fitness, including increasing your energy, improving your sleep, controlling your weight, strengthening your heart and improving your self-esteem and sense of well-being.

What Exercises Are Best?

Get a mix of aerobic (endurance), muscle-strengthening, and flexibility actives over the course of a week. Aerobic activity boosts feel-good chemicals (endorphins), fights pain, and improves mood and sleep. Strength training helps stabilize joints, and flexibility exercises help maintain joint range of motion.

Aerobic activity, such as walking, should be done for 30 minutes, five days a week. If you can't do 30 minutes all at once, you can break the activity into 10-minute intervals spread throughout the day. Once you're comfortable with 10 minutes, aim for 15.

Strengthening exercises can involve using home-made weights or exercise bars. Try to work muscle-strengthening exercise into your weekly routine so that all major muscles are worked on two days each week. Do slow, controlled movements, concentrating on proper form.

Flexibility and balance exercises include activities such as Tai chi or yoga, backward walking or standing on one foot (for balance). Try to do gentle stretches of flexibility exercises every day—you can mix them with muscle-strengthening exercises. Always stretch muscles while they are warm to reduce injury. Add in balance exercises to help reduce the risk of falls.

Get Better Sleep

Sleep restores your energy so that you can better manage pain. Only you know how much sleep your body needs, so get into the habit of listening to your body. Most people need approximately seven to nine hours of sleep per night. If you feel tired and achy after lunch every day, if feasible, take a brief nap (10 to 15 minutes). This can help restore your energy and spirits. If you have trouble sleeping at night, you can try relaxing quietly in the afternoon rather than taking a nap.

Practice Relaxation

People who are in pain experience both physical and emotional stress. Pain and stress have similar effects on the body. Muscles tighten, breathing becomes fast and shallow, and heart rate and blood pressure goes up. Relaxation can help you reverse these effects and give you a sense of control and well-being that makes it easier to manage pain.

There's no best way to learn how to relax, as long as you relax both your body and mind.

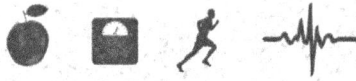

DON'T HAVE A HEART ATTACK!

Clinical studies, laboratory investigations and a number of surveys show certain personal characteristics and life-styles pointing to increased danger of heart attack (coronary heart disease). These danger signs are called "risk factors". The well-established risk factors are high blood pressure, high blood cholesterol, cigarette smoking and diabetes mellitus. Other factors that may increase or affect the risk for heart attack are obesity, a sedentary life-style, an aggressive response to stress, and certain drugs—prison life, basically.

In the past two decades, millions of Americans have learned about these risk factors and have tried to modify them favorably by seeking medical attention, and by changing their life-style. Many people have stopped smoking. The medical control of high blood pressure has greatly improved. The average cholesterol level of the population has decreased continually over the last two decades, probably due to changes in dietary habits and increased exercise.

This attempt to modify risk factors almost certainly has contributed to the declining death rate from heart disease in this country. Years ago, U.S. death rates from heart disease were still rising , but today the incidents from diseases of the cardiovascular system (including coronary heart disease) has fallen dramatically. Overall, heart-related problems have declined about 25 percent in the last decade. Some of this decrease undoubtedly is due to better medical care of heart attack victims, but it is likely that a sizable percentage is related to modification of risk factors.

The entire population has become more aware of the seriousness of heart disease and coronary heart problems. Because of this, CPR training has become much more mainstream.

There are a number of risk factors implicated in coronary heart disease. Some of these may raise coronary risk by accentuating the major risk factors already discussed. Others may act in ways not understood. And others may even be mistakenly linked to coronary risk.

Obesity predisposes individuals to coronary heart disease. Some of the reasons for this are known, others are not. The major causes of obesity are excessive intake of calories and inadequate exercise, when caloric intake is excessive, some of the excess is often saturated fat, which further raises the blood cholesterol. Thus, obesity contributes to higher coronary risk in a variety of ways—so get your lazy butt off your bed and exercise!

Most of the major risk factors are silent. They must be sought actively, and much of the responsibility for their detection lies with each of us as individuals. Regular checkups are particularly necessary if there is a family history of heart disease, high blood pressure, high cholesterol levels or diabetes, so if you fall into this category, make sure you notify your doctor.

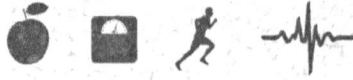

NEW THERAPY FOR HEART ATTACKS

New drugs can stop or limit the damage of a heart attack, but only if the patient gets help immediately, experts say. Once the flow of blood to a portion to the heart is blocked for several hours, the damage is irreversible.

Knowing the symptoms of a heart attack, which can be wide-ranging and confusing, is extremely important. So is knowing risk factors, such as obesity, diabetes, high blood pressure and family history.

Typical symptoms of a heart attack include a crushing pain in the chest, sweating, difficulty breathing, weakness and pain in the arms, particularly the left one. Symptoms one could attribute to something else can cause devastating delays in seeking medical treatment. These include feelings of indigestion, back shoulder and neck pain, and nausea. Early signs of trouble may appear during physical activity and disappear with rest. Any numbness or tingling of the fingers or toes, dizziness, shortness of breath of difficulty in breathing should not be ignored.

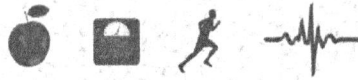

CONQUERING THE SMOKING HABIT

I'm not sure if there are any prisons that still allow smoking. However, as we all know, that doesn't stop prisoners from doing so if they want to bad enough. In addition, many of you will be released back into the free world and will have easy access to cigarettes.

Many smokers sincerely want to quit. They know cigarettes threaten their health, set a bad example for their children, and cost a ton of money.

Nobody can force a smoker to quit. It something each person has to decide for himself, and will require a personal commitment by the smoker. What kind of smoker are you? What do you get out of smoking? What does it do for you? It is important to identify what you use smoking for and what kind of satisfaction you feel that you are getting from smoking.

Many smokers use the cigarette as kind of a crutch in moments of stress or discomfort, and on occasion it may work; the cigarette is sometimes used as a tranquilizer. But the heavy smoker, the person who tries to handle severe problems by smoking heavily all day long, is apt to discover that cigarettes do not help him deal with his problems effectively.

When it comes to quitting, this kind of smoker may find it easy to stop when everything is going well, but may be tempted to start again in a time of crisis. Physical exertion, eating, drinking, or social activity in moderation may serve as useful substitutes for cigarettes, even in times of tension. The choice of a substitute depends on what will achieve the same effects without having any appreciable risk.

Once a smoker understands his own smoking behavior, he will be able to cope more successfully and select the best quitting approaches for himself and the type of lifestyle he leads.

Because smoking is a form of addiction, 80 percent of smokers who quit usually experience some withdrawal symptoms. These may include headaches, light-headedness, nausea, diarrhea, and chest pains. (I assure you this is nothing compared to the pains you will have when dying from cancer from smoking the death sticks.) Psychological symptoms, such as anxiety, short-term depression, and inability to concentrate may also appear. The main psychological symptom is increased irritability. People become so irritable, in fact, that they say they feel "like killing somebody." Yet there is no evidence that quitting smoking leads to physical violence.

Some people seem to lose all their energy and drive, wanting only to sleep. Others react in exactly the opposite way, becoming so over energized that they can't find enough activity to burn off their excess energy. Both these extremes, however, eventually level off. The symptoms may be intense for two or three days, but within 10 to 14 days after quitting, most subside. The truth is that after people quit smoking, they have more energy, they generally will need less sleep, and feel better about themselves.

Quitting smoking not only extends the ex-smoker's life, but adds new happiness and meaning to one's current life. Most smokers state that immediately after they quit smoking, they start noticing dramatic differences in their overall health and vitality.

Quitting is beneficial at any age, no matter how long a person has been smoking. The mortality ratio of an ex-smoker decreases after quitting. If the patient quits before a serious disease has developed, his body may eventually be able to restore itself almost completely.

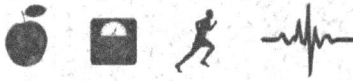

THE DANGERS OF DRUG USE

What Are the Dangers from Using Drugs?

Some people think everyone who takes drugs will end up dead. Others seem to think that drug use is not dangerous at all. The truth is somewhere in between...

Drug use can never by 100 percent safe, but it is not always as dangerous as people think.

The dangers of drug use depend on the drug, set and setting factors.

The drug bit is everything connected with the drug and how it is used. The set bit is everything connected with the person who is using the drugs. The setting bit is about what the person is doing at the time, where they are, the environment they live in, etc.

The basic principle is that drug dangers are a result of interactions between drug, set and setting.

The Drug

Drugs are not all the same. Different drugs have different dangers associated with them.

Some drugs (such as alcohol, heroin and tranquillizers) have a sedative effect which slow down the way the body and brain function. They can have a numbing effect that produces drowsiness if a lot is taken.

Other drugs (such as amphetamine, cocaine, crack and ecstasy) have a stimulant effect giving a rush of energy and making people more alert.

A third group of drugs (such as LSD and magic mushrooms and to a lesser extent cannabis and ecstasy) have a hallucinogenic effect. This means they tend to alter the way the user feels, sees, hears, tastes or smells.

Sedative drugs like alcohol and heroin can lead to fatal overdose if a lot is taken. They can also affect coordination making accidents more likely. Use of sedatives can also lead to physical dependence and withdrawal symptoms while others, drugs like cannabis, cannot.

Stimulant drugs can produce anxiety or panic attacks particularly if taken in large quantities. They can be particularly dangerous for people who have heart or blood pressure problems.

Hallucinogenic drugs sometimes produce very disturbing experiences and may lead to erratic or dangerous behavior by the user.

And of course, some drugs are legal to use and others are not. Being arrested and getting a conviction can lead to all sorts of problems.

√ Drug mixtures. Combining drugs can produce unpredictable and sometimes dangerous effects. In particular, mixtures of sedative drugs can be very dangerous. Many reported drug overdoses involve mixtures of alcohol and tranquilizers or opiates.

√ How a drug is taken. The method of use will influence the effect the drug has and it's possible dangers. Injecting drugs has a very quick and intense effect. Snorting or inhaling can also have a quick but slightly less intensive effect. Smoking drugs produces a slower, more subtle effect sometimes. The slowest effect of all is eating or drinking a drug.

Drug dangers also vary with the method used to take them:

√ Injecting is particularly risky because it is difficult to know how much is being taken. Injection also carries the risk of infection by blood borne diseases if any injecting equipment is shared. Highest profile recently has been given to HIV, the virus that leads to AIDS, but there are also risks from Hepatitis B and C, another very serious blood borne disease.

√ Eating or drinking a drug can be risky if people take a lot in one go. The effects tend to be slow, but once they come on it is too late to do anything about it. Examples are drinking too much alcohol in a short space of time or eating a lump of cannabis. In such cases people can suddenly feel very drunk or stoned and become very disoriented.

√ Snorting drugs like amphetamine or cocaine powder up the nose on a regular basis can lead to damage to the nasal membranes although this risk has sometimes been exaggerated.

There are more or less dangerous ways of inhaling solvents such as glues, gases and aerosols. Squirting solvents into a large plastic bag and then placing the bag over the head has led to death by suffocation. Squirting aerosols or butane straight down the throat had led to deaths through freezing the airways. Squirting into a rag or small bag then inhaling is not as dangerous, but still very dangerous.

Smoking a drug is relatively less dangerous method of use, although regular smoking can damage the respiratory system especially if the drug is smoked with tobacco, as is often the case with cannabis.

The Set

The effects and dangers of drugs are influenced by many things. Personal factors involving the person who is using the drugs can be just as important as the drugs being used.

The drug experience and the expectations of the user are important. Many young people experimenting with drugs for the first time will be unsure about what to do or what to expect. This ignorance and lack of experience can itself be dangerous.

The mental or psychological state of the drug user is very important. The mood people are in when they take drugs influences the effects and dangers of the drug use. If they are anxious, depressed or unstable they are more likely to have disturbing experiences when using drugs. They can become more anxious and disorientated, possibly aggressive, 'freak out' and do crazy things or take too much, etc. As a general rule, someone who is happy and stable is more likely to use more carefully and not be so badly affected.

Other things about the person which may affect drug dangers include:

√ If they have physical health problems like heart disease, high blood pressure, epilepsy, diabetes, asthma of liver problems, drug use could be more dangerous and possibly make their health problem worse.

√ The drug user's energy levels at the time of consuming drugs can also be important. If they are tired at the time of use, then it may have a different or more extreme effect than if they are fresh and full of energy.

√ If the user has a low body weight, the same amount of drugs may affect them more than heavier people. Also, people who have eating disorders like anorexia or bulimia can find that drug use makes their eating difficulties even worse.

√ Males and females can experience drugs in different ways. This is both because of their different physical make up and the different way people view male and female drug use. On average, women are of smaller body weight than men, have smaller livers as a proportion of body weight and a greater proportion of body fat. This means that, generally speaking, the same amount of drugs will have a greater effect on a woman than a man. Obviously this will not apply to a much larger than average woman or a much smaller than average man.

The effects and risks of drug use are also influenced by attitudes towards men and women taking drugs. Women are often seen as doubly bad if they take drugs. Male drug use is often seen as more acceptable than that of women and mothers, in particular, come in for a lot of criticism if they use drugs. Male drug users who are parents are not usually seen in the same sort of way. Sexism can also affect the experience of drug use and drug risk.

The Setting

The place where drugs are used and what people are doing at the time can influence how dangerous it is. For example, some young people take drugs in out-of-the-way places that are particularly dangerous, like canal banks, near motorways, in derelict buildings, etc.

Accidents are much more likely in these places, especially if the user is intoxicated. Also, if anything does go wrong, it is unlikely help will be at hand or that an ambulance could easily be called.

Even if the setting is not in itself inherently dangerous, there may be other types of risks associated with the place of use. Using or taking drugs into school has led to substantial numbers of young people being expelled from school with drastic affects on their future careers.

Driving a car or riding a bicycle or operating machinery while on drugs, will greatly increase the risks of accidents.

Drug use can lower inhibitions, increasing the likelihood of sexual encounters. Safer sex—for example, by using condoms—will be much more difficult if the person concerned is intoxicated. The risks of unwanted pregnancy, HIV and other STDs could be increased if people have sex while high on alcohol or drugs. Surveys have found that many young people have sexual encounters while under the influence of drugs, particularly alcohol and/or cannabis.

Another setting danger is that of people overexerting themselves when using ecstasy. Ecstasy gives a buzz of energy and is often used in clubs while dancing non-stop for long periods. In some situations people have danced for hours without a break in hot, crowded environments.

They run the risk of becoming dehydrated and getting heat exhaustion. In some cases this can be very dangerous and it has led to a number of deaths.

'Chilling out'—having a break from dancing, cooling off and sipping or drinking water or fruit juice (not alcohol) at regular intervals (around 1 pint per hour).

In Conclusion

There are many possible risks and dangers involved when using drugs. To fully understand potential risks and dangers you will need to think about drug, set and setting.

In addition, people may experience problems with drug use because of other people's perceptions and responses to them. Examples include conflict in family and other personal relationships, getting thrown out of school/college or work, getting a criminal record, getting into debt to pay for drugs, violence associated with drug dealing, etc.

Sharing Needles to Inject Drugs

Fast Facts:

- √ Sharing a needle or syringe to inject any type of substance (including steroids, etc.) puts you at risk of HIV and other infections found in the blood like hepatitis C. This applies whether injecting under the skin or directly into the blood stream.
- √ Sharing needles and syringes is not the only risk. Sharing water to clean injecting equipment, reusing containers to dissolve drugs, and reusing filters can also transmit HIV.
- √ To reduce transmission risk, avoid all shared needles and other injecting equipment, use a new or disinfected container and a new filter each time you prepare drugs, and use clean water when preparing drugs.

If you inject drugs, make sure you know how to do it safely to protect yourself from HIV and other infections.

How do you get HIV from injecting drugs?

During an injection, some blood goes into the needle and syringe. A needle and syringe that someone living with HIV has used can still contain blood with the virus in it after the injection. If you then use the same equipment without sterilizing it, you can inject the infected blood directly into your bloodstream.

Can I get HIV from any type of injecting?

Some people who inject drugs wrongly believe they are not at risk of HIV if they avoid injecting into a vein. You can also get HIV from injecting into the fat under the skin and injecting directly into a muscle.

Sharing a needle or syringe for any use, including injecting drugs under the skin, steroids, etc., can put you at risk of HIV and other infections found in the blood like hep C.

There are many ways you could get HIV from injecting drugs, including:

- √ preparing drugs with syringes that contain infected blood
- √ sharing water used to flush blood out of a needle and syringe
- √ reusing bottle caps, spoons, or other containers (cookers) to dissolve drugs into water and to heat drugs solutions
- √ reusing filters—normally small pieces of cotton or cigarette filters—used to filter out particles that could block the needle
- √ unsafe disposal of used needles or syringes where infected blood accidently gets into the body of another person.

If I use drugs, how can I reduce my risk of HIV?

If you inject drugs, don't share needles, syringes or other injecting equipment like spoons or swabs, as this exposes you to HIV and other viruses found in the blood like hepatitis C

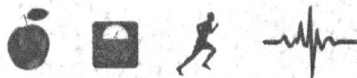

UNDERSTANDING RELAPSE

By Dr. Terrence T. Gorski

Relapse is more than just using alcohol and drugs. It is the progressive process of becoming so dysfunctional in recovery that self-medication with alcohol or drugs seems like a reasonable choice.

The relapse process is a lot like knocking over a line of dominoes. The first domino hits the second, which hits the third, and soon a progressive chain reaction has started. The sequence of problems that lead from stable sobriety to relapse are similar to those dominoes. There are two differences. First, each domino in the line (i.e. each problem that brings us closer to substance use) gets a little bit bigger and heavier until the last domino in the sequence is ten feet tall, four feet wide, and a foot thick. As this 10,000 pound domino begins to fall on us, it is too heavy for us to handle alone. The second difference is that the dominoes circle around behind us. So when the last domino falls, it hits us from being when we 1 re not looking.

So here we are, moving along in recovery. We tip over one small domino. No big deal! That domino hits the next, and then the next. A chain reaction gets started. The first dominoes are so small that we can easily convince ourselves that it's no big deal. We look the other way and start doing other things. All of a sudden a huge; domino falls on us from behind, crushing us to the floor, causing serious pain and injury in the process. We need to make the pain go away and we reach for an old, reliable solution—the magical substances that always helped us with our pain in the past. We've now started drinking and drugging.

The answer to avoiding relapse is not to take up weight training so you will be strong enough to lift that last domino off of your now crippled body. Part of the answer is to learn how not to tip over that first domino. Another part of the answer is to develop an emergency plan for stopping the chain reaction quickly, before the dominoes start so big and heavy that they become unmanageable.

The Relapse Process

The progression of problems that lead to relapse is called the relapse process. Each individual problem in the sequence is called a relapse warning sign. The entire sequence of problems is called a relapse warning sign list. The situations that we put ourselves in that cause or complicate the problems are called high risk situations.

It's important to remember that we don't start drinking or drugging because of the last problem in the sequence. We start drinking and drugging because the entire sequence of problems got out of control. Let's look at the steps of this process in more detail.

Step 1: Getting Stuck in Recovery: Many of us decide that alcohol or drugs is a problem, stop using, and put together some kind of recovery plan to help us stay sober. Initially we do fine. At some point, however, we hit a problem that we are unwilling or unable to deal with. We stop dead in our tracks. We are stuck in recovery and don't know what to do.

Step 2: Denying That We're Stuck: Instead of recognizing that we're stuck and asking for help, we use denial to convince ourselves that everything is OK. Denial makes it seem like the problem is gone, but it really isn't. The problem is still there. It just goes under ground where we can't see it. At some level we know that the problem is there, but we keep investing time and energy in denying it. This results in a buildup of pain and stress.

Step 3: Using Other Compulsions: To cope with this pain and stress, we begin to use other compulsive behaviors. We can start overworking, overeating, dieting, or over-exercising.

We can get involved in addictive relationships and distract ourselves by trying to experience the orgasm that shook New York City. These behaviors make us feel good in the short run by distancing us from our problems. But since they do nothing to solve the problem, the pain and stress comes back. We feel good now, but we hurt later. This is a hallmark of all addictive behaviors.

Step 4: Experiencing a Trigger Event: Then something happens. It's usually not a big thing. It's something we can normally handle without getting upset. But this time something snaps inside. One person described it this way: "It feels like a trigger fires off in my gut and I go out of control."

Step 5: Becoming Dysfunctional on the Inside: When the trigger goes off, our stress jumps up, and our emotions take control of our minds. To stay sober we have to keep intellect over emotion. We have to remember who we are (an addicted person), what we can't do (use alcohol or drugs), and what we must do (stay focused upon working a recovery program). When emotion gets control of the intellect we abandon everything we know, and start trying to feel good now at all costs. Relapse almost always grows from the inside out. The trigger event makes our pain so severe that we can't function normally. We have difficulty thinking clearly. We swing between emotional overreaction and emotional numbness. We can't remember things. It's impossible to sleep restfully and we get clumsy and start having accidents.

Step 6: Becoming Dysfunctional On the Outside: At first this internal dysfunction comes and goes. It's annoying, but it's not a real problem so we learn how to ignore it. On some level, we know something is wrong so we keep it a secret. Eventually we get so bad that the problem on the inside create problems on the outside. We start making mistakes at work, creating problems with our friends, families, and coworkers. We start neglecting our recovery programs. And things keep getting worse.

Step 7: Losing Control: We handle each problem as it comes along but look at the growing pattern of problems. We never really solve anything; we just put band-aids on the deep gushing cuts, put first-aid cream on seriously infected wounds, and tell ourselves the problem is solved. Then we look the other way and try to forget about the problems by getting involved in compulsive activities that will somehow magically fix us. This approach works for a while, but eventually things start getting out of control. As soon as we solve one problem, two new ones pop up to replace it. Life becomes one problem after another in an apparently endless sequence of crisis. One person put it like this: "I feel like I'm standing chest deep in a swimming pool trying to hold three beach balls underwater at once. I get the first one down, then the second, but as I reach for the third, the first one pops back up again." We finally recognize that we're out of control. We get scared and angry. "I'm sober! I'm not drinking! I'm working a program! Yet I'm out of control. If this is what sobriety is like— who needs it?"

Step 8: Using Addictive Thinking: Now we go back to using addictive thinking. We begin thinking along these lines: "Sobriety is bad for me, look at how miserable I am. Sober people don't understand me. Look at how critical they are. Maybe things would be better if I could talk to some of my old friends. I don't plan to drink or use drugs, I just want to get away from things for a while and have a little fun. People who supported my drinking and drugging were my friends. They knew how to have a good time. These new people who want me to stay sober are my enemies. Maybe I was never addicted in the first place. Maybe my problems were caused by something else. I just need to get away from it all for a while! Then I'll be able to figure it all out."

Step 9: Going Back to Addictive People, Places, and Things: Now we start going back to addictive people (our old friends), addictive places (our old hangouts), and addictive things (mind polluting compulsive activities). We convince ourselves that we're not going to drink or use drugs. We just want to relax. A client in one of my groups said he wanted to go to a bar so he could listen to music and relax while drinking soft drinks. An old timer in the group asked: "If you told me you were going to a whore house to say prayers, do you think I would believe you? Well, when you tell me you1 re going to a bar to drink cokes I have about the same reaction!"

Step 10: Using Addictive Substances: Eventually things get so bad that we come to believe that we only have three choices—collapse, suicide, or self-medication. We can collapse physically or emotionally from the stress of all our problems. We can end it all by committing suicide. Or we medicate the pain with alcohol or drugs. If these were your only three choices, which one sounds like the best way out? At this stage the stress and pain is so bad that is seems reasonable to use alcohol or drugs as a medicine to make the pain go away. The 10,000 pound domino just struck the back of our head, breaking our bones, and crushing us to the ground. We're dazed, hurt, and in tremendous pain. So we reach out for something, anything that will kill the pain. We start using alcohol and drugs in the misguided hope it will make our pain go away.

Step 11: Losing Control over Use: Once addicted people start using alcohol or drugs, they tend to follow one of two paths. Some have a short term and low consequence relapse. They recognize that they are in serious trouble, see that they are losing control, and manage to reach out for help and get back into recovery. Others start to use alcohol or drugs and feel such extreme shame and guilt that they refuse to seek help. They eventually develop progressive health and life problems and either get back into recovery, commit suicide, or die from medical complications, accidents, or drug-related violence.

Other Outcomes of the Relapse Process

Some relapse prone people don't drink. They may say "I'd rather be dead than drunk" and they either attempt or commit suicide. Others just hang in there until they have a stress collapse, develop a stress related illness, or have a nervous breakdown. Still others use half measures to temporarily pull themselves together for a little while only to have the problems come back later. This is called partial recovery and many people stay in it for years. They never get really well, but they never get drunk either

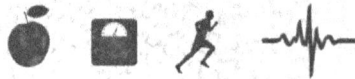

POST INCARCERATION SYNDROME & RELAPSE

By Dr. Terrence T. Gorski

Post-Incarceration Syndrome (PICS) is a serious problem that contributes to relapse in addicted and mentally ill offenders who are released from correction institutions.

Currently 60 percent of prisoners have been in prison before and there is growing evidence that PICS is a contributing factor to this high rate of recidivism.

The concept of Post-Incarceration Syndrome (PICS) has emerged from clinical consultation work with criminal justice system rehabilitation programs working with currently incarcerated prisoners and with treatment addiction programs and community mental health centers working with recently released prisoners.

This article will provide an operational definition of PICS, describe the common symptoms, recommended approaches to diagnosis and treatment, explore the implications of this serious new syndrome for community safety, and discuss the need for political action to reduce the number of prisoners and assure more humane treatment with our prisons, jails, and correctional institutions as a means of prevention. It is my hope that this initial formulation of a PICS Syndrome will encourage researchers to develop objective testing tools and formal studies to add to our understanding of the problems encountered by released inmates that influence recovery and relapse.

Operational Definition

PICS is a set of symptoms that are present in many currently incarcerated and recently released prisoners that are caused by being subjected to prolonged solitary confinement and severe institutional abuse.

The severity of symptoms is related to the level of coping skills prior to incarceration, the length of incarceration, the restrictiveness of the incarceration environment, the number and severity of institutional episodes of abuse, the number and duration of episodes of solitary confinement, and the degree of involvement in educational, vocational, and rehabilitation programs.

PICS is a mixed mental disorder with five clusters of symptoms:

1. Institutional Personality Traits resulting from the common deprivations of incarceration, a chronic state of learned helplessness in the face of prison authorities, and antisocial defenses in dealing with a predatory inmate milieu,

2. Post-Traumatic Stress Disorder (PTSD) from both pre-incarceration trauma and trauma experienced within the institution,

3. Antisocial Personality Traits (ASPT) developed as a coping response to institutional abuse and a predatory prisoner milieu, and

4. Social-Sensory Deprivation Syndrome caused by prolonged exposure to solitary

confinement that radically restricts social contact and sensory stimulation.

5. Substance Use Disorders caused by the use of alcohol and other drugs to manage or escape the PICS symptoms.

6. PICS often coexists with substance use disorders and a variety of affective and personality disorders.

Symptoms of Post Incarceration Syndrome (PICS)

Below is a more detailed description of five clusters of symptoms of PICS:

1. Institutionalized Personality Traits. Institutionalized Personality Traits are caused by living in an oppressive environment that demands: passive compliance to the demands of authority figures, passive acceptance of severely restricted acts of daily living, the repression of personal lifestyle preferences, the elimination of critical thinking and individual decision making, and internalized acceptance of severe restrictions on the honest self-expression thoughts and feelings.

2. Post-Traumatic Stress Disorder (PTSD). Post-Traumatic Stress Disorder (PTSD) is caused by both traumatic experiences before incarceration and institutional abuse during incarceration the includes the six clusters of symptoms:

   √ intrusive memories and flashbacks to episodes of severe institutional abuse;

   √ intense psychological distress and physiological reactivity when exposed to cues triggering memories of the institutional abuse;

   √ episodes of dissociation, emotional numbing, and restricted affect;

   √ chronic problems with mental functioning that include irritability, outbursts of anger, difficulty concentrating, sleep disturbances, and an exaggerated startle response.

   √ persistence avoidance of anything that would trigger memories of the traumatic events;

   √ hypervigilance, generalized paranoia, and reduced capacity to trust caused by constant fear of abuse from both correctional staff and other inmates that can be generalized to others after release.

3. Antisocial Personality Traits. Antisocial Personality Traits are developed both from preexisting symptoms and symptoms developed during incarceration as an institutional coping skill and psychological defense mechanism. The primary anti personality traits involve the tendency to challenge authority, break rules, and victimize others. In patients with PICS these tendencies are veiled by the passive aggressive style that is part of the institutionalized personality. Patients with PICS tend to be duplicitous, acting on a compliant and passive aggressive manner with therapists and other perceived authority figures while being capable with direct threatening and aggressive behavior when alone with peers outside of the perceived control of those in authority. This is a direct result of the internalized coping behavior required to survive in a harshly punitive correctional institution that has two sets of survival rules: passive aggression with the guards, and actively aggressive with predatory inmates.

4. Social-Sensory Deprivation Syndrome. The Social-Sensory Deprivation Syndrome is caused by the effects of prolonged solitary confinement that imposes both social isolation and sensory deprivation. These symptoms include severe chronic headaches, developmental regression, impaired impulse control, dissociation, inability to concentrate, repressed rage, inability to control primitive drives and instincts, inability to plan beyond the

moment, inability to anticipate logical consequences of behavior, out or control obsessive thinking, and borderline personality traits.

5. Reactive Substance Use Disorders. Many inmates who experience PICS suffer from the symptoms of substance use disorders. Many of these inmates were addicted prior to incarceration, did not receive treatment during their imprisonment, and continued their addiction by securing drugs on the prison black market. Others developed their addiction in prison in an effort to cope with the PICS symptoms and the condition causing them. Others relapse to substance abuse or develop substance use disorders as a result of using alcohol or other drugs in an effort to cope with PICS symptoms upon release from prison.

PICS Symptoms Severity

The syndrome is most severe in prisoners incarcerated for longer than one year in a punishment orientation environment, who have experienced multiple episodes of institutional abuse, who have had little or no access to education, vocational training, or rehabilitation, who have been subjected to 30 days or longer in solitary confinement, and who have experienced frequent and severe episodes of trauma as a result of institutional abuse.

The syndrome is least severe in prisoners incarcerated for shorter periods of time in rehabilitation oriented programs, who have reasonable access to educational and vocational training, and who have not been subjected to solitary confinement, and who have not experienced frequent or severe episodes of institutional abuse.

Reasons to be Concerned about PICS

There is good reason to be concerned because about 40 percent of the total incarcerated population are released each year. The number of prisoners being deprived of rehabilitation services, experiencing severely restrictive daily routines, being held in solitary confinement for prolonged periods of time, or being abused by other inmates or correctional staff is increasing.

The effect of releasing this number of prisoners with psychiatric damage from prolonged incarceration can have a number of devastating impacts upon American society including the further devastation of inner city communities and the destabilization of the blue-collar and middle class districts unable to reabsorb returning prisoners who are less likely to get jobs, more likely to commit crimes, more likely to disrupt families. This could turn many currently struggling lower middle class areas into slums.

As more prisoners are returned to the community, behavioral health providers can expect to see increases in patients admitted with the Post Incarceration Syndrome and related substance use, mental, and personality disorders. The National network of Community Mental Health and Addiction Treatment Programs need to begin now to prepare their staff to identify and provide appropriate treatment for this new type of client.

The nation's treatment providers, especially addiction treatment programs and community mental health centers, are already experiencing a growing number of clients experiencing PICS. This increase is due to a number of factors including: the increasing size of the prisoner population, the increasing use of restrictive and punishing institutional practices, the reduction of access to education, vocational training, and rehabilitation programs; the increasing use of solitary confinement and the growing number of maximum security and super-max type prison and jails.

Both the number of clients suffering from PICS and the average severity of symptoms is expected to increase over the next decade. In 1995 there were there were 463,284 prisoners released back to the community. Based upon conservative projections in the growth of the prisoner population it is projected that in the year 2000 there will be 660,000 prisoners returned to the community, in the year 2005 there will be 887,000 prisoners returned to the community, and in the year 2010 1.2 million prisoners will be released. The prediction of greater symptom severity is based upon the growing trend toward longer periods of incarceration, more restrictive and punitive conditions in correctional institutions, decreasing access to education, vocational training, and rehabilitation, and the increasing use of solitary confinement as a tool for reducing the cost of prisoner management. There was 626,000 released in 2018 from being incarcerated.

Clients with PICS are at a high risk for developing substance dependence, relapsing to substance use if they were previously addicted, relapsing to active mental illness if they were previously mentally ill, and returning to a life of regression, violence and crime. They are also at high risk of chronic unemployment and homelessness.

Post Release Symptom Progression

This is because released prisoners experiencing PICS tends to experience a six stage post release symptom progression leading to recidivism and often are not qualified for social benefits needed to secure addiction, mental health, and occupation training services.

Stage 1 of this Post Release Syndrome is marked by helplessness and hopelessness due to inability to develop a plan for community reentry, often complicated by the inability to secure funding for treatment or job training;

Stage 2 is marked by an intense immobilizing fear;

Stage 3 is marked by the emergence of intense free-floating anger and rage and the emergence of flashbacks and other symptoms of PTSD;

Stage 4 is marked by a tendency toward impulse violence upon minimal provocation;

Stage 5 is marked by an effort to avoid violence by severe isolation to avoid he triggers of violence;

Stage 6 is marked by the intensification of flashbacks, nightmares, sleep impairments, and impulse control problems caused by self-imposed isolation. This leads to acting out behaviors, aggression, violence, and crime, which in turn sets the stages for arrest and incarceration.

Currently 60 percent of prisoners have been in prison before and there is growing evidence that PICS is a contributing factor to this high rate of recidivism.

Reducing the Incidence of PICS

Since PICS is created by criminal justice system policy and programming in our well-intentioned but misguided attempt to stop crime, the epidemic can be prevented and public safety protected by changing the public policies that call for incarcerating more people, for longer periods of time, for less severe offenses, in more punitive environments that emphasize the use of solitary confinement, that eliminate or severely restrict prisoner access to educational, vocational, and rehabilitation programs while incarcerated.

The political antidote for PICS is to implement public policies that:

Fund the training and expansion of community based addiction and mental health programs staffed by professionals trained to meet the needs of criminal justice system clients diverted into treatment by court programs and released back into the community after incarceration;

Expand the role of drug and mental health courts that promote treatment alternatives to incarceration;

Convert 80 percent of our federal, state, and county correctional facilities into rehabilitation programs with daily involvement in educational, vocational, and rehabilitation programs;

Eliminate required long mandated minimum sentences;

Institute universal prerelease programs for all offenders with the goal of preparing them to transition into community based addiction and mental health programs;

Assuring that all released prisoners have access to publicly funded programs for addiction and mental health treatment upon release.

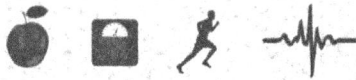

A RELAPSE PREVENTION PLAN
By Dr. Terence T. Gorski

People who relapse aren't suddenly taken drunk. Most experience progressive warning signs that reactivate denial and cause so much pain that self-medication with alcohol or drugs seems like a good idea. This is not a conscious process. These warning signs develop automatically and unconsciously. Since most recovering people have never been taught how to identify and manage relapse warning signs, they don't notice them until the pain becomes too severe to ignore.

There are nine steps in learning to recognize and stop the early warning signs of relapse.

Step 1: Stabilization

Relapse prevention planning probably won't work unless the relapser is sober and in control of themselves. Detoxification and a few good days of sobriety are needed in order to make relapse prevention planning work. Remember that many patients who relapse are toxic. Even though sober they have difficulty thinking clearly, remembering things and managing their feelings and emotions. These symptoms get worse when the person is under high stress or is isolated from people to talk to about the problems of staying sober. To surface intense therapy issues with someone who has a toxic brain can increase rather than decrease the risk of relapse. In early abstinence go slow and focus on the basics. The key question is "What do you need to do to not drink today?"

Step 2: Assessment

The assessment process is designed to identify the recurrent pattern of problems that caused past relapse and resolve the pain associated with those problems. This is accomplished by reconstructing the presenting problems, the life history, the alcohol and drug use history and the recovery relapse history.

By reconstructing the presenting problems, the here and now issues that pose an immediate threat to sobriety can be identified and crisis plans developed to resolve those issues.

The life history explores each developmental life period including childhood, grammar school, high school, college, military, adult work history, adult friendship history, and adult intimate relationship history. Reviewing the life history can surface can surface painful unresolved memories. It's important to go slow and talk about the feelings that accompany these memories.

Once the life history is reviewed, a detailed alcohol and drug use history is reconstructed. This is best done by reviewing each life period and asking four questions: (1) How much alcohol or drugs did you use? (2) How often did you use it? (3) Want did you want alcohol and drugs to accomplish? (4) What were the real consequences, positive and negative, of your use? In other words, did the booze and drugs do for you what you wanted it to do during each period of your life?

Finally, the recovery and relapse history is reconstructed. Starting with the first serious attempt at sobriety each period of abstinence and chemical use is carefully explored. The major goal is to find out what happened during each period of abstinence that set the stage for relapse. This is often difficult because most relapsers are preoccupied with their drinking and drugging and resist thinking or talking about what happened during periods of abstinence.

Comprehensive assessments have shown that most relapsers get sober, encounter the same recurring pattern of problems, and use those problems to justify the next relapse. As one person put it "It is not one thing after the other, it is the same thing over and over again!"

A 23 year old relapser named Jake reported drinking about a six pack of beer every Friday and Saturday night during high school. He did it in order to feel like he was part of the group, relax and have fun. At that stage in his addiction the beer did exactly what he wanted it to do.

That all changed when he left school and went to work as a salesman. He had to perform in a high pressure environment and felt stressed. The other salesmen were competitive and no matter what he did they wouldn't let him belong. He began drinking bourbon every night to deal with the stress. He wanted to feel relaxed so he could cope better at work. He consistently drank too much and woke up with terrible hangovers that caused new problems with his job.

Every time Jake would attempt to stop drinking he would feel isolated and alone and become overwhelmed by the stress of his job. Even when with others at Twelve Step Meetings he felt like he didn't belong and couldn't fit in. As the stress grew he began to think "If this is sobriety, who needs it?" Each relapse was related with his inability to deal with job related pressures.

By comparing the life history, the alcohol and drug use history, and the recovery relapse history, Jake could see in a dramatic way the recurrent problems that cause him to relapse. The two major issues were (1) the need to drink in order to feel like he belonged and (2) the need to drink in order to cope with stress.

It wasn't surprising that Jake discovered that during every past period of abstinence he became isolated, lonely and depressed. The longer he stayed sober, the worse it got. The stress built up until he felt that he didn't take a drink to relax he would go crazy or collapse.

Step 3: Relapse Education

Relapsers need to learn about the relapse process and how to manage it. It's not a bad idea to get their family and Twelve Step Sponsors involved. The education need to reinforce the four major messages: First, relapse is a normal and natural part of recovery from chemical dependence. There is nothing to be ashamed or embarrassed about. Second, people are not suddenly drunk. There are progressive patterns or warning signs that set them up to use again. These warning signs can be identified and recognized while sober. Third, once identified, recovering people can learn to manage the relapse warning signs while sober. And Fourth, there is hope. A new counseling procedure called relapse prevention therapy can teach recovering people how to recognize and manage warning signs so a return to chemical use becomes unnecessary.

When Jake entered relapse prevention therapy he felt demoralized and hopeless. That began to change when he heard his first lecture that described the typical warning signs that precede relapse to chemical use. He felt like someone had read his mail. "Since someone understands what causes me to get drunk," he thought, "perhaps they know what to do in order to stay sober."

Step 4: Warning Sign Identification

Relapsers need to identify the problems that caused relapse. The goal is to write a list of personal warning signs that lead them from stable recovery back to chemical use.

There is seldom just one warning sign. Usually a series of warning signs build one on the other to create relapse. It's the cumulative effect that wears them down. The final warning sign is simply the one that breaks the camel's back. Unfortunately many of relapsers think it's the last warning sign that did it. As a result they don't look for the earlier and more subtle warning signs that set the stage for the final disaster.

When Jake first came into relapse prevention therapy he thought that he was crazy. "I can't understand it," he told his counselor, "Everything was going fine and suddenly, for no reason at all 1 started to overreact to things. I'd get confused, make stupid mistakes and then not know what to do to fix it. I got so stressed out that I got drunk over it."

Jake, like most relapsers, didn't know what his early relapse warning signs were and as a result didn't recognize the problem until it was too late. A number of procedures are used to help recovering people identify the early warning signs of relapse.

Most people start by reviewing and discussing The Phases and Warning Signs of Relapse (available from Independence Press, POB HE, Independence, MO 64055). This warning sign list describes the typical sequence of problems that lead from stable recovery to alcohol and drug use. By reading and discussing these warning signs, relapsers develop a new way of thinking about the things that happened during past periods of abstinence that set them up to use. They learn new words with which to describe their past experiences.

After reading the warning signs they develop an initial warning sign list by selecting five of the warning signs that they can identify with. These warning signs become a starting point for warning sign analysis. Since most relapsers don't know what their warning signs are they need to be guided through a process that will uncover them. The relapser is asked to take each of the five warning signs and tell a story about a time when they experienced that warning sign in the past while sober. They tell these stories both to their therapist and to their therapy group. The goal is to look for hidden warning signs that are reflected in the story.

Jake, for example, identified with the warning signs "Tendency toward loneliness." He told a story about a time when he was sober and all alone in the house because his wife had left with the children. "I felt so lonely and abandoned," he said. "I couldn't understand why she would walk out just because we had a disagreement. She should be able to handle it better than she does."

The group began to ask questions and it turned out that Jake had frequent arguments with his wife that were caused by his grouchiness because of problems on the job. It turned out that these family arguments were a critical warning sign that occurred before most relapses. Jake had never considered his marriage to be a problem, and as a result never thought of getting marriage counseling.

Jake not had identified three warning signs: (1) the need to drink in order to feel like he belonged, (2) the need to drink in order to cope with stress, and (3) the need to drink in order to cope with marital problems. In order to be effectively managed, each of these warning signs would need to be further clarified.

I then had Jake write these three warning signs using a standard format and identify the irrational thoughts, unmanageable feelings and self-defeating behavior that accompanied each. He wrote:

(1) I know I'm in trouble with my recovery when I'm feeling lonely and unable to fit in with other people. When this happens I tend to think that I am no good and nobody could

ever care about me. When this happens I tend to feel lonely, angry and afraid. When this happens I have an urge to hide myself away so I don't have to talk with anyone.

(2) I know I am in trouble with my recovery when I feel unable to cope with high levels of job related stress. When this happens I tend to think that I need to try harder in order to get things under control or else I will be a failure. When this happens I tend to feel humiliated and embarrassed. When this happens I drive myself to keep working even though I need to rest.

(3) I know I am in trouble with my recovery when I get irrationally angry at my wife. When this happens I tend to think that I am a terrible person for treating her that way, but part of me believes she deserves it. When this happens I tend to feel angry and ashamed. When this happens, forget that the incident every happened, put it behind us and get on with our marriage.

(4) With this detailed description of the relapse warning signs Jake was ready to move on to the fifth step of relapse prevention planning.

Step 5: Warning Sign Management

Understanding the warning signs is not enough. We need to learn how to manage them without resorting to alcohol or drug use. This means learning nonchemical problem solving strategies that help us to identify high risk situations and develop coping strategies. In this way relapsers can diffuse irrational thinking, manage painful feelings, and stop the self-defeating behaviors that lead to alcohol or drug use.

This is done by taking each relapse warning sign and developing a general coping strategy. Jake, for example developed the following management strategy for dealing with his job related stress.

Warning Sign: I know I am in trouble with my recovery when I feel unable to cope with high levels of job related stress.

General Coping Strategy: I will learn how to say no to taking on extra projects, limit my work to 45 hours per week, and learn how to use relaxation exercises and meditation to unwind.

The next step is to identify ways to cope with irrational thoughts, unmanageable feelings, and self-defeating behaviors that accompany each warning sign. Jake developed the following coping strategies:

Irrational Thought: I need to try harder in order to get things under control or else I will be a failure.

Rational Thought: I am burned out because I am trying too hard. I need time to rest of I will start making more mistakes.

Unmanageable Feelings: Humiliation and embarrassment.

Feeling Management Strategy: Talk about my feelings with others. Remind myself that there is no reason to be embarrassed. I am a fallible human being and all people get tired.

Self-defeating Behavior: Driving myself to keep working even though I know I need to rest.

Constructive Behavior: Take a break and relax. Ask someone to review the project and see if they can help me to solve the problem.

Now Jake is ready to move unto the sixth step of recovery planning. A recovery plan is a schedule of activities that puts relapsers into regular contact with people who will help them to avoid alcohol and drug use. They must stay sober by working the Twelve Step Program and attending relapse prevention support groups that teach them to recognize and manage relapse warning signs. This is why I called relapse prevention planning a "Twelve Step Plus" approach to recovery.

Jake needed to build something into his recovery program to help him deal with job related stress. He decided to enter into counseling with a counselor who specialized in stress management, understood chemical dependency and had a background as an employee assistance counselor. By doing this Jake was forced to regularly discuss his problems at work and review how he was coping with them. By identifying job relater problems early, he could prevent getting overwhelmed by small problems that became overwhelming.

Step 6: Inventory Training

Most relapsers find it helpful to get in the habit of doing a morning and evening inventory. The goal of the morning inventory is to prepare to recognize and manage warning signs. The goal of the evening inventory is to review problems and progress. This allows relapsers to anticipate high risk situations and monitor for relapse warning signs. Relapsers been to take inventory work seriously because most warning signs are deeply entrenched habits that are hard to change and tend to automatically come back whenever certain problems or stresses occur. If we weren't alert we may not notice them until it's too late.

Step 7: Family Involvement

A supportive family can make the difference between recovery and relapse. We need to encourage our family members to get involved so they can recover from codependency. With this foundation of shared recovery we can begin talking with our families about past relapses, the warning signs that led up to them, and how the relapse hurt the family. Most importantly we can work together to avoid further relapse.

If we had heart disease we would want our family to be prepared for an emergency. Chemical dependency is a disease just like heart disease. Our families need to know about the early warning signs that lead to relapse. They must be prepared to take fast and decisive action if we return to chemical use. We can work out in advance, when we are in a sober state of mind, the steps they should take if we return to chemical use. Our very life could depend on it.

Step 8: Follow Up

Our warning signs will change as we progress in recovery. Each stage of recovery has unique warning signs. Our ability to deal with the warning signs of one stage of recovery doesn't guarantee that we will recognize or know how to manage the warning signs of the next stage. Our relapse prevention plan needs to be updated regularly; monthly for the first three months, quarterly for the first two years, and annually thereafter.

Available now! A Guide To Relapse Prevention For Prisoners, by Charles Hottinger. "The BOP requires you to have a relapse prevention plan. This book provides the information and guidance that can make a real difference in the preparation of a comprehensive relapse prevention plan. Discover how to meet the parole board's expectation using these proven and practical principles. Included is a blank template and sample relapse prevention plan to assist in your preparation." To order, send $15.00 plus $5.00 s/h to:

The Cell Block
PO Box 1025
Rancho Cordova, CA 95741.

On the other hand, a comprehensive reentry book is Life With A Record, ten hard hitting chapters outline the purpose of making a Strategic Reentry Plan and making peace with supervisors, family, your community and your future. explores the most commonly confronted issues and attitudes that sabotage reentry. It provides tools that cut across functions of discrimination, in corporations, political life and throughout society. It opens the door to empowerment, reminding ex-offenders that change and long term freedom begins with a commitment to daily growth. Addressing the whole reentry process, Life With a Record is "must" reading for anyone preparing to leave prison and face the world. It's an ideal book for ex-offenders with decades of experience as well as first time prisoners who need help jump starting their new life. Written by well-known reentry technician Anthony Tinsman. Softcover, 8"x10", 360 pages. Order your copy today $27.99 plus $7 s/h to:

Freebird Publishers

Box 541

North Dighton, MA 02674

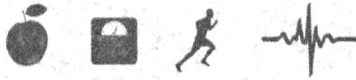

THE SECRET TO HEALTH

Have you ever read the book The Secret, by Rhonda Byrne? On the back of the book it says. "It has been passed down through the ages, highly coveted, hidden, lost, stolen, and bought for vast sums of money. This centuries-old Secret has been understood by some of the most prominent people in history: Plato, Galileo, Beethoven, Edison, Carnegie, Einstein—along with other inventors, theologians, scientists, and great thinkers...Now The Secret is being revealed to the world.

"As you learn The Secret, you will come to know how you can have, be, or do anything you want. You will come to know who you really are. You will come to know the true magnificence that awaits you in life."

Now, in my search for wisdom and knowledge in many areas, I've noticed a common element in each. In short, it is the essence of The Secret; this includes when it comes to your health. Here is an excerpt from the book...

Dr. John Hagelin, Quantum Physicist and Public Policy Expert: Our body is really the product of our thoughts. We're beginning to understand in medical science the degree in which the nature of thoughts and emotions actually determines the physical substance and structure and function of our bodies.

Dr. John Demartini: We've known in the healing arts of a placebo effect. A placebo is something that supposedly has no impact and no effect on the body, like a sugar pill.

You tell the patient that this is just as effective, and what happens in the placebo sometimes has the same effect, if not greater effect, than the medication that is supposed to be designed for that effect. They have found out that the human mind is the biggest factor in the healing arts, sometimes more so than the medication.

As you are becoming aware of the magnitude of The Secret, you will begin to see more clearly the underlying truth of certain occurrences in humankind, including in the area of health.

The placebo effect is a powerful phenomenon. When patients think and truly believe the tablet is a cure, they will receive what they believe, and they will be cured.

Dr. John Demartini: If somebody is in a situation where they're sick and they have an alternative to try to explore what it is in their mind creating it, versus using medicine, if it's an actual situation that could really bring death to them, then obviously the medicine is a wise thing to do, while they explore what the mind is about. So you don't want to negate medicine. Every form of healing has a place.

Healing through the mind can work harmoniously with medicine. If pain is involved, then medicine can help to eliminate that pain, which then allows the person to be able to focus with great force on health. "Thinking perfect health" is something anybody can do privately with themselves, no matter what is happening around them.

Lisa Nichols: The Universe is a masterpiece of abundance. When you open yourself to feel the abundance of the Universe, you'll experience the wonder, joy, bliss, and all the great things that the Universe has for you—good health, good wealth, good nature. But when you shut yourself off with negative thoughts, you'll feel the discomfort, you'll feel the aches, you'll feel the pain, and you'11 feel as if every day is painful to get through.

Dr. Ben Johnson, Physician, Author, and Leader in Energy Healing: We've got a thousand different diseases and diagnosis out there. They're just the weak link. They're all the result of one thing: stress. If you put enough stress on the chain and you put enough stress on the system, then one of the links breaks.

All stress begins with one negative thought. One thought that went unchecked, and then more thoughts came and more, until stress manifested. The effect is stress, but the cause was negative thinking, and it all began with one little negative thought. No matter what you might have manifested, you can change it...with one small positive thought and then another.

Dr. John Demartini: Our physiology creates disease to give us feedback, to let us know we have an imbalanced perspective, or we're not being loving and grateful. So the body's signs and symptoms are not something terrible.

Dr. Demartini is telling us that love and gratitude will dissolve all negativity in our lives, no matter what form it has taken. Love and gratitude can part seas, move mountains, and create miracles. And love and gratitude can dissolve any disease.

Michael Bernard Beckwith: The question frequently asked is, "When a person has manifested a disease in the body temple or some kind of discomfort in their life, can it be turned around through the power of 'right' thinking?" And the answer is absolutely, yes.

Laughter is the Best Medicine

Cathy Goodman, A Personal Story: I was diagnosed with breast cancer. I truly believed in my heart, with my strong faith, that I was already healed. Each day I would say, "Thank you for my healing." I believed in my heart I was healed. I saw myself as if cancer was never in my body.

One of the things I did to heal myself was to watch very funny movies. That's all we would do was laugh. We couldn't afford to put any stress in my life, because we knew stress was one of the worst things you can do while you're trying to heal yourself.

From the time I was diagnosed to the time I was healed was approximately three months. And that's without any radiation or chemotherapy.

This beautiful and inspiring story from Cathy Goodman demonstrates three magnificent powers in operation: The power of gratitude to heal, the power of faith to receive, and the power of laughter and joy to dissolve disease in our bodies.

Cathy was inspired to include laughter as part of her healing, after hearing about the story of Norman Cousins.

Norman had been diagnosed with an "incurable" disease. The doctors told him he had just a few months to live. Norman decided to heal himself. For three months all he did was watch funny movies and laugh, laugh, laugh. The disease left his body in those three months, and the doctors proclaimed his recovery a miracle.

As he laughed, Norman released all negativity, and he released the disease. Laughter really is the best medicine.

Dr. Ben Johnson: We all come with a built-in basic program. It's called "self-healing." You get a wound, it grows back together. You get a bacterial infection, the immune system comes and takes care of those bacteria, and heals it up. The immune system is made to heal itself.

Bob Proctor: Disease cannot live in a body that's in a healthy emotional state. Your body is casting off millions of cells every second, and it's also creating millions of new cells at the same time.

Dr. John Hagelin: In fact, parts of our body are literally replaced every day. Other parts take a few months, other parts a couple of years. But within a few years we each have a brand new physical body.

If our entire bodies are replaced within a few years, as science has proven, then how can it be that degeneration or illness remains in our bodies for years? It can only be held there by thought, by observation of the illness, and by the attention given to the illness.

Think Thoughts of Perfection

Think thoughts of perfection. Illness cannot exist in a body that has harmonious thoughts. Know there is only perfection, and as you observe perfection you must summon that to you. Imperfect thoughts are the cause of all humanity's ills, including disease, poverty, and unhappiness. When we think negative thoughts we are cutting ourselves off from our rightful heritage. Declare and intend, "I think perfect thoughts. I see only perfection. I am perfection."

I banished every bit of stiffness and lack of agility right out of my body. I focused on seeing my body as flexible and as perfect as a child's, and every stiff and aching joint vanished. I literally did this overnight.

You can see that beliefs about aging are all in our minds. Science explains that we have a brand new body in a very short time. Aging is limited thinking, so release those thoughts from your consciousness and know that your body is only months old, no matter how many birthdays you have chalked up in your mind. For your next birthday, do yourself a favor and celebrate it as your first birthday! Don't cover your cake with sixty candles, unless you want to summon aging to you. Unfortunately, Western society has become fixated on age, and in reality there is no such thing.

You can think your way to the perfect state of health, the perfect body, the perfect weight, and eternal youth. You can bring it into being, through your consistent thinking of perfection.

Bob Proctor: If you have a disease, and you're focusing on it, and you're talking to people about it, you're going to create more diseased cells. See yourself living in a perfectly healthy body. Let the doctor look after the disease.

One of the things people often do when they have an illness is talk about it all the time. That's because they're thinking about it all the time, so they're just verbalizing their thoughts. If you are feeling a little unwell, don't talk about it—unless you want more of it. Know that your thought was responsible and repeat as often as you can, "I feel wonderful. I feel so good," and really feel it. If you are not feeling great and somebody asks you how you are feeling, just be grateful that the person has reminded you to think thoughts of feeling well. Speak only the words of what you want.

You cannot "catch" anything unless you think you can, and thinking you can is inviting it to you with your thought. You are also inviting illness if you are listening to people talking about their illness. As you are listening you are giving all of your thought and focus to illness, and when you give all your thought to something, you are asking for it. And you are certainly not helping them. You are adding energy to their illness. If you really want to help that person, change the conversation to good things, if you can, or be on your way. As you walk away, give your powerful thoughts and feelings to seeing that person well, and then let it go.

Lisa Nichols: Let's say you have two people, both stricken with something, but one chooses to focus on joy. One chooses to live in possibility and hopefulness, focusing on all the reasons why she should be joyful and grateful. Then you have the second person. Same diagnosis, but the : second chooses to focus on the disease, the pain, and the "woe is me."

Bob Doyle: When people are completely focused on what is wrong and their symptoms, they will perpetuate it. The healing will not occur until they shift their attention from being sick to being well. Because that's the law of attraction.

Patience Mulford: Let us remember, as far as we can, that every unpleasant thought is a bad thing literally put in the body.

Dr. John Hagelin: Happier thoughts lead to essentially a happier biochemistry. A happier, healthier body. Negative thoughts and stress have been shown to seriously degrade the body and the functioning of the brain, because it's our thoughts and emotions that are continuously reassembling, reorganizing, re-creating our body.

No matter what you have manifested in regards to your body, you can change it—inside and out. Start thinking happy thoughts and start being happy. Happiness is a feeling state of being. You have your finger on the "feeling happy" button. Press it now and keep your finger pressed down on it firmly, no matter what is happening around you.

Dr. Ben Johnson: Remove psychological stress from the body, and the body does what it was designed to do. It heals itself.

You don't have to fight to get rid of a disease. Just the simple process of letting go of negative thoughts will allow your natural state of health to emerge within you. And your body will heal itself.

Michael Bernard Beckwith: I've seen kidneys regenerated. I've seen cancer dissolved. I've seen eyesight improve and come back.

I have been wearing reading glasses for about three years before I discovered The Secret.

One night as I was tracing the knowledge of The Secret back through the centuries, I found myself reaching for my glasses to see what I was reading. And I stopped in my tracks. The realization of what I had done struck my like a lightning bolt.

I had listened to society's message that eyesight diminishes with age. I had watched people stretch their arms out so they could read something. I had given my thought to eyesight diminishing with age, and I had brought it to me. I hadn't done it deliberately, but I had done it. I knew that what I had brought into being with thoughts I could change, so I immediately imagined myself seeing as clearly as when I was twenty-one years old. I saw myself in dark restaurants, on planes, and at my computer, reading clearly and effortlessly.

And I said over and over, "I can see clearly, I can see clearly." I felt the feelings of gratitude and excitement for having clear vision. In three days my eyesight had been restored, and I now do not own reading glasses. I can see clearly.

When I told Dr. Ben Johnson, one of the teachers from The Secret, about what I had done, he said to me, "Do you realize what had to happen to your eyes for you to do that in three days?" I replied, "No, and thank goodness I didn't know, so that thought was not in my head! I just knew I could do it, and I could do it fast." (Sometimes less information is better i)

Dr. Johnson eliminated an "incurable" disease from his own body, so the restoration of my eyesight seemed like nothing to me, compared with his own miracle story. In fact, I expected my eyesight to come back overnight, so three days was no miracle in my mind. Remember, time and size do not exist in the Universe. It is as easy to heal a pimple as a disease. The process is identical; the difference is in our minds. So if you have attracted some affliction to you, reduce it in your mind to the size of a pimple, let go of all negative thoughts, and then focus on the perfection of health.

Nothing is Incurable

Dr. John Demartini: I always say the incurable means "curable from within."

I believe and know that nothing is incurable. At some point in time, every so-called incurable disease has been cured. In my mind, and in the world I create, "incurable" does not exist. There is plenty of room for you in this world, so come join me and all who are here. It is the world where "miracles" are everyday occurrences. It is a world overflowing with total abundance, where all good things exist not, within you. Sounds like heaven, doesn't it? It is.

Michael Bernard Beckwith: You can change your life and you can heal yourself.

Morris Goodman, Author and International Speaker: My story begins on March 10, 1981. This day really changed my whole life. It was a day I'll never forget. I crashed an airplane. I ended up in the hospital completely paralyzed. My spinal cord was crushed, I broke the first and second cervical vertebrae, my swallowing reflex was destroyed, I couldn't eat or drink, my diaphragm was destroyed, I couldn't breathe. All I could do was blink my eyes.

The doctors, of course, said I'd be a vegetable the rest of my life. All I'd be able to do is blink my eyes. That's the picture they saw of me, but it didn't matter what they thought. The main thing was what I thought. I pictured myself being a normal person again, walking out of that hospital.

The only thing I had to work with in the hospital was my mind, and once you have your mind, you can put things back together again.

I was hooked to a respirator and they said I would never breathe on my own again because my diaphragm was destroyed. But a little voice kept saying to me, "Breathe deeply, breathe deeply." And finally I was weaned from it. They were at a loss for an explanation. I could not afford to allow anything to come into my mind that would distract me from my goal or from my vision.

I had set a goal to walk out of the hospital on Christmas. And I did. I walked out of the hospital on my own two feet. They said it couldn't be done. That's a day I will never forget.

For people who are sitting out there right now and are hurting, if I wanted to sum up my life and sum up for people what they can do in life, I would sum it up in six words:

"Man becomes what he thinks about."

Morris Goodman is known as The Miracle Man. His story was chosen for The Secret because it demonstrates the unfathomable power and unlimited potential of the human mind. Morris knew the power within him to bring about what he chose to think about. Everything is possible. Morris Goodman's story has inspired thousands of people to think, imagine, and feel their way back to health. He turned the greatest challenge of his life into the greatest gift.

Since the film The Secret was released, we have been inundated with miracle stories of all types of diseases dissolving from people's bodies after they watched The Secret. All things are possible when you believe.

On the subject of health I would like to leave with you these illuminating words from Dr. Ben

Johnson: "We are now entering the era of energy medicine. Everything in the Universe has a frequency and all you have to do is change a frequency or create an opposite frequency. That's how easy it is to change anything in the world, whether that's disease or emotional issues or whatever that is. This is huge. This is the biggest thing that we have ever come across."

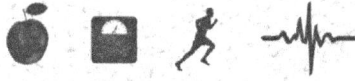

SPIRITUAL PRACTICES FOR INMATES
By Dennis Klocek

Every human being, no matter how old they are, or what their situation, has a part of themselves who remembers how life used to be before things got crazy. No amount of misunderstandings, mistakes, ridicule, taunts, humiliations or abuse can erase the memories stored in this part of every single human.

We could say that there is an inner being in every person who is doing this remembering at all times. This inner being who is doing the remembering is the very kernel and core of our humanness.

This core being lives in an inner timeless world. In the timeless world our inner being lives among memories of how it was when someone was running things in our universe besides crazy people. The inner being in us is constantly living in this timeless world where there is some peace of mind at all times, even though things in the regular time driven world often seem to be getting more and more insane all the time.

The whole concept of doing time in prison hinges on the fact that crazy things do happen to everyone in this world at some time or another. Some individuals react to this fact in more radical ways than others do. Then society takes something away. That thing which is taken away is access to the true nature of time. The true nature of time is freedom.

In their inner being each human is given time as a free gift of the Creator. At rock bottom this is the real sore spot about doing time in prison. Humans have a fundamental resentment about their time (freedom) being taken away or being controlled by others. This resentment plays into things even outside the walls of the prison.

Things like the minimum wage and slave labor or even having a boss who is a jerk have this fundamental resentment at their root. The key to surviving this chronic resentment about freedom and time requires that the angry resentful part of ourselves get in touch with the free inner part of ourselves, that is the free being who is continually living in a timeless world. Remembering what life was like before things got out of control helps the better person in us ask the reactive person in us some basic questions like, "How did it become like this in my life?" or, "What would I wish to do better?" or, "How can I survive this without doing something radical to someone?"

These questions cannot really be answered just like that. But the secret and profound value in these questions is not in asking them just once, but in asking them of ourselves on a regular rhythmic basis. Asking questions of ourselves rhythmically in time actually forms a spiritual practice. The sad fact of the matter is that the one who remembers how the world was when things made sense may now be buried under tons of anger so deep as to make us want to do even more radical things. This of course only will bring a reaction from you- know- who.

Then even more craziness will pour into life from the vast torrent of general insanity, which prevails in the world. Experience shows that getting radically reactive against people is not a good option even though it seems very tempting when the world is closing in on us.

So a big task is how to get in contact with the timeless inner being who is constantly remembering how it was before life got unpredictable and then direct them to forget the craziness so that the part of ourselves which is stuck here in this situation filled with danger and abuse and pain can remember how it was before things got so out of control. Of course, this is easier said than done. Usually, all of the crap stored in our soul rises to the surface of the mind as soon as any kind of remembering is done. Then the whole thing starts over, again and again. So the real secret technique is to regularly ask significant, tough questions of ourselves as if we really didn't expect an answer, like we were talking to the wall or to the bed or to the toilet. Ask the hard questions regularly but do not expect any answers. We can form a practice of asking the same questions every day at the same time every day. Asking questions like this is like stretching exercises done before and after a session lifting weights. They can serve as a warm up for the heavy lifting about to be done and a cool down so that we are not totally sore the next day.

Heavy lifting for the soul is the inner work we do by learning to control our mind. We could call the work of controlling the mind, soul gym. The goal of soul gym is to build mental muscles to be able to withstand the abuse and the humiliation and resentment which can make doing time in prison a living hell mentally and emotionally. It is like the emotional difference between just serving your time and being put in solitary. One is a royal pain but the other is dangerous and crazy making. Without working on ourselves, everyday inside the walls can be like a descent into the deepest, loneliest darkness imaginable. Without daily work on ourselves our souls can be pressed flat by the intense burden of time. However, through working on ourselves we can actually form a different, more conscious relationship to time. To get around the darkness of doing time it is useful to develop another relationship to time itself. When things start to hit the fan it is beneficial to remember the fact that our inner being, the one who remembers how things were in the spiritual world, is always living in a timeless realm. If we can get access to that realm and to that inner being when things are creating major disruptions in our soul, then our perception of time begins to change. Actually, time remains as it is, it is our perception of time, which we can change to our benefit.

There are some fundamental things, which keep our inner being, the being of freedom that lives in a timeless way, buried under piles of resentment. The first and foremost is our inability to pay attention and concentrate the mind. A simple exercise to strengthen this is to practice watching the second hand of the clock tick off thirty seconds without thinking of any other thing except watching the second hand tick off the seconds. If no watch is available then counting backward from 30 at one-second intervals is the same. For people with either a lot of time on their hands or who are slaves to a timeclock, this is a precise and very beneficial mental exercise. There are a number of important things, which can be learned from this exercise. The first is that in the beginning it is damn near impossible to do. It is so deceptively simple and yet so difficult to accomplish. The beauty of it is that it is so short and doesn't cost anything and when we fail there is an almost infinite supply of minutes available to continue the work. Well, we could ask, why do an exercise, which is almost impossible to do? Won't it just led to frustration and then more resentment?

The secret of this and any other mental exercise is that the outcome of the exercise is unimportant. Whether we succeed or not is truly irrelevant. No one is giving us a reward for doing the exercise or watching over our shoulder to see that we do it right. The truly great part of concentration exercises is that we are the only one who knows what we are doing. The best attitude for concentrating the mind is that no matter what happens, whether I succeed or I fail, I will just do the same 30 second exercise at the same time the next day. If I manage to get one 30 second exercise done then I am free to try another repetition in the soul gym. After a few reps of the 30-second concentration exercise, as a cool down I can ask myself, "Is there anything today which I can be grateful for?" We should ask this without really expecting an answer. If I think of something to be grateful for then the gratitude will eventually help me to overcome depression. If I cannot think of anything to be grateful for then just asking the question is steadying and cooling for the mind. After asking the question spend a few minutes listening into the silence of timelessness.

Find a time during your day in which it will be easy to do these things at the same time every day. Each day do a few repetitions of the 30-second concentration exercise and then ask the question and listen a little bit into the silence. The whole thing should take about five to ten minutes, total. But it is time well spent. During the whole exercise period no one except yourself is dictating how you should be using your time. It is time spent in complete freedom whether the exercise works or not. The great secret of training the mind is that the time spent doing any mental exercise, successful or not is time spent in complete freedom. This freedom is born out of an impulse in our own soul to take back control of our own minds. The real benefit in this exercise is in remembering daily to ask the question and do the exercise. The forces built up by making many repetitions of this exercise can someday be available to us when our inner peace is threatened by some circumstance, which is out of our control. This exercise can make us free to not have to react.

Once this idea begins to take root in the soul it is usually followed by a wish to actively search for the inner being in us who remembers how it was before things got out of control. No other person, not even "the Man", can trash this quality time which we are spending with ourselves in these exercises. This is true even if the exercise we are attempting to do is a complete disaster. The exercise is working in us even if we only remember to do it without actually doing it. The goal is to try anew each day to form the impulse to develop concentration whether or not the exercise works, or whether we missed it yesterday or even whether or not we can actually ever do it. Buddha said, "Act but do not be attached to the fruits of your actions."

After a month or so a subtle mood comes over the time spent doing the exercise. When we are doing the exercise there is a feeling as if we are having a talk with someone we trust. This is not a big time revelation with light shows and funky smoke and voices speaking to us. It is just a subtle feeling of being in a regular conversation with someone who we know will never lie to us. This feeling is the calling card of the inner being who remembers what it was like before things got crazy in our lives.

When this feeling shows up we can begin to do another very effective exercise to develop a new way seeing the world. We can practice looking at the everyday common things, which are around us in a new way. We practice looking at the bed, the sink, or our clothes and trying each day to notice something that we hadn't seen before about that thing. It helps to keep a list to make sure that every day something different is noticed. When we can no longer notice anything new about the thing we are observing then we can pick another thing to observe. This exercise has a funny effect on time. We can become so absorbed in thinking about and observing common, boring things that time seems to melt away. If this exercise is added to the 30 second exercise and the gratitude exercise and then listening to the silence of timelessness, then a very absorbing practice can result. An exercise like new seeing can open whole worlds to a mind locked shut with bitterness, anger, blaming and resentment. This exercise is fundamentally the kind of activity, which grew into the study of birds, which saved the sanity, and the humanity of the birdman of Alcatraz. Through an exercise like new seeing the soul is led back into having an interest in life and in developing itself through a living, active thinking. After this exercise of new seeing a good question to ask yourself is "How has my life become like this?" Like the gratitude question this question is followed with another session of listening into the silence of timelessness.

With the addition of this practice the total time spent in developing the mind can now be ten or fifteen minutes a day. The ideal would be to spend 15 minutes in the morning before starting any of the day's activities. The sense of freedom in the mind from these exercises when practiced regularly can offset years of crazy living, anger and resentment. Once again it is not the success of a particular practice, which is of value. It is the doing of the practice even when it is failing dismally which moves the mind slowly towards the timeless state of the inner being who remembers.

A final simple exercise which makes the others blend into a seamless whole and gives them much more power is to add a practice of reviewing the day backwards at the end of each day. This is most effective if no judgements are made of anything, which happened during the day. To begin with, simply remembering what you ate for each meal backwards will provide a good start on this one. Start by visualizing dinner then lunch then breakfast. Do not try to remember too much detail but simply glide over each event as if you were watching a movie in reverse. When you encounter something negative try to see it as if you were watching someone else's life and not yours. If dinner was not really edible try to visualize it as if someone else were eating it. Try to make no judgements but simply visualize the facts of what happened in their reverse order.

This takes some practice to do successfully but since we are trying to not let success be the determining factor here, once again it is the effort to do this rhythmically which allows for the most effective practice. This exercise may take ten or fifteen minutes to do in the evening. It is most enlivening and powerful if it is done just as you are going off to sleep. The total time spent each day doing the morning and evening exercises might equal a half an hour. These are 30 minutes in which you yourself are the shaper of your own destiny and the warden of your own experience of time.

People inside the walls understandably feel that they are the only ones doing time. However, among esoteric teachers throughout the ages it has always been felt that most people are doing time in their lives even outside the walls of a prison. We could even say that most people are being done by time. The real prison for most humans whether inside or outside of the walls is in their own minds. The great philosopher Rousseau said "Man is born free, but everywhere he is in chains."

For those inside the physical walls, their own minds must bear the most terrible daily impact of the threats and abuses of the culture of incarceration. However, in the realm of the spirit the inherent freedom of a person's mind cannot be put into a prison. The freedom of the one who remembers how it was before everything went crazy is available to anyone who is willing to control their own thoughts. This requires not a successful practice but a regular practice in order to discipline the mind and strengthen the spirit. Time spent in disciplining the mind every morning can give the soul a sense of purpose even in an environment, which is aimed at seeming purposeless. The fruits of a morning practice are a gradual feeling of hope for the coming day. The hope appears magically where there was nothing but despair and pain. The fruits of a practice continued every evening are that the soul eventually develops an inner strength and repose in the face of life's many trying circumstances. This lends a poise and resolve to the soul, which can help us to overcome many difficulties by helping us to not accelerate die reaction process in threatening situations. With these feelings a person can eventually see that everyone is in the prison of their own minds and belief structures. Whether inmate or guard or warden or governor each person must experience the purging of the soul which is brought on by the bitter wisdom of powerlessness. The bitter wisdom of being in a condition in which others have the power is the greatest and most effective medicine that there is to heal the heart of its tendency to rebel and get crazy. Of course it is the very thing which makes the heart rebel and want to get crazy. This fundamental paradox lies at the root of human freedom and is the secret treasure of meditators the world over. The secret is that you can't put the human spirit in prison.

Eventually the morning and evening rhythms of these practices meet each other in an experience, which the Rosicrucian's called sacred sleep. Sacred sleep brings to birth in human beings the consciousness that can remember how life was before free time was taken away from us and everything became crazy. Sacred sleeping helps us to learn the tough lessons which life must deal out to us without resentment or blaming. In sacred sleep the practices done upon awaking and just before going off into sleep begin to awaken in the soul a sense of belonging to something much larger than the present condition which we find ourselves in. We awaken in the morning with thoughts of how it could be if we had control over our reactions and we go to sleep remembering the events of the day in a mood of serenity. Through inner work and sacred sleeping our soul begins to participate in ever-higher dimensions of freedom even though our body may be bound by walls of societal ignorance and caught up in the furious tides of reaction found in the culture of incarceration.

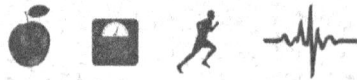

WHAT YOUR DOCTOR DOES NOT WANT YOU TO KNOW

Did you know that Doctors are one of the leading causes of DEATH in the USA? And I'm talking about Doctors in the free world, not just prison doctors.

An article published in the Journal of The American Medical Association (one of the most respected in the industry) shows that in the US there are approximately:

- √ 12,000 deaths per year from unnecessary surgery
- √ 7,000 deaths each year from medication errors in hospitals
- √ 20,000 deaths caused from other errors in hospitals
- √ 80,000 deaths caused annually from infections in hospitals
- √ 106,000 deaths caused annually from adverse effects of medications

This adds up to nearly a quarter of a million people that die each year due to iatrogenic causes (i-at-ro-gen-ic, adj.: induced inadvertently by a physician or surgeon or any medical treatment or diagnostic procedures); third only to heart disease and cancer! (Of course the numbers will vary every year, but you get the idea.)

Four times as many people die in one year from doctors mistakes than died in the entire Vietnam War and more than TEN times the amount of American soldiers that have died in the Iraq war. These are just deaths in hospitalized patients and does not include disabilities and disorders received from iatrogenic causes.

10 HORRIFYING THINGS DOCTORS DON'T TELL YOU!

As a modern culture, we tend to put our faith wholeheartedly in doctors. They're the experts, and more often than not we take their advice without question. But what we don't take into account is that many of these doctors either don't have a clue, or actively withhold information that could be putting your life in jeopardy. And if you think that sounds sensationalist, take a look at these facts—facts that doctors know about but which they conveniently forget to mention.

10. Cancer Isn't Always Cancer

The worst possible outcome of a trip to the doctor is a diagnosis of the Big C. We're so terrified of it that even the word is taboo in some places, and the medical community lives by one maxim: early diagnosis. The earlier you find the cancer, the more easily you can treat it. But such enthusiasm can easily lead to false positives, and treating something that isn't there can be dangerous.

9. Some Vaccines Fail

In 2012, the US saw the worst outbreak of whooping cough since 1955. And that's strange, considering that we've been vaccinating against it for over 50 years. Whooping cough is caused by two types of bacteria, Bordetella pertussis and Bordetella parapertussis, but the vaccine—the DTaP—is only designed to fight the first one, B. Pertussis. Which doesn't seem too bad. Getting rid of half the problem is better than doing nothing, right?

Not quite. In all these years of exclusively pounding away at one of the causes, the second type of bacteria has been flourishing, to the point that receiving the vaccine causes B. parapertussis lung infections to grow 40 times as large as they would normally. And recently, the vaccine has also been less effective on the things it's actually supposed to treat. In 2011, the CDC nearly doubled their recommendations for the vaccine, saying you need three initial shots of DTaP followed by three additional shots if you expect it to work.

That's because vaccines can actually strengthen viruses. They can rewire the human genome (and you can dismiss links to autism as alarmist nonsense) but vaccines can stimulate mutations in the viruses they fight. China found that out in the worst possible way when their Hepatitis B vaccines caused the virus to begin mutating twice as fast as it normally would. We've been seeing the same thing happen with the flu virus—vaccines basically just fuel the virus's instinct to survive.

8. Prescription Drugs Can Cause Diabetes

Type 2 diabetes is caused when your body either doesn't make enough insulin or can't effectively use all the insulin it makes. The result is a buildup of glucose, or sugar, in the bloodstream, which starts damaging nerves and blood vessels over time. About 2.3 million Americans have type 2 diabetes, and the numbers rise every year.

It turns out that some of the most commonly prescribed drugs, like antidepressants, might be causing it. In 2011, there were 46.7 million prescriptions given out to treat depression in the UK alone. When researchers as the University of Southampton looked at the numbers, they found that people who took two of the most common types of antidepressants, SSRIs and tricyclic antidepressants, were twice as likely to develop diabetes. And sure, those findings were released in 2013, but we've known about the link since 2008 and yet millions more are prescribed on a monthly basis.

And it gets worse—some of the most common drugs used to treat ADHD in children can triple the risk of type 2 diabetes. More often than not, that's a lifelong condition, and kids don't even get the choice to refuse.

7. Some Medications Increase Cancer Risk

Now that we've assuaged some of your worries about cancer, let's go ahead and kick everything back up again.

Blood pressure medications can almost triple your risk of aggressive breast cancer. In the US alone, about 58.6 million people take medication for high blood pressure, so you'd think the cancer link would be more well-known.

The study that discovered this relationship looked at 1,763 women with breast cancer. Those who used a particular type of blood pressure medicine—calcium channel blockers—were 2.5 times more likely to develop cancer. The risk is greater in elderly women over the age of 55 and it likely happens because calcium channel blockers prevent cells from dying. If cells can't complete their normal life cycle, they go rogue and become cancerous.

But even that wouldn't be a problem if the medication weren't so grossly over-prescribed. In a review of one hospital, 150 out of 161 doctors prescribed calcium channel blockers to their patients. But how many of those doctors told their patients about the risks? Only eight!

That's a potentially deadly lapse in duty.

6. Aspirin Can Cause Internal Bleeding

One of the more common pieces of advice from doctors is that you should take a low dose of aspirin every day. The idea is that it serves as a maintenance treatment to prevent blood clots, which can cause heart attacks and strokes. But what they don't tell you is the small fact that doing so can trigger massive internal bleeding.

Researchers found out that, out of 10,000 people, a daily dose of aspirin prevented 46 people from dying over the course of 10 years. But they also found that 49 people out of the same 10,000 experienced major internal bleeding, and another 117 started bleeding in their gastrointestinal tract. So there may be some benefits, but there may be an even higher chance that something will go horribly wrong.

On top of that, aspirin doesn't actually work for everyone. Some people have aspirin-related platelets, which negates any positive effect you might get from aspirin. But since we have no way to test for that, doctors never know if they're recommending a dud treatment or not.

5. Heartburn Drugs Have Deadly Side Effects

One of the main problems with medications is that, while they usually do a decent job of treating what they're supposed to treat, they often cause horrible side effects. And even though it's the doctor's job to tell people about those side effects, sometimes that just doesn't happen. For example, proton pump inhibitors, a type of heartburn drug marketed under the brand names Nexium and Prilosec, have been linked to bone decay, birth defects, and an inability to absorb vitamin B12, which can lead to permanent neurological damage.

Despite that, Nexium was the single most prescribed drug in 2012, and in many cases it doesn't even work. It's usually prescribed to treat Barrett's esophagus, which is when excess stomach acid burns the lining of the esophagus, but the pills don't do a thing for the condition. Pediatricians have even started prescribing these meds to infants, even though it's been proven that doing so can actually cause permanent intestinal disorders.

4. "Safe" X-Rays Still Cause Cancer

It's a well-known fact that gamma radiation and X-rays carry the risk of kickstarting cancer. Now, we're constantly exposed to radiation just by being alive, so there's a general guideline for "safe exposure" to X-rays, which the medical profession sticks to when they look for broken bones or give you a mammogram. Radiation is measured in units called sieverts, and every year you're exposed to about 2.4 millisieverts, just from general background radiation; by contrast, a mammogram only gives you about 0.7 millisieverts.

The difference, though, is that medical X-rays pop that radiation into you in the space of minutes, whereas it takes a whole year to absorb your typical background radiation. And it's a huge difference, even with low-radiation "safe" X-rays. In the UK, diagnostic x-rays cause about 700 cases of cancer each year. And it could be even worse than that—some researchers claim that the majority of cancer cases were either caused of aggravated by medical X-rays.

And to top it all off, women who get X-rays when pregnant have been found more likely to give birth to children with cancer. And a CT scan is the go-to diagnostic tool for young children, which, you guessed it, is just another type of X-ray.

3. Doctors Get Paid When You Buy Certain Drugs

Conspiracy theorists aren't shy about proclaiming the evils of Big Pharma. But conspiracy theory is one thing, and documented proof is a whole different beast. When the Harvard Law

School took a closer look, they realized that they didn't have to dig very deep at all to discover that doctors are paid handsomely to prescribe certain drugs, even when those drugs turn out to be harmful.

One of the most publicized cases was Dr. Joseph L. Biederman, who began diagnosing two-year-old toddlers with bipolar disorder and prescribing strong antipsychotics that were never approved by the FDA for children under 10. The manufacturer of the antipsychotics paid him $1.6 million. Then there's Dr. Alan F. Schatzberg, who began prescribing an abortion drug to treat depression—he owned $4.8 million of stock in the company that produced the drug.

And then you have Dr. Charles B. Nemeroff, who received $500,000 to advertise as safe a drug than can cause seizures and paralysis. The fact is, doctors are allowed to prescribe any drug for any illness, no matter what the drug was originally intended to treat. We're not saying all doctors take money to prescribe questionable treatments—but how do you know which ones do?

2. Pandemic Scares Are Over-Hyped

Who can forget the swine flu pandemic in 2009 and 2010? When the World Health Organization called for a state of global emergency, the world went haywire. Lines for the vaccine stretched for blocks, and doctors everywhere told people to seek immediate treatment.

Over the course of about 10 months, pharmaceutical companies raked in about $10.5 billion in 2010 from vaccine sales. Doctors tied to the vaccine's manufacturers were 8.4 times more likely to recommend the vaccine to their patients. And not only recommend they were more likely to publicly hype the dangers of the flu in the media, which immeasurably contributed to the state of panic.

And strangely, doctors who were being paid by pharmaceutical companies were also more likely to volunteer information to the press. That doesn't seem like much of a difference, but it's these quoted experts that we tend to believe in a news article. In the end, about 17,000 people died from swine flu, as opposed to the 46,000 that die every year from the normal flu. Surely the low numbers were due to the mass vaccinations—rather than, say, the fact that the disease was just a common mutation artificially inflated to terror-inducing proportions.

1. Registered Sex Offenders And Violent Criminals

Your doctor doesn't have to disclose his criminal history, and usually that wouldn't be considered a problem. Between the strict admission policies of most medical schools and the vague notion that hospitals probably screen their employees, who would even think to ask? Well, maybe you should.

In November 2013, the UK's General Medical Council, or GMC, released a database with the criminal histories of physicians in the United Kingdom. It turned out that almost 800 practicing doctors held criminal records, including 31 who were arrested for assault and 330 arrested for drunk driving. The rest of them? Crimes range from theft to drug trafficking, and they're under zero obligation to let their patients know about it.

And it's not exactly rare. There's the rapist surgeon working in Miami, and the New York doctor who was caught trying to meet a young boy for sex, and a Scottish physician who had reams of child pornography stored on his computer.

Where "better" for these criminal doctors to work than...a prison, perhaps? Who's really taking care of YOU?

TIPS FOR HOW TO ADVOCATE FOR YOURSELF MEDICALLY

Be the Master of Your Own Paperwork

Keeping good records (1) helps you track your medical condition and your communications with your doctor; (2) provides proof of any shortcoming in your access to proper medical care; and (3) creates a record that you have followed the prison's rules for solving problems and the courts' requirement that you "exhaust all remedies" before filing a lawsuit, if you choose to do so.

A. Keep Copies of Your Prison Records

B. It is very important to keep all copies of all documents related to the problem you are trying to resolve. If you don't already have them, you may wish to request copies of your medical or administrative complaint records from the prison. Important documents to keep include medical records; x-rays; co-pays; administrative grievances; letters to family members, prison officials, and advocates about your medical condition or care; request forms; etc. If possible, make a second copy of these documents and send them to someone you trust outside of the prison, such as a family member or friend.

C. You can request your medical records be provided to you or anyone of your choice by filling out and filing an "Authorization For Release Of Protected Health Information" form (in CA it's form CDCR 7385). We recommend that you complete this form and share it with a trusted friend on the outside before you have any medical emergencies. You can limit which records are released by specifying a time period or medical issue. That person can turn the document into the prison immediately if they wish to access your records now, or they can hold on to it for later use. Prison staff will be much more likely to speak with your family member or friend about your medical care if they have this signed release.

D. Keep a Diary

E. It can also be helpful to keep a journal or medical diary of your experiences. Write down as much detail as you can, such as date and time of the event or appointment, names and positions of people involved, medications prescribed or taken, symptoms experienced, forms submitted, etc. For recording symptoms, it is important to describe them precisely and accurately. This helps you obtain proper diagnosis and treatment, as well as to record a timeline of your condition. Constructing a timeline of the problem and your attempts to resolve it can help you better track your health and will make it much easier to file an effective grievance and, should you choose, a lawsuit. If possible, it is a good idea to periodically make copies of this journal (even handwritten copies) and send them to someone whom you trust.

F. Show Prior, Outside Medical Records to Prison Medical Officials

G. If you had a medical condition before entering the prison, you may be able to provide prison medical officials with records of your previous care. This can be helpful in convincing the prison to continue the same type of level or care. To do this, you will need to call or write your outside medical care provider to request a copy of that office's medical records release form. A family member or supporter on the outside may be able to help you obtain this form. Complete, sign, and return the form to the outside medical provider's office. You can limit which records are released by specifying a time period or medical issue. The outside medical office will then mail or fax your records to the location that you requested. If you wish, you may ask that your medical records be released directly to your prison doctor or the prison's Chief Medical Officer. However, you may wish to have the records sent to a family member outside of the prison so that they can make a copy before providing them to the prison doctors.

H. File Administrative Grievances

I. Filing a "Request For Interview" form seeks to resolve an issue through scheduling informal interviews with staff, asking a question of a staff member, or requesting items or services. Staff members sometimes view this form as less than confrontational than a grievance and can be more likely to respond in a helpful way.

If your request is unclear, staff may refuse to answer your question or respond productively. When filing the form, your request should clearly state the issue and the service you would like and specify any documents attached to the form. Once you file the "Request For Interview" form, a staff member is required to respond to it. If you do not like the response you receive, you can file a second Request with the staff member's supervisor.

Once you've tried the more informal "Request For Interview" route, you may consider submitting a formal grievance form that documents your complaints. On this form, you can specify your issues, document problems, and request certain solutions from the prison staff. All incarcerated people have the right to file a grievance on any issue or concern related to confinement and to request relief. Most prisons have a time limit when filing a grievance, so make sure you meet the time limit set by your prison.

Although formal grievances often do not result in the desired response, following the proper grievance procedure shows that you have attempted to follow the prison's rules for resolving problems. Additionally, if you ever try to file a law suit, the first step is to file a grievance to demonstrate that you have "exhausted your administrative remedies."

When writing your grievance, be sure to clearly describe your situation. The following questions are to guide your writing:

- √ What are your condition(s) and/or symptom(s)?
- √ When did each event occur?
- √ Who was involved?
- √ What have you done so far to achieve solutions?

Providing evidence to support your claim can be very helpful. If you attach any proof, such as copies and forms, specify that you are including documents and indicate which ones.

You may also want to consider being interviewed by a staff member, as it will allow the prison to ask you any clarifying questions that can further support your grievance.

If your grievance is successfully submitted and processed, the form will be given a log number. Sometimes, however, prison staff "misplaces" a grievance before you receive the log number. To create evidence that you submitted a grievance, you can submit a "Request" form along with your submission of your original grievance, and if possible within the timeline, make a copy of the grievance for your records. On your "Request" you will want to indicate what the grievance said, when you submitted it, and which member of the prison staff is responsible for delivering it. That is, a "Request" form can be used to request that a specific staff member turns in your grievance and it can act as a receipt for your grievance, especially if you're in a prison where the "Request" forms have to be signed by an officer. With these two steps, even if you are not given a log number for your grievance, you will have evidence that you submitted it because you will have both your own copy of the grievance and your goldenrod/copy of the "Request" form that you attached to it. This can help you to comply with the time limits for filing a grievance or to track failures of prison staff to log the grievance.

A. Follow Up Verbal Communications with Written Communications

If you or your outside supporter verbally speaks with someone regarding your problem, it is a good idea to follow up these conversations with a brief letter in order to create a record of your efforts to resolve the issue. For example, if your outside supporter calls the prison and speaks to an officer about your situation, ask them to write a follow-up letter or e-mail to the prison official summarizing the conversation. You can then ask your outside supporter to send you a copy for your records, and you can ask them to keep a copy for their own records. See the example below.

Dear Officer Smith,

I am writing to follow up on our telephone conversation, which happened on April 3, 2018, at approximately 2:30pm, regarding my son, John Doe, XI2345. During this call, I notified you that my son has been waiting three weeks for the results of his chest x-ray. You told me you would look into this matter and try to help him get an appointment with his yard doctor. Thank you for your attention to this matter. If you have further questions, please contact me at (916) 911-1515.

Sincerely,

Jane Doe

Advocating To Prison Officials

You and your outside supporters, whether they are family or concerned friends, may find it helpful to contact prison administrators on your behalf. Contacting prison officials puts them on notice that you are experiencing a problem and that they have a responsibility to address your concerns. As you probably know, incarcerated people sometimes report that they suffer retaliation from staff as a result of speaking about the violation of their rights. Use your discretion to determine whether this is the most effective action in your case.

Whenever you or your supporters contact officials about your condition, keep copies of the correspondence or follow-up letters summarizing and phone conversations with these individuals. If you are keeping a medical diary, make sure to keep track of all contacts with officials, including dates of contact/call/ correspondence, name of the person contacted, and a brief summary of the conversation.

A. Contact the Office of the Ombudsman

The Office of the Ombudsman reports directly to the Secretary of your state prison. The Ombudsman's mission states that the office works independently as an intermediary to provide individuals with a confidential avenue to address complaints and resolve issues at the lowest possible level and proposes policy and procedural changes when systemic issues are identified.

When contacting the Office of the Ombudsman, provide as much of the following information as possible:

- √ Your name and prison number
- √ Location of prison
- √ A phone number, if possible
- √ Brief description of the situation
- √ The log numbers of relevant grievances
- √ An overview of what had been done to resolve the issue

You can also contact other prison officials. You may consider writing directly to your prison's warden of chief medical officer as well.

Get Help From Outside The Prison System

You and your outside supporters, whether they are family or concerned friends, may find it helpful to contact other government officials on your behalf. Contacting other government officials can sometimes help because they may be able to influence the prison administration As you probably know, incarcerated people sometimes report that they suffer retaliation from staff as a result of speaking out about a violation of their rights, so use your discretion to determine whether this is the most effective action in your case.

As always, if you decide to contact officials, be sure to keep copies of any correspondence and write follow-up letters.

Here are Some questions to consider in an effective advocacy letter:

- √ What is the nature of the problem?
- √ How long has this problem been happening?
- √ How is the problem affecting you? Why is this problem creating a difficult situation for you?
- √ What attempts have you made to solve the problem and how has the prison responded to your efforts?
- √ What do you want to happen in order to resolve the problem?
- √ Do you have copies of any supporting documents that will help to further explain your situation?

A. Contact the Office of the Inspector General

Office of the Inspector General (OIG), which is independent from the Department of Corrections (DOC), was established to investigate problems in the DOC. They describe themselves as being responsible for "rigorously investigating and auditing the DOC to uncover criminal conduct, administrative wrongdoing, poor management practices, waste, fraud, and other abuses by staff, supervisors, and management." In order "to bring public transparency into the operation of the state's correctional system, the OIG posts the findings of every audit and large-scale investigation on their website." The OIG does not provide legal advice.

Complaints are handled in one of the following ways. (1) Your complaint may be referred back to the DOC Office of Internal Affairs if they have not previously investigated the issue. (2) Even if the complaint has been investigated by the DOC'S Internal Affairs, the OIG may still send the complaint back again for further investigation. (3) The OIG may investigate the complaint directly. (4) The complaint may be referred to law enforcement authorities if the complaint involves criminal misconduct. (5) If the OIG finds after a preliminary review that there is insufficient evidence to support your claim, your inquiry may be closed without further action

The OIG also claims that it will investigate allegations of retaliation against persons who have filed complaints with their office. However, it operates limited resources and cannot assure anyone's protection from retaliatory acts.

California prisoners may contact the following:

Office of the Inspector General
Placerville Road, Suite 110
Sacramento, CA 95827
(916) 830-3600
Toll-free: (800) 700-5952

B. Contact Elected Representatives

You or your supporters may also write to member of the state legislature, who are responsible for overseeing the DOC. You will have to find the appropriate person to contact in your state.

File Complaints with State Medical licensing Agencies

If you have concerns about specific prison health staff, you may consider filing complaints with the appropriate state licensing boards. These agencies are designed to monitor medical professionals in order to protect the public (which includes incarcerated people) and ensure that medical professionals are providing care consistent with their licenses. There is no guarantee that by filing a complaint you will get the specific care you desire or that the medical staff person will be reprimanded. However, by filing with the appropriate board, you are creating a record and lodging an official complaint with outside state agencies about the difficulties incarcerated people experience getting adequate medical care at your prison (where you are housed). This can help other prisoners later. You will have to research the appropriate agency's address in your state.

NOTE:

The following Chapters are excerpts from The Jailhouse Lawyer's Manual. References have been omitted in this version. For a complete copy of The Jailhouse Lawyer's Manual visit: jlm.law.columbia.edu

Columbia University School of Law

435 West 116th Street
New York, NY 10027
212-854-1601

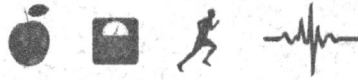

YOUR RIGHT TO
ADEQUATE MEDICAL CARE

A. Introduction

The U.S. Constitution requires prison officials to provide all state and federal prisoners as well as pretrial detainees (people in jail waiting for trial) with adequate medical care. If you think your right to medical care might have been violated, this Chapter will help you determine whether you have a legal claim for which you can get relief.

Part B of this Chapter explains your right to medical care under the U.S. Constitution and state law. Part C provides specific examples of when you may have medical care rights. Some examples include: when you have a diagnosed medical condition, when you want an elective procedure (a voluntary, non-emergency operation), when you need psychiatric care, when you are exposed to second-hand smoke, and when you need dental care. Part D is about special medical issues for women prisoners, including the right to basic medical and gynecological care, abortions, and accommodations for pregnant women. Part E talks about your right to receive information about your medical treatment before being treated and your right to keep your medical information confidential in prison. Part F explains the possible ways to seek relief in state and federal courts if your rights have been violated.

This Chapter will focus on federal law and some New York state laws. If you are a state prisoner, your right to adequate medical care might also be protected by your state's statutes, regulations, and tort law. The New York Correction Law and the Official Compilation of Codes, Rules, and Regulations of the State of New York explain the right to adequate medical care for New York state prisoners. If you are in prison in another state, be sure to research the law in that state.

The rights of prisoners with mental illnesses, infectious diseases, or disabilities present special issues not included in this chapter.

It is important that you speak up about any medical issue that you have. If you end up going to court to pursue your right to adequate medical care, a judge will ask for evidence that you tried to obtain medical care in a variety of ways within the prison first. Usually, you must prove "exhaustion" by showing that you went through the grievance procedures of your prison system before going to court. Also, it is a good idea to record all of your requests for medical care and complaints to guards and medical professionals. A record of your requests and complaints can help prove that prison officials ignored your medical needs, which can be important if you bring a claim of "deliberate indifference" (discussed in Part B(1)). Keeping a record will also allow you to show that prison officials were aware of your medical problems (the "subjective component," discussed in Part B(1)(b)). In summary, be sure to tell the prison officials around you about your health concerns as soon as they come up, and keep a log of everything you did to get the medical care you need.

If, after reading this Chapter, you think you are not receiving adequate medical care, you should first try to protect your rights through the administrative grievance procedures that your prison has set up for grievances (complaints). Courts are likely to dismiss your case if you do not "exhaust" (use up) all of the options available through your institution first. To learn more about inmate grievance procedures and the exhaustion requirement.

B The Right to Adequate Medical Care

1. Constitutional Law

The Eighth Amendment of the Constitution protects prisoners from cruel and unusual punishment. In 1976, the Supreme Court said in Estelle v. Gamble that a prison staff's "deliberate indifference" to the serious medical needs of prisoners is cruel and unusual punishment forbidden by the Eighth Amendment. Thus, if prison officials treated your serious medical needs with "deliberate indifference," they violated your constitutional right to be free from cruel and unusual punishment.

You must prove two things to show that prison officials treated your serious medical needs with "deliberate indifference" (and therefore violated your constitutional rights). You must first prove that your medical needs were sufficiently serious (the "objective" part). Second, you must prove that prison officials knew about and ignored "an excessive risk to your health or safety" (the "subjective" part). Since deciding Estelle, courts have tried to clarify how prisoners can prove these two things. This Chapter explains each part separately below.

Note that the Constitution does not guarantee comfortable prisons; prison conditions may be "restrictive and even harsh." However, the medical care you receive should meet an acceptable standard of care in terms of modern medicine and beliefs about human decency.

(a) The Objective Part: Sufficiently Serious Medical Need

To establish the first part (the "objective" part) of an Eighth Amendment claim based on prison officials' deliberate indifference to your medical needs, you must show that your medical needs were sufficiently serious. Courts define serious medical need as "one that has been diagnosed by a physician as mandating treatment or one that is so obvious that even a lay person would easily recognize the necessity of a doctor's attention." To decide if a medical need is serious, the Second Circuit (which governs New York, Connecticut, and Vermont) considers several factors including, but not limited to, the following:

(1) whether a reasonable doctor or patient would perceive the medical need in question as "important and worthy of comment or treatment,"

(2) whether the medical condition significantly affects daily activities, and

(3) whether "chronic and substantial pain" exists.

Under the Prison Litigation Reform Act (PLRA), a medical need is only sufficiently serious if it involves physical injury. For example, in one case a patient with HIV was denied his medication for several days.

His illness was clearly serious, but it was determined that missing a few days of medication caused him no physical harm. Generally, though, if your medical condition is extremely painful, your medical need could be considered sufficiently serious. For example, in Hemmings v. Gorczyk, prison medical staff diagnosed a ruptured tendon as a sprain and refused for two months to send the prisoner to a specially trained doctor; however, the Second Circuit later found that the prisoner's condition was painful enough to be sufficiently serious. The general trend seems to be that the courts will consider injuries to be sufficiently serious if they significantly change a prisoner's quality of life. The Second Circuit has held that the denial of care has to be objectively serious enough to create a condition of urgency—a situation where death, permanent injury, or extreme pain appears likely to occur or has occurred. Other circuits have similarly high requirements for what counts as a serious injury or denial of care.

Recent court decisions have emphasized pain and disability when evaluating prisoners' medical needs. Drug or alcohol withdrawal is a serious medical need. Transsexualism or gender identity disorder (GID) has been recognized as a serious medical need in some cases. There might also be a serious cumulative effect from the repeated denial of care for minor problems. Where medical treatment is delayed, courts look at whether the effects of the delay or interruption—not the underlying medical condition—are objectively serious enough to present an Eighth Amendment question. Whether a medical need is serious" should be determined on a case-by-case basis and not only by a prison's serious need list. Prisons are not allowed to have a rigid list of serious medical needs without allowing some flexibility in individual prisoner evaluations. In addition, a treatment that a hospital or prison considers to be elective (voluntary and non-emergency) may still be a serious medical need.

(b) The Subjective Part (Prison Officials Knew of and Disregarded a Risk)

After proving that your medical need was sufficiently serious, you must also prove that prison officials purposely allowed you to go without necessary medical help. This is the second part of your Eighth Amendment claim (the "subjective" part). It is difficult to prove that prison officials knew about your serious medical need and meant to deny you necessary medical care. Part 3 of this Chapter explains the different ways you can prove that prison officials knew about and disregarded your serious medical need.

You have to prove two things to show that a prison official knew about and disregarded your serious medical need. First, the official has to have known facts that could have shown or proven that your health was in danger. Second, after the official was aware of the threat to your health, the official must actually have believed that your health was in danger. Courts have struggled to determine exactly how much knowledge a prison official must have in order to meet this standard. In general, the standard is very high, as you will see from the cases discussed below.

2. Courts Defer to Prison Health Officials' Medical Judgment

It can be difficult to win a deliberate indifference claim when the prisoner and the prison officials have different opinions about what medical treatment is best for the prisoner. For example, a prison doctor might give a prisoner X medication for his medical condition, but the prisoner believes Y medication is better. As long as both X and Y medications are approved for treating the prisoner's disease, the prisoner will probably not win in court because the court will defer to (respect) the prison doctor's professional medical judgment that X was best for the prisoner. Even if you have your own outside doctor who says something different from the prison doctor, prison officials may rely upon their own doctor's judgment.

A difference in opinion over medical treatment, or even an error in medical judgment, is not likely to win a case. But that does not mean that you can never challenge a prison doctor's decisions; a medical professional's erroneous treatment decision can lead to deliberate indifference liability if the decision was made in the absence of professional judgment. Thus, the prison health official must actually use legitimate medical judgment.

While general prison medical procedures might be fine for most prisoners, forcing some prisoners to abide by those procedures might constitute deliberate indifference to those particular prisoners' medical conditions. For example, the Second Circuit has held that a statewide prison medical policy that denied Hepatitis C treatment to prisoners with any substance abuse problems within the past two years might lead to deliberate indifference if applied to a particular prisoner. The prison followed the policy despite "the unanimous, express, and repeated recommendations of plaintiff's treating physicians, including prison physicians," to depart from the policy in the plaintiff's case.

3. Common Types of Deliberate Indifference

Listed below are some common situations in which courts have found prison medical staff to be deliberately indifferent to prisoners' serious medical needs. They include:

(1) Ignoring obvious conditions;
(2) Failing to provide treatment for diagnosed conditions;
(3) Failing to investigate enough to make an informed judgment;
(4) Delaying treatment;
(5) Interfering with access to treatment;
(6) Making medical decisions based on non-medical factors; and
(7) Making a medical judgment so bad it falls below professional medical standards.

(a) Ignoring Obvious Conditions

One way to prove that prison officials were deliberately indifferent to your serious medical needs is to show that the problem was so obvious that they should have been aware of a serious and substantial risk to your health. Even if the prison official did not notice the risk (injury, disease, physical condition, etc.), the official can be held liable if the risk to the prisoner was very obvious. In Brice v. Virginia Beach Correction Center, the court found that a prison guard may have ignored a serious and substantial risk (and thus may have been deliberately indifferent) when a prisoner received no medical care after a fight, even though the prisoner's mouth was bleeding and he complained of horrible pain. In Phelps v. Kapnolas, the court said that a prison official disregarded an obvious risk by putting a prisoner in solitary confinement with inadequate food when the official should have known such a small amount would cause pain and distress.

In Phillips v. Roane County, Tenn., the Sixth Circuit ruled that correctional officers at the Roane County Jail were responsible for the death of a female prisoner. Medical examiners testified that the prisoner died from untreated diabetes. According to the court, prison authorities were aware of her deteriorating condition during the two weeks before her death, as she complained of vomiting, chest pain, fatigue, nausea, and constipation. Their failure to take her to a hospital was considered deliberate indifference to her medical needs.

The risk to the prisoner must be very obvious because courts frequently find that the prison official is not responsible when he did not know enough about a prisoner's condition. In Reeves v. Collins, prison guards were not liable when they forced a prisoner to work, even after he had warned them that he had a previous back injury, was doubled over, and was complaining of excessive pain. He was later taken to the infirmary and diagnosed with a double hernia. The court decided that the guards had not disregarded a substantial risk because even if the guards had checked the prisoner's medical records (which they did not), they would not have learned of the prisoner's history of hernias due to a mistake in the records.

In Sanderfer v. Nichols, the court found that a prison doctor was not responsible for her failure to treat a patient's hypertension after he died of a heart attack. Although the plaintiff's medical records included a history of hypertension, the doctor was not liable because the plaintiff complained only of bronchitis when he met with the doctor. The prisoner never told the doctor that hypertension was a problem for him, and his blood pressure later was checked on three occasions and was normal. This means that it is very important that you speak up and tell prison officials about your health problems.

If you are making an Eighth Amendment claim that prison officials were deliberately indifferent to your serious medical needs, you should tell the court all of the reasons your medical needs should have been obvious to prison officials.

(b) Failing to Provide Treatment for Diagnosed Conditions

The easiest way to establish prison officials' deliberate indifference to your medical needs is to prove that a prison doctor diagnosed you with a serious medical condition and prescribed treatment for you, but you never received that treatment. In Hudson v. McHugh, the prisoner was transferred from a halfway house to a county jail but was not given his medicine.[42] After eleven days without it, despite repeated requests to the jail's medical personnel, he had a seizure. The Seventh Circuit held that this was the most obvious kind of case in which a prisoner could raise a claim: This is the prototypical case of deliberate indifference, an inmate with a potentially serious problem repeatedly requesting medical aid, receiving none, and then suffering a serious injury. It is important to note that not only was the prisoner denied his medicine, but he also requested it several times before he became dangerously ill. If you are making an Eighth Amendment claim that prison officials were deliberately indifferent to your serious medical needs, you should tell the court about your requests for medical treatment to show that officials knew of your needs.

(c) Failing to Investigate Enough to Make an Informed Judgment

If a court finds that prison officials never made an informed decision about your medical care, you may be able to establish an Eighth Amendment claim of deliberate indifference to your medical needs on this basis. Prison officials may not have made an informed decision about your medical care if, in response to your complaints of a medical problem, they did not properly treat you, did not investigate the cause of your medical condition, did not order diagnostic tests, did not send you to a specialist, or did not consult your medical records before stopping medication.

(d) Delaying Treatment

You can also establish an Eighth Amendment claim of deliberate indifference to your serious medical needs by proving that (1) prison officials delayed your treatment, and (2) that delay caused serious consequences. Whether or not to delay treatment is sometimes an issue of professional opinion, but some delays are very serious and may prove deliberate indifference. If you suffered from a serious injury that prison officials knew about, but you had to wait a very long time before getting medical treatment, you may be able to bring a claim. Denial of or delay in access to medical personnel, or in providing treatment, can be deliberate indifference. In determining whether or not a delay constitutes deliberate indifference, two factors are taken into account:

(1) the seriousness of the prisoner's medical need, and

(2) whether the delay was objectively serious enough to present an Eighth Amendment question.

Remember that prison officials may have had a valid reason for delaying your non-emergency medical treatment. For example, if no prison official who could properly take care of your non-emergency medical needs was on duty, delaying your treatment is probably justified.

Security concerns may also justify denying your request for a particular medical treatment. For instance, in Schmidt v. Odell, the court rejected the plaintiff's claim that failure to provide him with a wheelchair was a constitutional violation. The court found that having a wheelchair among the jail's population could pose a legitimate security risk. The court concluded that this was sufficient to show that the refusal to provide a wheelchair did not alone violate the Eighth Amendment. However, the court noted that the prison's delay in providing a shower chair appears to have resulted not only in the unnecessary infliction of pain, but also in a needless indignity that a jury could find was inconsistent with the Eighth Amendment.

Even when there is no apparent reason for delay in treatment, a court might not find that officials acted with deliberate indifference if the delay does not cause a great deal of harm. In Smith v. Carpenter, the court said that it was proper for a jury to consider the fact that a prisoner did not suffer any bad effects after officials refused to give him treatment for his HIV-related illness for periods of five and seven days; the jury found no deliberate indifference. In Jolly v. Badgett, the prisoner had epilepsy, a condition that causes seizures and high blood pressure. He took medication to prevent the life-threatening consequences of this disease, but officials refused to allow the prisoner to leave his cell to get water to take his medication until two hours after his prescribed time. The court found that officials did not act with deliberate indifference because there was no evidence that the officials knew the delay would have a dangerous effect.

In general, if there is a legitimate reason for a delay in your treatment, or if you cannot prove officials knew that the treatment needed to be given to you immediately, you will have a hard time establishing deliberate indifference on the basis of delayed treatment.

(e) Interfering with Access to Treatment

You can also establish an Eighth Amendment claim of deliberate indifference to your serious medical needs by showing that prison officials interfered with your ability to obtain medical treatment. Prison guards and/or prison medical staff can prevent prisoners from getting treatment in many different ways, including:

(1) Denying you access to medical specialists who are qualified to address your health problem;

(2) Allowing you to see a specialist but then refusing to carry out the specialist's recommendations (or refusing to carry out the recommendations of a specialist who directed treatment before you were incarcerated); or

(3) Refusing to carry out or simply ignoring medical orders.

For example, in Brown v. Coleman, the court found deliberate indifference because, although the prison medical staff repeatedly recommended surgery for a prisoner, officials with no medical training ignored the recommendations. In Martinez v. Mancusi, the court found that the prisoner could bring a claim against prison officials who had used force to remove him from a hospital where he was recovering from leg surgery. Prison officials ignored the doctor's instructions that the prisoner could not walk and removed the prisoner, who was partially paralyzed, without the doctor's permission. This caused the surgery to be unsuccessful. The prisoner was also denied the pain medication his surgeon prescribed him and thus was left in constant pain. In Woodall v. Foti, a prisoner with suicidal tendencies had received treatment for manic depression before being incarcerated. The prisoner's diagnosis was confirmed by the prison doctor. The prisoner claimed his condition worsened when he was denied treatment by the sheriff, who placed him in solitary confinement. On appeal, the court found that if these facts were true, the sheriff's actions could establish deliberate indifference because he interfered with the prisoner's access to medical treatment.

Refusing to treat a prisoner unless the prisoner complies with an official's order can also be considered deliberate indifference. In Harrison v. Barkley, a prison dentist refused to fill a prisoner's cavity unless the prisoner allowed the dentist to pull another one of the prisoner's teeth because the policy of the prison was to pull teeth that were in poor condition. Although the tooth was rotten, the prisoner did not want it removed because it was not painful and he only had a few teeth left. The court said that in a situation like this one, the dentist's actions constituted deliberate indifference. Similarly, in Benter v. Peck, a district court in Iowa found that doctors treating prisoners have a responsibility to provide them the medical care that they need. In that case, the doctor had allowed the prison to withhold eyeglasses from a prisoner who could not function without them in order to force him to pay for the glasses. The court held that withholding the prescription glasses from the prisoner rose to the standard of deliberate indifference.

(f) Making Medical Decisions Based on Non-Medical Factors

If the prison health staff is making medical decisions about you based on non-medical factors, you may also be able to establish an Eighth Amendment claim of deliberate indifference to your serious medical needs. Prisons should not decide what medical treatment you get based on factors like the prison's lack of staff or lack of interpreters, the prison's budgetary restrictions, because you are about to be released, or because they want to punish you. In particular, widespread "deficiencies in staffing, facilities, or procedures that make unnecessary suffering inevitable" may support a finding of deliberate indifference. In other words, you can establish that prison officials were deliberately indifferent to your medical needs even if they ignored your needs because of problems that were part of the prison system (its staffing, facilities, or other non-medical policies). Interestingly, a San Francisco judge refused to send a convicted robber to jail, citing the poor medical care the man would receive and equating a prison sentence to a death sentence. While this was an extremely unusual situation, the case law may still help you develop a lawsuit based on problems that are affecting everyone's medical care at your prison.

(g) Medical Judgment So Bad It's Not Medically Acceptable

You also can establish that prison officials were deliberately indifferent to your serious medical needs if you believe that your prison's health staff is making medical decisions that are so bad that no trained health professional would ever make the same decisions. For example, in 2004, a federal court in California ordered a prison to arrange for a medical evaluation of a prisoner's eligibility for a liver transplant. Prison officials had refused to allow the evaluation, but the prisoner would die without a transplant. The court stated that the prison's failure to identify any alternative treatment that would save the prisoner's life supported the prisoner's deliberate indifference claim. The court noted that:

In order to prevail on a claim involving choices between alternative courses of treatment, a prisoner must show that the course of treatment the doctors chose was medically unacceptable in light of the circumstances and that they chose this course in conscious disregard of an excessive risk to plaintiff's health.

A medically unacceptable treatment may be "an easier and less effective treatment" or simply no treatment at all. Showing that prison health staff failed to follow professional medical standards or prison medical care procedures can help you make this deliberate indifference claim. These standards or protocols can serve as evidence that the prison official knew of the risk posed by particular symptoms or conditions and deliberately ignored that risk.

4. Medical Negligence

(a) Medical Negligence Is Not Unconstitutional

You cannot win a federal constitutional claim of deliberate indifference by alleging only that prison medical staff acted negligently, no matter how often or repeatedly they were negligent. However, you still may be able to make a state tort claim of negligence, which is described in the next Subsection. Negligence is when a person fails to exercise care that a "reasonable person" would exercise to protect someone at risk. Medical negligence is often called medical malpractice. Again, the Eighth Amendment does not protect prisoners from medical malpractice.

At one time, negligence was grounds for liability. After the Supreme Court's holding in Farmer v. Brennan, however, mere negligence—even repeated negligence—cannot by itself constitute deliberate indifference. Therefore, in a class action suit brought by prisoners in Ohio, the court held that if the prisoners could only prove the prison doctor was repeatedly negligent in his treatment, but not that he was "subjectively aware of a substantial risk of serious harm," then the prisoner had not stated an Eighth Amendment claim. Even if it is possible that an official's action led to the death of a prisoner, negligence alone is not enough to bring a federal constitutional claim. Repeated acts of negligence can be evidence that a prison official is ignoring a substantial risk, but acts of negligence by themselves, without any other claim, cannot count as deliberate indifference.

(b) State Law Negligence Claims Are Possible

If you believe that you were injured because prison medical staff acted negligently, you cannot make an Eighth Amendment deliberate indifference claim, but you can still make a negligence claim under state law. To prove negligence under state law, you must prove that (1) the defendant (your prison) owed a duty of care to you; and (2) that this duty was "breached," meaning that the prison was responsible for some aspect of your well-being and did not honor its responsibility. Therefore, you must ask whether the prison's medical practitioner did for you what a reasonable health professional would have done for you in the same circumstances.

You can find many of the duties a prison owes its prisoners listed in state laws. Thus, a New York prisoner could use the state corrections law to prove that New York prisons have a duty to "provide reasonable and adequate medical care to the prisoners." State case law also provides clear definitions of what duties a prison owes its prisoners. In New York, in order to prove a medical malpractice claim, the prisoner must prove a departure from accepted practice and that this departure was the "proximate cause" of the injury. To prove proximate cause, you must show that the injury would not have occurred without the departure from accepted practice. The court of claims also recognizes medical negligence as a cause of action. A state may be liable for ministerial neglect if employees fail to comply with the prison's own administrative procedures for providing medical care to prisoners. If you want to make a state tort claim of medical negligence or medical malpractice

C. Specific Health Care Rights

This Part covers different situations in which you may have a right to medical treatment and includes examples of cases that might be useful to you. If you have specific questions about the rights of prisoners with mental illnesses or infectious diseases, make sure you also look at Chapter 29 of the JLM, Special Issues for Prisoners with Mental Illness and Chapter 26 of the JLM, Infectious Diseases: AIDS, Hepatitis, and Tuberculosis in Prisons. If you need to learn more about disability discrimination.

1. Treatment for Diagnosed Conditions

To decide whether or not you have an Eighth Amendment claim for lack of treatment for diagnosed medical illnesses and conditions, there are several things you must consider. As discussed above, you must prove both the objective and subjective parts of deliberate indifference. This involves proving that the medical condition was sufficiently serious and proving that prison officials knew about the risk to your health and ignored it.

In the following examples, courts found that diagnosed medical conditions were sufficiently serious. In Montalvo v. Koehler, the court found that a prison's failure to provide shower and sleeping facilities to a prisoner confined to a wheelchair was sufficiently serious because it posed a risk of serious bodily injury to the prisoner. Also, in Koehl v. Dalsheim, a court found that prison officials were deliberately indifferent when they confiscated a prisoner's eyeglasses. The double vision, headaches, and severe pain that the prisoner experienced without his eyeglasses were sufficiently serious. Failure to treat a serious hip condition requiring surgery, an infected and impacted wisdom tooth, and a hernia have all been found to establish a prison's deliberate indifference to prisoners' serious medical needs.

The following are examples of harm that the courts did not consider to be sufficiently serious. In Holmes v. Fell, the court held that a prisoner's allergic reaction to a tuberculosis test, which caused swelling and a scar on the prisoner's arm, did not meet the sufficiently serious standard. In fact, simple exposure to tuberculosis does not meet the standard when there is no reason to believe that the prisoner will actually catch the disease. In McGann v. Coombe, the court held that prison officials were not deliberately indifferent when they refused to provide orthopedic footwear for the arthritis and gout in a prisoner's feet, but instead prescribed medication for the condition that was causing the foot problems. In addition, the Eighth Amendment is not violated when prison officials refuse to treat penile warts or an old injury that has healed but still causes pain.

2. Elective Procedures

Generally, you will not be able to win on a claim that prison officials violated your Eighth Amendment rights based on their refusal to perform an elective procedure on you. An elective procedure is an optional procedure that you would benefit from but that is not immediately necessary for your survival or relative well-being. Remember that the Supreme Court has held that the Constitution does not promise comfortable prisons and that conditions may be restrictive and even harsh.

However, prison officials are not allowed to call a necessary procedure "elective" just to avoid having to provide it. Furthermore, if your condition gives you continual pain or discomfort for a long period of time, you may be able to bring a claim that your condition is sufficiently serious to warrant an elective procedure, even though the condition may not require immediate attention. Lengthy delays in providing prisoners with elective surgery for certain medical conditions can be unacceptable. Courts seem to recognize that there are some situations that, while not serious enough to be considered emergencies, are too serious to be considered elective; however, you may have to get a court order before you are allowed to be treated in such a situation.

3. Exposure to Second-Hand Smoke

Prisoners have the right to be free from exposure to excessive second-hand smoke. Courts previously rejected prisoners' claims of cruel and unusual punishment resulting from exposure to environmental tobacco smoke (ETS) because plaintiffs had not yet suffered serious injuries. However, in Helling v. McKinney, the Supreme Court rejected the argument that "only deliberate indifference to current serious health problems of inmates is actionable under the Eighth Amendment" by comparing forced exposure to ETS to live electrical wires or communicable diseases. The Court concluded that prison officials may violate the Eighth Amendment's prohibition of cruel and unusual punishment if they deliberately expose prisoners to high levels of ETS.

To satisfy the objective part of the Eighth Amendment under Helling, you will have to show you are exposed to ETS levels that "pose an unreasonable risk of serious damage to your future health" in a way that violates contemporary standards of decency. To obtain an injunction against further ETS exposure, you do not need an actual physical injury to show an Eighth Amendment violation.

Note that claiming prison officials are deliberately indifferent to the risk of future harm is different from claiming deliberate indifference to current harm. You can claim that ETS exposure affects your current health, but you have to prove you have a serious medical need made worse by the exposure. In Talal v. White, the Sixth Circuit found that a state prison violated the objective component of the Helling test by forcing a non-smoking prisoner with a serious medical need to share a cell with a prisoner who smoked. However, the non-smoking prisoner had to provide a lot of evidence: (1) he documented that he suffered from ETS allergy, sinus problems, and dizziness and (2) he showed that the prison medical staff had recommended that he have a non-smoking cell partner. Note two issues relevant to the subjective standard of deliberate indifference: whether your prison has adopted a smoking policy and how that policy is administered.

4. Other Environmental Health and Safety Cases

Other environmental and safety conditions have also been found to violate the Eighth Amendment. Inadequate ventilation and deprivation of outdoor exercise have been found to violate the Eighth Amendment. In addition, excessive heat, excessive cold, polluted water, toxic or noxious fumes, exposure to sewage, lack of fire safety, inadequate food or unsanitary food service, inadequate lighting or constant lighting, exposure to insects, rodents and other vermin, exposure to asbestos, and exposure to the extreme behavior of severely mentally ill prisoners have all been found to violate a prisoner's Eighth Amendment rights.

5. A Prisoner's Right to Psychiatric Care

This Section gives you a short summary of your right to psychiatric (mental health) care, including your right to refuse treatment.

You have the same right to mental health care that you have to physical health care. Most courts recognize that there is no difference between a prisoner's right to physical treatment and his right to mental health treatment. However, your right to mental health care may only include treatment that is necessary and that will not cost an unreasonable amount of money or take an unreasonable amount of time. Nonetheless, some courts have held that an increased level of care is necessary for mental health patients. For example, courts may require a minimum number of acute-care (active, short-term care for a severe injury or illness), intermediate-care beds, and specialized physicians on staff at all times. In 2011, the United States Supreme Court upheld a "remedial order" (a court order requiring someone to comply with a duty) issued by a court in California that requires prisons to provide adequate resources to prisoners with mental disorders.

If you believe your right to mental health care has been violated, you can make an Eighth Amendment claim of deliberate indifference against prison officials. For example, the relatives of a Georgia prisoner who committed suicide sued the state for deliberate indifference. The prisoner had a history of mental illness and took anti-depressants, but the prison psychiatrist stopped his medications. When a prison official learned the prisoner was thinking about suicide, the official did not do anything. The court found that these events could establish deliberate indifference to the prisoner's health in violation of the Eighth Amendment.

(a) Right to Refuse Psychiatric Treatment

You also have a limited right to refuse mental health treatment. In Washington v. Harper, the Supreme Court used a "rational basis test" (a test to determine whether the government's action was reasonably related to a legitimate goal) to decide whether a prison could require a prisoner to undergo psychiatric treatment. The Court held that if the prison's actions are reasonably related to legitimate prison interests, then the action is proper. Given the requirements of the prison environment, the Due Process Clause permits the State to treat a prison inmate who has a serious mental illness with antipsychotic drugs against his will, if the inmate is dangerous to himself or others and the treatment is in the inmate's medical interest.

If you refuse to take the prescription drugs that the prison doctor gives you for mental illness, the prison must go through certain procedures before they can force you to take the medication. To satisfy the Constitution's Due Process Clause, a prison must have:

(A) medical finding, that a mental disorder exists which is likely to cause harm if not treated...and the medication must first be prescribed by a psychiatrist, and then approved by a reviewing psychiatrist, which ensures that the treatment in question will be ordered only if it is in the prisoner's medical interest.

In other words, before a prison can give you medication against your will, a psychiatrist must prescribe medication, and a second psychiatrist must agree that (1) you need the medication and (2) your mental disorder is likely to be dangerous if untreated.

In Washington v. Harper, the Court held the state's policy of medicating unwilling patients was constitutional because it met these requirements. In Washington, the decision to administer drugs against the patient's will had to be made by a committee including a neutral psychiatrist and a neutral psychologist, neither of whom were currently treating the prisoner. The prison superintendent could accept or reject the committee's decision, and the prisoner had the option to ask a court to review the committee's decision.

You are also entitled to certain due process protections, including a hearing, before prison authorities can transfer you to a psychiatric hospital. In Vitek v. Jones, the Supreme Court held it unconstitutional to subject a prisoner to behavior modification treatment without a legitimate reason.

In addition, you should be aware that different psychiatric programs are used to treat prisoners who were convicted of sex offenses. Sometimes, prisoners who have not been convicted of sex offenses can still be classified as sex offenders. Thus, prison officials can prevent those prisoners from getting parole by claiming that the prisoners did not complete a required therapeutic program. Courts disagree on whether a hearing is required before prison officials can make this classification.

6. Right to Dental Care

The right to adequate medical care has been extended to include dental care in some cases. The Second Circuit has held that a claim regarding inadequate dental care, like one involving medical care, can be based on various factors, such as the pain suffered by the plaintiff,...the deterioration of the teeth due to a lack of treatment,...or the inability to engage in normal activities. Recently, because of a federal class action lawsuit, the California Department of Corrections and Rehabilitation (CDCR) agreed to provide dental care for all prisoners.

Like inadequate medical care, dental care is also governed by the deliberate indifference and seriously needs analysis.

To prove an Eighth Amendment claim of inadequate dental care, you have to show both deliberate indifference, like in other inadequate medical care claims, and that the denial caused you substantial harm.

In practice, courts often note that there is a difference between preventive dental care, such as cleanings or fluoride treatments, and dental emergencies, such as cavities. In Dean v. Coughlin, the court held that prison officials had violated the Eighth Amendment when they refused to provide serious dental treatments such as fillings and crowns. However, the court also found that prisoners had no right to preventive care. If you are interested in preventive care, it is constitutional for prisons to require that you pay for such care yourself.

But, note that in some circumstances, limiting care to pulling teeth that could be saved may be unconstitutional. In Chance v. Armstrong, the court held that when the prison decided to pull the prisoner's teeth instead of repair them only because this option was cheaper, the action violated the Eighth Amendment because afterwards the prisoner was in great pain for six months, could not chew properly, and lost his teeth.

D. Medical Care for Female Prisoners

1. Accessing Medical Care

Like male prisoners, female prisoners have a constitutional right under the Eighth Amendment to adequate medical care. Female prisoners should read this entire Chapter, not only this Part, to understand prison health care rights. This Part of the Chapter only explains special medical issues and procedures for women, like gynecological examinations, abortion, and pregnancy.

Though state and federal laws guarantee you a right to the medical services described in this Part, prisons do not always provide these services, so it is important to know your rights. You should consult your prison's regulations about medical care as well as federal and state law. For New York, the regulations about prison health care are found in Part 7651 of Title 9 (Executive) of the Codes, Rules and Regulations. If your prison or the corrections department in your state does not have such regulations, you should find out if your institution has a health care manual or if your state's corrections department has an operations manual. In Texas, each correctional facility must have a written Health Services Plan describing procedures for regularly scheduled sick calls, emergency services, long-term care, and other medical services. In California, health care provisions are found in Chapter Nine of the Department Operations Manual of the California Department of Corrections.

Many female prisoners have an increased risk of chronic health problems, such as HIV, hepatitis, asthma, gynecological diseases, nutrition problems, and convulsive seizure disorders. Federal law requires all federal prisoners to receive a medical examination within twenty-four hours after arriving in prison. You should be tested for sexually transmitted infections (STIs) and tuberculosis (TB) during this exam. Some courts have ruled that certain state prisons must also perform these tests. Many states have TB screening plans, which require screening of prisoners in facilities of certain sizes or after a prisoner has been held for a certain period of time. Read Chapter 26 of the JLM, "Infectious Diseases: AIDS, Hepatitis, and Tuberculosis in Prison," for more information. While prisons have a duty to perform these exams, many female prisoners do not receive a medical exam after being admitted. You should also receive check-ups and diagnostic tests, but, again, some prisons do not follow the law.

2. Abortion

According to Roe v. Wade, every woman has the right to decide whether to have an abortion or to go forward with a pregnancy. However, states are allowed to place restrictions or limitations on a woman's right to an abortion, like requiring parental consent for minors, as long as they do not place an "undue burden" on a woman's right to choose. Courts decide what kind of obstacles might count as an undue burden.

If you are a pregnant federal prisoner, federal regulations require that prison officials offer you medical, religious, and social counseling before you have an abortion. You may accept or decline this counseling, and officials should allow you to make the final decision on whether or not to have an abortion. Once you have received the offer of counseling, and have notified the prison in writing that you wish to have an abortion, the prison must arrange for the abortion.

If you are a state prisoner, your rights will mostly depend on the abortion laws in your state. In New York, abortions are allowed if a doctor has a reasonable belief that the abortion is necessary to preserve your life or the abortion occurs in the first twenty-four weeks...of the pregnancy.

Some states, like California and New York, have codes that say that female prisoners have the same right to an abortion as any other woman in the state. In other states, there may be additional restrictions on prisoners seeking abortions. You should first look at your state code or prison regulations. Few courts have ruled on the issue of whether prisons may treat female prisoners differently than other women in the state when it comes to the right to get an abortion. In Monmouth County Correctional Institutional Inmates v. Lanzaro, the Third Circuit held that female prisoners have the same right to an abortion as non-prisoner women in the same state. The court found that requiring a woman to get a court-ordered release for an elective abortion was an undue burden on her constitutionally-protected right to have an abortion, as well as a violation of her Eighth Amendment right to medical treatment in prison. The court classified an elective abortion as a serious medical need where denial or undue delay in providing the procedure could cause the prisoner's condition to become irreparable. The court also found that a prison is not required to pay for a prisoner's abortion, but if you request an abortion and are entitled to one under state law, then a prison official is required to transport you to a clinic.

Some courts have decided that restrictions on elective abortions violate the Fourteenth Amendment, but not the Eighth Amendment. In Roe v. Crawford, the Eighth Circuit considered the constitutionality of a Missouri Department of Corrections (MDC) policy prohibiting transportation of pregnant prisoners off-site for elective, non-therapeutic abortions. The court found that the MDC policy was unconstitutional under the Fourteenth Amendment, and that women prisoners do not lose their right to abortions once incarcerated. However, in a different case, the Fifth Circuit upheld a prison policy requiring prisoners to get a court order for abortions because the policy was implemented reasonably and was rationally connected to the legitimate penological objectives prison security served.

Note that if you ask for an abortion but never get one because of prison officials' negligence, you probably do not have a constitutional claim. In Bryant v. Maffucci, for example, a pretrial detainee requested an abortion, but because of administrative inefficiency and unreasonable delays by prison officials the abortion was scheduled too late to be performed. The court found that the prison officials were not deliberately indifferent, only negligent, so their conduct was not in violation of the Eighth Amendment. Similarly, in Gibson v. Matthews, the Sixth Circuit found that prison officials were merely negligent when they incorrectly estimated the due date of a pregnant prisoner and thus denied her access to abortion facilities.

3. Pregnancy

Your treatment during pregnancy is important. Prisons should (but might not) have policies and procedures for risk assessment and treatment of pregnant prisoners, diet and nutrition, prenatal care, and counseling.

In New York State, you have a right to "comprehensive prenatal care...which shall include, but is not limited to, regular medical examinations, advice on appropriate levels of activity and safety precautions, nutritional guidance, and HIV education. Shortly before you are about to give birth, you should be moved from the jail or prison to some other location a reasonable time before the anticipated birth of your child, and provided with comfortable accommodations, maintenance and medical care. You will be returned to the prison or jail "as soon after the birth of your child as the state of your health will permit. In California, a pregnant prisoner in a local detention facility has a right to receive necessary medical services from the physician of her choice, but she must pay for any private doctors. California has recently amended its state regulations concerning pregnant prisoners. These rules provide for routine physical examinations as well as mandatory nutritional guidelines to be followed by prison facilities when caring for pregnant prisoners. In particular, the use of leg and waist restraints is subject to stringent requirements.

In determining whether prison officials violated your Eighth Amendment rights by denying you medical care, courts generally consider the amount of time left before you reach the full term of your pregnancy, the symptoms of labor that you has exhibited, any previous or potential complications with your pregnancy, and the reaction of prison officials to the your condition and requests. In a federal case in Wisconsin, a woman prisoner charged prison nurses with violating her Eighth Amendment rights by failing to bring her to the hospital when she was in labor. The prisoner gave birth in her prison cell. The court denied summary judgment and held that a reasonable jury could conclude that the nurses had shown deliberate indifference toward the pregnant prisoner because the nurses ignored the prisoner's request to go to the hospital and they only examined her through the small tray slot in the cell door, rather than conducting a more comprehensive exam.

Pregnant prisoners have also had some success in lawsuits alleging negligence against prisons. One court found a prison liable for the wrongful death of a premature baby born to a prisoner because the prison was negligent. Prison officials did not follow the prison's procedures, failed to diagnose the labor despite complaints of bleeding and abdominal pain, and did not bring the prisoner to a hospital until it may have been too late to prevent the premature birth.

Shackling pregnant prisoners in labor is unfortunately still common, and many departments of corrections and the Federal Bureau of Prisons allow the use of restraints during labor. This may be changing, however. California has banned shackling you by the wrists or ankles during labor, delivery, and recovery, unless it is necessary for the safety and security of you, the staff, or the public. Similarly, New York does not allow the use of restraints on you during delivery. A D.C. court has struck down a practice of shackling women in their third trimester with leg shackles, handcuffs, a belly chain, and a black box. The court held these practices violated the Eighth Amendment; leg shackles alone provide sufficient security during the third trimester and even these must be removed during labor and for a short period thereafter.

The Eighth Circuit also recently ruled that that a reasonable jury could find that a prison officer violated the Eighth Amendment by shackling a prisoner after she went into labor. According to the court, a jury could infer that the officer recognized that the shackles interfered with the prisoner's medical care, could be an obstacle in the event of a medical emergency, and caused unnecessary suffering at a time when the prisoner would have likely been physically unable to flee. The court also wrote in a footnote that a jury could determine the officer was aware of the risks involved in labor because they were obvious.

E. Your Right to Informed Consent and Medical Privacy

1. Informed Consent

Before you are treated, you should ask your doctor or other prison health staff what to expect from a medical procedure and its risks and alternatives. Depending on your state, you may have both a statutory and constitutional right to receive this information and agree to treatment before you are treated. Giving "informed consent" means that you agree to your particular medical treatment after your doctor has told you about the purpose of the treatment, it's possible side effects, and other alternative treatments.

In New York, if you did not give informed consent before you received a medical treatment (meaning that you did not agree to the treatment or were never fully told of the treatment's risks and alternatives), you can bring a state law claim against your doctor or other prison officials for acting without your informed consent. To prove that you did not give your informed consent, you must show (1) that your doctor did not tell you about the risks of the treatment and the alternative treatments available, (2) that a reasonable patient in your position would not have agreed to the treatment if he had been fully informed, and (3) that the lack of consent caused your injury. You must have been injured as a result of the lack of informed consent in order for your claim to succeed.

You may also be able to bring a similar constitutional claim. In Pabon v. Wright, the Second Circuit held that your constitutionally protected interest in refusing medical treatment under the Fourteenth Amendment includes the related right to such information as a reasonable patient would deem necessary to make an informed decision regarding medical treatment. In order to succeed on this claim, you must meet a different test. Specifically, you will have to show (1) that government officials failed to provide you with the kind of information that a reasonable patient would need to make an informed decision, (2) that you would have refused the medical treatment if you had been so informed, and (3) that the officials failed to provide you with information with deliberate indifference to your right to refuse medical treatment. However, a prison official can still forcibly give you medical treatment even if you do not consent as long as the official reasonably determines that it "furthers a legitimate penological purpose"—for example, one related to prison security.

2. Medical Privacy

You have constitutional privacy rights protecting your medical information. You are entitled to confidentiality of information about your medical condition and treatment. But like all prisoners' rights, your privacy rights are limited by the needs of prison administration and depend on the circumstances.

Courts have long recognized the general right to privacy in one's medical information: 'There can be no question that...medical records, which may contain intimate facts of a personal nature, are well within the ambit of materials entitled to privacy protection. The Third Circuit has held that you have a Fourteenth Amendment privacy interest in your medical information because it is among those rights that are not inconsistent with your status as a prisoner or with the legitimate penological objectives of the corrections system. Similarly, in Powell v. Schriver, the Second Circuit held that you do have a constitutional right to keep previously undisclosed medical information confidential as long as the disclosure is not reasonably related to a legitimate penological interest.

In 1996, Congress passed the Health Insurance Portability and Accountability Act (HIPAA), which contains significant protections for prisoners' medical privacy rights. Under the final

HIPAA privacy rule, identifiable health information pertaining to you has been deemed protected health information, or (PHI). A hospital providing prison health care may disclose PHI to a correctional institution or a law enforcement official having lawful custody of a prisoner only if the correctional institution or law enforcement official represents that disclosing such protected health information is necessary for:

(1) the provision of health care to such individuals;

(2) the health and safety of such individual or other prisoners;

(3) the health and safety of officers, employees, or others at the correctional institution;

(4) the health and safety of such individuals and officers or other persons responsible for the transport of prisoners or their transfer from one institution, facility, or setting to another;

(5) the health and safety of law enforcement on the premises of the correctional institution; or

(6) the administration and maintenance of the safety, security, and good order of the correctional institution.

A prison hospital is allowed to share protected health information to entities outside the hospital if the entity says that the protected health information is necessary for any of the purposes listed above. Furthermore, a prison hospital may reasonably rely upon any such representations from public officials regarding your health. However, when you are released from custody—including probation, parole, and supervised release—you are no longer categorized as an inmate, and these permitted use and disclosure provisions no longer apply.

You should also note that some courts have held prison officials liable for disclosing a prisoner's confidential medical information, not because they violated the prisoner's privacy rights but because by disclosing the information, the officials put the prisoner in danger. In Anderson v. Romero, for example, the court indicated that prison employees would violate a prisoner's Eighth Amendment rights against cruel and unusual punishment if, knowing that an inmate identified as HIV positive was a likely target of violence by other inmates yet indifferent to his fate, the employees gratuitously revealed his HIV status to other inmates and a violent attack upon him ensued.

F. Actions You Can Bring When You Are Denied Medical Care

Now that you know your rights, it is important to be able to enforce them. This Part describes the actions you can bring when your right to adequate medical care is violated. Remember that in almost every instance, your case will be helped by attempting to go through your institution's complaint process.

1. Remedies for State Prisoners

(a) 42 U.S.C. § 1983 Actions

Section 1983 is a federal statute that allows you to bring a lawsuit when your federal constitutional rights have been violated. When persons acting under state authority (for example, prison guards, prison doctors, and prison administrators) violate your right to adequate medical care, you may use Section 1983 to bring a lawsuit in federal court. (b) Tort Actions

As discussed in Part B of this Chapter, the federal constitutional standard established by Wilson and Farmer cannot be proven by claiming only negligence. If the facts of your case are not enough to prove a constitutional violation, but only show negligence, you may want to consider bringing a tort action against state officials instead of a constitutional claim to succeed on a negligence claim you must prove three things:

(1) "Duty of Care"—that the defendants had a duty of care towards you;

(2) "Breach of Duty"—that the defendants failed to meet that duty; and

(3) "Injury"—that you were injured as a result of that failure.

There are several ways to prove that the prison has a duty of care towards you. First, as discussed above, Estelle v. Gamble held that prison officials have a duty to provide adequate medical care. Second, a state statute may declare, or require, a prison's duty of care. Many states have statutes that require prison officials to provide adequate medical care. For example, in New York, Section 70(2)(c) of the New York State Correction Law directs Department of Corrections and Community Supervision officials to maintain and operate correctional facilities with due regard to...the health and safety of every person in the custody of the Department" There are also common law (law made through judge's opinions, rather than by statute) claims of medical malpractice and negligence actions that you may bring.

The most common method of proving that a defendant breached a duty is to have an expert provide testimony that the defendant did not use the usually accepted procedures. For example, in Stanback v. State, the plaintiff's expert testified that an x-ray of plaintiff's knee would have revealed his torn ligament. However, prison doctors only offered ace bandages, braces, and painkillers and did not x-ray the knee for over three years. Expert testimony is not always necessary. In Rivers v. State, the court held that a medical expert's testimony is not required where a lay person, relying on common knowledge and experience, can find that the harm would not have occurred in the absence of negligence. In other words, if an ordinary person could have used common sense to find out that negligence must have occurred, you do not need an expert witness. Thus, no expert testimony was necessary in Rivers to prove that a doctor was negligent when he performed a hernia operation on a prisoner's right side, even though the patient required the operation on his left side and the hernia was visible on the left side. As previously noted in Part B of this Chapter, there are differences between medical malpractice and medical negligence claims. The need for an expert is linked to this distinction: if you decide to file a medical malpractice claim, you may need an expert witness to support your claim that a reasonable medical practitioner would not have caused the injury you claim was caused.

Finally, you must prove that the breach of duty was the direct cause of your injury. This element is not usually difficult to prove, but if you interfere with your treatment in any way, you may fail to prove direct causation. For example, in Brown v. Sheridan, the plaintiff lost his case when the court found that he did not receive immediate treatment because of his own failure to disclose the nature of his injury, and that defendants took reasonable steps to ascertain and monitor plaintiff's condition. The court noted that the prisoner did not openly display symptoms of his injury, and refused to cooperate with psychiatric care that could have aided defendants in discovering and treating his injury sooner. Also, in Marchione v. State, the plaintiff, who was given medication for hypertension and became permanently impotent as a result, lost on his negligence claim because he did not report his symptoms in time. At trial, medical experts found that the impotence would have occurred if not treated within eight hours after the onset of symptoms. Although the prisoner noticed the symptoms by ten o'clock in the morning, he did not indicate his situation was an emergency and delayed making a specific report of his symptoms until the evening.

An advantage to filing a state tort claim is that you only need to establish negligence, which is easier than establishing deliberate indifference. A disadvantage to filing a state tort claim is that you can only get money damages, while Section 1983 claims provide both "declaratory relief" (a judgment that is binding on both parties in the present and the future) and "injunctive relief" (a court order that prohibits or commands action to undo some wrong or injury) in addition to money damages. Furthermore, a negligence action may only be filed in state court, while a Section 1983 claim can be filed in either federal or state court.

(c) Article 78 Proceedings in New York State

In New York, there is a legal procedure called an Article 78 proceeding that allows you to challenge a decision made by a state official. If you are denied medical care, you can bring a complaint under Article 78 to require the prison to provide that care. In an Article 78 proceeding, you can recover only limited money damages. To be successful, you must be able to show that the prison authorities were deliberately indifferent to your serious medical needs. The statute of limitations requires that the proceeding be brought within four months of the denial or you cannot bring the claim. Administrative remedies must be exhausted before beginning an Article 78 proceeding

2. Remedies for Federal Prisoners

(a) Bivens Actions Under 28 U.S.C. § 1331

A Bivens action is the federal prisoner's equivalent to a state prisoner's Section 1983 action. In a Bivens action, you must prove that the prison doctor or official showed deliberate indifference to your serious medical needs. For more on Bivens actions,

(b) Federal Tort Claims Act

Under the Federal Tort Claims Act (FTCA), you can obtain relief if a prison doctor or official was negligent. In other words, you can sue the federal government if something a government employee did or failed to do while working for the government harmed you. Courts look to see whether the behavior would be a tort in the state where the behavior occurred. If it is a tort in that state, you can sue the federal government.

If the injury was caused by intentional behavior, however, a claim cannot be brought under the FTCA. For example, an allegation of assault and battery (considered purposeful behavior under the law) could not be brought as an FTCA claim. If the act or omission that caused your injury arose from a discretionary duty, you cannot sue under the FTCA.

If you do meet FTCA suit requirements, you must bring it against the United States, not the federal employees who caused your injury. If you name employees as defendants, the FTCA authorizes the court to substitute the United States as the sole defendant.

(c) Choosing Between a Bivens Claim and an FTCA Action

If you are a federal prisoner, you may have the choice of bringing either a Bivens suit or an FTCA claim. While it is easier to bring a successful FTCA action because it allows suit for mere medical malpractice, there are several advantages to bringing a Bivens action not available under the FTCA. First, while you cannot bring an FTCA action for an intentional tort, you can bring a claim for an intentional tort in a Bivens suit against an individual. Second, under the FTCA you can only sue the federal government, while in a Bivens action you can sue the individuals who mistreated you. Third, under the FTCA you can only receive compensatory damages (money equal to the cost of repairing or compensating the actual injury you suffered), while in a Bivens suit you may receive punitive damages (extra money awarded as a penalty against the wrongdoer). Fourth, in an FTCA action, you cannot later sue the individuals who injured you, but in a Bivens action, if you are unable to collect on the judgment against the individual employees, you can bring a suit against the government. Finally, a judge hears an FTCA suit, but a jury hears a Bivens suit.

If your injury occurred because of a violation of your constitutional rights and also from a tort, you can bring both an FTCA and a Bivens action. If you do not wish to bring both, you can choose between them.

G. Conclusion

The Constitution and state law protect your right to adequate medical care. Part B explained what you need to prove to show you have been denied adequate medical care in violation of the Eighth Amendment. You must show that you suffered serious harm because you did not receive medical treatment (the objective test), and that the prison official who denied you treatment "knew of and ignored an excessive risk to your health or safety" (the subjective test). Part C talked about how courts treat certain common prisoner health complaints. Part D explained specific health rights for female prisoners. Part E explained your right to receive information before you are treated and your right to keep your medical records confidential. Part F talked about the different ways you can go to court if your rights have been violated. Because this Chapter focused on federal and New York state law, you will need to research the law in your own state if you are in a prison outside of New York.

If you believe you are not receiving adequate medical care, the first step is to assert your rights through your institution's grievance procedure. If your problem is not addressed, you will have preserved your right to bring a lawsuit in court. You can only bring your lawsuit in federal court, or state court in New York (an Article 78 proceeding), after you are unsuccessful or do not receive a favorable result through the inmate grievance procedure.

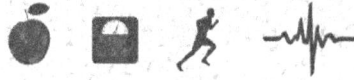

INFECTIOUS DISEASES:
AIDS, HEPATITIS, AND TUBERCULOSIS IN PRISON

A. Introduction

This Chapter explains your legal rights with respect to infectious diseases in prison. This Chapter has information both for prisoners who already have an infectious disease (like HIV/AIDS, tuberculosis, hepatitis B, hepatitis C, or Methicillin-resistant Staphylococcus aureus (MRSA)), and for prisoners who want to avoid getting an infectious disease. Part B gives you some basic facts about infectious diseases. Section (1)(a) of Part B also describes how women may have different symptoms of HIV/AIDS. Part C explains the general standard used to determine whether a prison policy is constitutional. Part D is about medical testing for infectious diseases in prisons, including whether a prison can force you to get tested or have others tested. Part E discusses disease prevention and segregation issues. Part F discusses the role of confidentiality and what you can expect in terms of keeping your health status private in prison. Part G deals with treatment options and your legal rights to those options. Part H discusses issues of discrimination. Part I discusses sentencing issues. Part J discusses planning for your release if you have an infectious disease. Finally, Appendix A lists resources for further information, counseling, and support for you and your family.

You should also read other chapters of the JLM to understand your legal rights, especially Chapter 16, Using 42 U.S.C. § 1983 and 28 U.S.C. § 1331 to Obtain Relief From Violations of Federal Law, Chapter 36, Special Considerations for Sex Offenders, Chapter 28, Rights of Prisoners with Disabilities, Chapter 23, Your Right to Adequate Medical Care, and Chapter 35, Getting Out Early: Conditional & Early Release.

There are more court cases about HIV/AIDS than about tuberculosis, hepatitis B, hepatitis C, and MRSA. Because judges always look at the specific facts of each case, try to find cases about your disease. But, you also can try to make comparisons between different diseases and explain how the diseases are very similar, including how they are spread and their effects on prisoners. For example, if you want to use a case about AIDS and argue the law should also apply to hepatitis C, you should try to explain your reasons as clearly as possible.

This Chapter is only a summary of the many issues about infectious diseases in the prison system. You probably will have to do more research elsewhere. For example, this Chapter only includes HIV/AIDS, tuberculosis, hepatitis (the most common infectious diseases in prison), and MRSA, but there are many other diseases. Scientists are always discovering new information about infectious diseases, so some of this information may not be correct in the future.

B. Background Information on Infectious Diseases

1. HIV and AIDS

HIV, the Human Immunodeficiency Virus, is the virus that causes AIDS. AIDS stands for

Acquired Immunodeficiency Syndrome. Over time, the HIV virus weakens your immune system so your body cannot fight off infection properly. You may develop various infections—known as "opportunistic" infections—that take advantage of your body's weakened condition.

About half of people with HIV develop AIDS within ten years of getting HIV. How long it takes for HIV to develop into AIDS is different for each person. Medical treatments can slow down how fast HIV weakens your body. As HIV gets worse and becomes AIDS, people become sick with serious illnesses and infections.

Being HIV-positive does not mean that you have AIDS. It is very important that you consult a doctor to find out if you are infected with HIV or if you have developed AIDS so that you can receive the proper medical treatment. The only way you can know for certain whether you are infected is to be tested.

An estimated 1.2 million people in the United States were living with HIV as of 2013, and, in 2015 alone, 18,303 people in the United States were diagnosed with AIDS. The estimated rate of confirmed AIDS cases in state and federal prisons between 1999 and 2008 was more than two times higher than in the general population. In 2014, approximately 710 prisoners in New York State prisons were HIV positive and 1,284 prisoners had AIDS—excluding prisoners in New York City.

HIV is most commonly spread by having unprotected anal, vaginal, or oral sex with a person with HIV; by sharing needles or injection equipment with a drug user who has HIV; from an HIV-infected mother to her baby, before or during birth or through breast-feeding; and through unsanitary tattooing or body piercing procedures.

You cannot get HIV by working with or being around someone who has HIV, or by sharing a cell with another prisoner who has HIV. You also cannot get HIV from sweat, spit, tears, clothes, drinking fountains, telephones, toilet seats, or through everyday activities like sharing a meal. HIV is also not transmitted through insect bites or stings, donating blood, or through closed-mouth kissing (although there is a very small chance of getting it from open-mouthed or "French" kissing with someone who is HIV positive because of possible blood contact through open wounds, warts, etc.).

If you are currently HIV negative, you can help avoid getting HIV by taking the following steps:

(1) Never share needles or syringes if you inject drugs;

(2) Never share needles or syringes if you get a tattoo or body piercing;

(3) Do not share equipment used to prepare and inject drugs (works);

(4) Use a latex condom—not a lambskin condom—every time you have sex, including anal and oral sex;

(5) Never share razors or toothbrushes because of the risk of contact with someone else's blood.

Taking these precautions can help protect you from contracting the HIV infection.

(a) Women and HIV/AIDS

Symptoms of HIV are often different for women than for men. Because these symptoms are typically not associated with HIV, many women go undiagnosed until the virus progresses to AIDS. Early signs for a woman with HIV include gynecological disorders, especially pelvic inflammatory disease (PID), infections, such as human papillomavirus (HPV), that can cause cervical dysplasia, and chronic yeast infections. HIV-positive women also have a higher risk of developing cervical cancer. If you are HIV-positive, getting a complete gynecological exam, including an inspection of the cervix (colposcopy), and a pap smear every six months, is important to detect any problems early. If you believe you may be infected with HIV or AIDS, try to get tested.

Appendix A includes several organizations and sources of information about HIV and AIDS. If you are HIV-positive, it is important that you be tested for tuberculosis, a very contagious and serious disease, because HIV-positive people have a much higher risk of getting tuberculosis.

2. Tuberculosis

Tuberculosis (TB) is a disease caused by bacteria that are spread through the air. When you breathe in the bacteria, they usually settle in and attack your lungs, but the bacteria can also move to and attack other parts of your body. Outside of prison, TB does not spread that easily. In prison, however, TB spreads much more easily because of overcrowding and poor ventilation. People born outside the United States (especially in Latin America, the Caribbean, Africa, Asia, Eastern Europe, or Russia) are also more likely to have been infected with the bacteria. Additionally, people who have spent time in places where TB is common, like homeless shelters, hospitals, and prisons, are also more likely to have a TB infection.

It is important to know that being infected with the TB bacteria is not the same as having TB disease. If you have "TB infection" (latent TB), you will have no symptoms and you cannot spread TB to others. But if you do not get medical treatment, your TB infection can develop into "TB disease" (active TB). If you have active TB, you can have symptoms like a bad cough lasting more than three weeks, pain in your chest, coughing up blood or phlegm, weakness or fatigue, weight loss, no appetite, chills, a fever, or night sweating.

TB is particularly dangerous for HIV-positive people because of their weakened immune systems. In fact, TB is one of the leading causes of death for HIV-positive people. Although an estimated 11.2 million people in the United States have latent TB, only about five to ten percent will develop active TB disease if left untreated. If you have HIV, however, you should be aware that people with both HIV and TB bacteria are much more likely to develop active TB than HIV-negative people.

Be sure to consult other sources and prison medical professionals if you think you have TB. Active TB disease can be treated and cured if you get medical care, take prescription medication, and follow your doctor's orders.

3. Hepatitis B and Hepatitis C

Hepatitis is a disease that attacks the liver. There are different types of hepatitis, but the most common types among prisoners are hepatitis B and hepatitis C.

(a) Hepatitis B

In 2014, there were about 19,200 new hepatitis B infections in the United States. About 1,800 people die each year from liver disease related to hepatitis B. The hepatitis B virus, like HIV, is spread by having sex with infected persons without a condom, through sharing needles (works) when shooting drugs, through workplace exposure to infected needles or other sharp objects, or from an infected mother to her baby during birth. You can avoid getting hepatitis B by taking the same precautions as you would for HIV. For more information on HIV prevention, see Part B(1) of this Chapter.

People who have hepatitis B often do not have any symptoms, but can still spread the virus to other people. If you do have symptoms, you may develop yellow eyes and skin, tiredness, loss of appetite, dark urine, abdominal pains, and nausea. There are vaccines to protect you from hepatitis B, but once you get hepatitis B, there is no cure. You should still get medical attention, however, because there are medical treatments to help your symptoms. If you have hepatitis B, you should get tested for HIV and hepatitis C.

(b) Hepatitis C

Hepatitis C virus (HCV) causes hepatitis C. In 2014, there were an estimated 30,500 new hepatitis C virus infections in the United States, and there were about 2.7-3.9 million chronically or permanently infected persons. Almost 80% of infected persons do not show any signs or symptoms of hepatitis C. Many people infected with hepatitis C may not show any symptoms for twenty or thirty years. Hepatitis C symptoms include yellow skin, dark urine, fatigue, abdominal pain, and loss of appetite. Most people (around 70%) with chronic HCV infection have some liver damage. If you have hepatitis C, you should not drink alcohol because alcohol can make your liver damage worse.

While few people outside of prison have HCV, a very high percentage of prisoners are infected with HCV. To avoid getting hepatitis C, you should:

(1) Never shoot drugs (if you cannot stop, never reuse or share syringes, water, or works);

(2) Never share toothbrushes, razors, or other personal care items;

(3) Avoid getting a tattoo or body piercing if there is a chance that someone else's blood is on the tools or the artist or piercer does not follow good health practices;

(4) Avoid having unprotected sex.

Though the likelihood of spreading hepatitis C through sexual intercourse is not known, the likelihood of spreading hepatitis C through direct contact with infected blood is extremely high. If you have hepatitis C, you should be tested for HIV and hepatitis B.

4. Methicillin-resistant Staphylococcus Aureus (MRSA)

Staphylococcus (staph) is a kind of bacteria that can cause various infections, including everything from minor skin problems to serious, fatal infections. Methicillin-resistant Staphylococcus aureus, or MRSA, is a kind of staph not easily treatable with the antibiotics that normally cure a staph infection. Many people carry staph bacteria in their nasal passages without getting sick. The illness can develop if the bacteria enter the skin, often through a scratch, scrape, or other minor wound. Most cases of MRSA happen in healthcare settings like hospitals, but MRSA is also more likely to spread in crowded living conditions, including in dormitories, athletic facilities, and correctional facilities.

The first symptom of MRSA is usually a skin infection easily mistaken for a pimple, boil, or insect bite. The infection may be painful, swollen, red, or produce pus. It can develop into a large abscess or blister. MRSA is usually treatable, by either draining the wound or taking antibiotics. Do not drain the wound yourself, since this can cause the infection to spread. The infection may return even after treatment.

MRSA and other staph infections can be spread to other people through direct physical contact or, less commonly, through contact with an infected surface or object. You can reduce the risk of infection by keeping wounds clean, dry, and covered. It is also important to keep shared surfaces clean, wash your hands often (especially after touching a wound), and avoid sharing personal items like razors and clothing. If you suspect you have MRSA, it is especially important to seek treatment if you have HIV or another immune system problem, because a MRSA infection may lead to more serious problems.

C. Constitutional Rights in a Prison Setting

The rest of this Chapter discusses your rights to treatment for and protection from infectious diseases in prison. It also explains when and how a correctional facility can limit your rights to treatment and protection. This Part explains the general legal standard that courts use to determine if a prison policy is constitutionally valid. Knowing the rule will help you better understand the court decisions in this Chapter.

In general, correctional facilities can limit your constitutional rights if the prison's actions are reasonably related to a legitimate penological (meaning, prison-related) interest. To decide if a prison policy has a legitimate penological interest, courts look at four factors:

(1)   The existence of a valid, rational connection between the prison policy and a legitimate state interest;

(2)   The existence of alternative means of exercising the right being limited;

(3)   The impact that allowing exercise of the right will have on guards, other prisoners, or the allocation of prison resources; and

(4)   Whether the prison policy or regulation is an exaggerated response to prison concerns, as shown by the ready availability of alternative means of exercising the right.

These four factors are often referred to as the Turner standard, since the Supreme Court first stated this standard in Turner v. Safley.

So, if you think a prison policy illegally violates your constitutional rights, you may want to argue that there is no legitimate penological interest which justifies the violation, or, at least, that the interest is not "reasonably related" to the actions or policy of the prison officials. You can also try to argue that there are other ways of accomplishing the same governmental goal without compromising your constitutional rights.

D. Legal Rights Concerning Testing for Infectious Diseases

1. Involuntary Testing

Mandatory testing policies vary widely among states. States may also have different policies for different diseases. For example, a state may require prisoners to take a TB test but not an HIV test. If you are outside New York State, you should check your state's laws to find out what its testing policies are. Because courts find that the prevention of disease is a legitimate state interest, courts generally allow prisons to test prisoners for infectious diseases, even without a prisoner's consent.

(a) HIV Testing

In New York State prisons, you normally cannot be tested for HIV without your consent (which means that you will not be tested unless you voluntarily agree). But, if you are convicted of certain sex offenses, you can be tested for HIV against your will if the victim requests that you be tested. You will learn your test results and the results will also be sent to the victim, and possibly to the victim's immediate family, guardian, physicians, attorneys, and medical or mental health providers. Past and future contacts of the victim may also be notified if there has been a risk of HIV transmission to that contact. Your test results cannot be used against you in a civil or criminal proceeding related to the events that were the basis of your conviction.

Federal prisons, unlike New York state prisons, can require a prisoner to undergo HIV testing, although federal prisons do not test all prisoners. If you have a sentence of six months or more, and if medical personnel think you might be infected with HIV, they may require you to take an HIV test. If you refuse the test, you might receive an incident report for failing to follow an order. Also, if you refuse HIV testing, you may not be able to file a claim for failure to receive adequate medical care for that condition. Additionally, federal prisons conduct mandatory random testing once a year. If you test positive, the prison cannot subject you to disciplinary action based solely on your results, though you may be punished if you have performed an act that could transmit the disease. Also, federal prisons test prisoners being considered for release, parole, good conduct time release, furlough, or placement in a community-based program. If you refuse to be tested, prison staff may result file an incident report for refusing an order. If you test positive, the prison cannot deny you participation in activities and programs just because of the result.

Outside of New York, many states have involuntary HIV testing when you enter prison, during custody, and/or upon your impending release. Involuntary HIV testing has been challenged on the basis of the Eight Amendment's prohibition against cruel and unusual punishment, the Fourth Amendment's prohibition against unreasonable searches and seizures, the right to privacy, and the Equal Protection Clause of the Fourteenth Amendment. However, courts tend to uphold involuntary testing on the grounds that it is reasonably related to a legitimate penological interest.

(b) TB Testing

While HIV cannot be passed from person to person by casual contact, TB is spread through the air. So, prison TB testing policies often differ from prison HIV testing policies. In New York State, Department of Corrections and Community Supervision (DOCCS) policy requires all prisoners entering prison to be tested for TB. The TB screening includes a chest x-ray and a skin test, where a small amount of purified protein derivative (PPD) is injected beneath your skin and observed for a reaction. After the initial test, you will be re-tested yearly. If you refuse testing, medical personnel will counsel you as to the benefits of the test. If you still refuse, then you will be placed in medical keeplock (also known as tuberculin (TB) hold) for up to a year until you have received three negative chest x- rays or you agree to be tested. While in TB hold, you are only allowed one hour of solitary exercise per day and three showers a week. You lose your telephone privileges but can receive visits from lawyers.

Courts have generally upheld the New York State DOCCS TB testing policy against challenges claiming violation of the Fourth Amendment protection against unreasonable searches or the Eight Amendment prohibition against cruel and unusual punishment because they consider the policy to be reasonably related to preventing the spread of tuberculosis in correctional facilities. Additionally, some courts have upheld mandatory TB testing or confinement in TB hold even if the test is against the prisoner's religious beliefs. However, DOCCS TB policy states that accommodations for those with religious objections to tuberculin skin test may be made if they can be done without putting the health of other inmates and staff at significant risk. According to the policy, if you refuse the PPD test on religious grounds, you are placed in TB hold while the legitimacy of your objection is determined. If the Chief Medical Officer determines that you sincerely hold a religious belief that prohibits PPD testing, he may request that you take a blood test and chest x-ray instead of the skin test. You will remain in TB hold until the results of the blood test, chest x-ray, and physical examination indicate that you do not have latent TB.

If the TB test is against your religious beliefs and you want to challenge the policy as a violation of your First Amendment right to free exercise of religion, you should try to show how the policy, as applied to your particular circumstances, does not make sense. If you have submitted to the test in the past or are willing to undergo a chest x-ray, you might strengthen your chances of succeeding. Although courts do not always validate inmates' Eight Amendment claims, you may also be able to argue that being placed on TB hold is a violation of your Eight Amendment right to be free from cruel and unusual punishment. This is especially true if your prison's ventilation system does not prevent the air that circulates in your cell from reaching other prisoners or staff. In such a case, you might be able to argue that the keeplock policy does not make sense as applied to you because the air from your cell can still reach others through the ventilation system, which means that the keeplock policy does not help protect others' safety.

If you are in a federal prison, you must undergo a PPD test and possibly a chest x-ray when you enter the facility. If you refuse both tests, the prison will conduct them without your consent. Refusing to be tested may result in an incident report, although you will not be placed in medical isolation unless there is a clinical indication for such measures.

(c) Hepatitis B and Hepatitis C

New York State does not require HCV testing for all prisoners, but does test all prisoners who are determined to be at high risk. You are considered to be at high risk of HBV or HCV if you have a history of any of the following: HIV infection, intravenous drug use, intranasal cocaine use, sexually- transmitted diseases, blood transfusions before July 1992, hemodialysis, infusion of clotting factor before 1987, tattoos or body piercing with non-sterile equipment, solid organ transplants, or symptoms of hepatitis.

In New York State, during your initial health screening, you will be offered a hepatitis B vaccine if you are not currently infected but are at high risk, unless your medical history suggests otherwise. You are considered at high risk if: you are eighteen years old or younger and not immune; you have had more than one sex partner in six months; you recently had a sexually transmitted disease; you are male and have had sex with other men; you inject drugs; you have been exposed to blood or blood contaminated products; you have had household contact with persons suffering from chronic hepatitis B infection; you are a hemodialysis patient; you take clotting factor concentrates (you are a hemophiliac); or you have chronic hepatitis C and are not immune. The vaccine consists of three doses over six months.

If you are in a federal prison, you will be screened to determine if you are likely to be infected by HBV or HCV. Similar to the TB policy in the federal prison system, refusal to submit to the test will result in an incident report for failure to follow an order.

(d) MRSA

The Federal Bureau of Prisons recommends that all prisoners should be checked for skin infections at their initial intake screening and also after returning from a hospitalization. Prisoners at high risk for MRSA infections (including those with HIV, diabetes, or open wounds) are supposed to be screened at all routine medical examinations.

2. Right to Testing upon Request

(a) HIV Testing

Many states provide HIV tests for prisoners upon request. If you are denied a test, you might consider challenging the denial as a violation of the correctional facility's own policy. In New York State prisons, you will be offered a test when you first enter the facility. Also, anonymous testing (where you do not include your identity) is available through the Criminal Justice Initiative (CJI).

If you are a federal prisoner, you can request HIV testing, but only once per year. More than one federal court does not recognize a constitutional right to HIV testing, especially if you cannot allege specific exposure to HIV. But, even in those courts, you may have an Eight Amendment claim if you belong to a high-risk group and are denied an HIV test, since such a denial would prevent you from getting proper medical care. Additionally, if you meet the prison's specified criteria for HIV testing and are still refused a test, you may also have a claim. You should check to see how the courts in your jurisdiction have decided this issue.

(b) Hepatitis B

If you are in a federal prison, you can request a hepatitis B test after consulting with a Bureau of Prisons' health care provider. However, you can only ask to be tested once per year.

(c) MRSA

If you have a skin infection that may be caused by MRSA, the wound may be tested if your doctor feels it is necessary to prevent further infection.

3. Consequences of Testing Positive for HIV in New York

States have different rules about what happens after a prisoner tests positive for HIV. In New York, in order to track HIV/AIDS better and to increase prevention of HIV infection, the state assembly adopted the HIV Reporting and Partner Notification (HIVRPN) law, which became effective in 2000. This law requires doctors and other medical providers (including the laboratories doing the tests) to report to the Department of Health the names of people infected with HIV, HIV-related illness, or AIDS. The information is supposed to remain confidential.95 However, New York regulations allow for HIV status to be revealed to employees or agents of the Division of Probation and Correctional Alternatives, Division of Parole, Commission of Correction, or any local probation department. Disclosure of HIV status is only allowed to the extent that the individuals who receive such information are authorized to access records containing such information to carry out their functions, powers, and duties. If you are diagnosed with an HIV-related illness, your medical care provider will ask for the names of your spouse, sexual partners, and/or needle-sharing partners. If you provide those names, those individuals will receive notice they are at risk of being infected with HIV, and they will be offered counseling and HIV testing. Your name will not be given to them. You have the right to refuse to give that information at no legal penalty (civil or criminal).

E. Legal Rights and Prevention of Infectious Diseases

1. Prevention and Prison Policy

The government has a duty to provide medical care to the people it incarcerates. This duty may also include protecting prisoners from infectious diseases, such as TB. But, it is also very important to take the necessary precautions to protect yourself and others from disease. If you have anal, vaginal, or oral sex, it is extremely important to use latex condoms in order to protect yourself against HIV infection and other sexually-transmitted diseases. This is particularly vital in the prison system, where a higher proportion of the population is HIV-positive. Very few jails or prisons provide condoms for prisoners. A few jails in Los Angeles, New York City, Philadelphia, San Francisco, and Washington, D.C. supply condoms on a limited basis, and Mississippi and Vermont offer condoms to prisoners.

Prisons have some duty to prevent MRSA's spread once they know infection is present within the prison. As a prisoner, you have limited options to enforce this duty. An Eight Amendment claim for failing to protect a prisoner from contracting MRSA would have to show the prison's "deliberate indifference" to the prisoner's serious medical needs. Courts generally hold that prisons do not have to take every possible measure to prevent MRSA's spread. As long they take reasonable steps, you cannot make a constitutional claim by showing the prison could have done more.

2. Segregation of Prisoners with Infectious Diseases

(a) Mandatory Segregation

(i) Mandatory Segregation of Prisoners with TB

Prisons may want to segregate (separate) prisoners with infectious diseases from other prisoners to prevent the disease's spread. This type of segregation is often mandatory and involves separate housing. New York law allows prison officials to separate prisoners if a contagious disease becomes widespread. But, New York law also states that all who are sick shall receive all necessary care and medical assistance," and that all such prisoners should be transferred back to the general population as soon as possible.

Because TB can be spread through the air, the law often treats people with TB differently. Prisons can usually isolate prisoners who are suffering from TB to prevent the spread of a contagious disease. New York City law even allows non-incarcerated persons infected with TB to be detained in a hospital in certain circumstances. DOCCS TB policy requires prisoners with contagious TB to be placed in respiratory isolation. While in respiratory isolation, you are only allowed to leave the area for certain medical treatment and you will have to wear a surgical mask.

(ii) Mandatory Segregation of Prisoners with HIV

Because HIV does not spread as easily as TB, New York state prisons and federal prisons do not determine housing or program assignments based upon HIV status alone. New York prisons are not allowed to automatically segregate HIV-positive prisoners. New York state courts have found that mandatory segregation violates your right to privacy specifically, your right to medical confidentiality because housing in an AIDS unit tells other prisoners and staff that you are HIV-positive. If you are a federal prisoner who has HIV or AIDS, the prison can only separate you if prison officials have reasonable evidence that you pose a health risk. For more information on confidentiality issues, see Part F of this Chapter, and for information regarding discriminatory treatment based on your health status, see Part H of this Chapter.

Although New York prisons may not automatically segregate HIV-positive prisoners, some states require that all HIV-infected prisoners live separately. Many courts outside of New York have upheld prisons' decisions to segregate HIV-positive prisoners. Courts generally view segregation as a reasonable means to limit other prisoner's exposure to HIV, and courts consider preventing the spread of HIV to be a legitimate interest of prisons. Additionally, at least one federal court of appeals found that there is a high risk of transmitting HIV in prison. The prison in question did not present evidence of actual HIV transmission, but the court thought that the mere presence of high-risk behavior like intravenous drug use, sex, and violent exchanges was enough to establish a significant risk of transmitting HIV. The court also rejected the prisoners' suggestions to either hire more corrections officers or to identify prisoners who were both HIV-positive and also likely to engage in high-risk conduct. The court found that these two suggestions were unreasonable and created an "undue hardship" on the prison facility. The court's ruling might make it more difficult to argue that your segregation is unconstitutional.

(iii)Mandatory Segregation of Prisoners with MRSA

Prisons may segregate prisoners who have active MRSA infections to prevent the spread of the infection to others through contact. The Federal Bureau of Prisons generally recommends, however, that prisoners do not need to be housed separately if they have MRSA wounds that are either not draining or that can be easily covered with bandages. As the infection becomes more serious or develops into MRSA pneumonia, separate housing is recommended or required. A prison may have the right to threaten you with solitary confinement if you refuse to accept the prison's prescribed treatment for your MRSA infection.

(iv) Segregation Requested by Prisoners

If you are afraid of contracting an infectious disease, read Part B of this Chapter to get a sense of the steps that you can take to protect yourself. In general, prisoners who are afraid of getting infectious diseases from other prisoners have not been able to successfully sue prison officials. Some prisoners have tried to get prisons to segregate other prisoners who are infected with a communicable disease, but these prisoners have been generally unsuccessful. Prisoners who already are infected have also been unsuccessful when they request that the prison give them a single cell or vaccinate other prisoners so that they do not spread their diseases. Courts will generally support a prison's decision not to segregate prisoners with HIV-related illnesses.

Although prisons may have a legal responsibility to protect prisoners from exposure to communicable diseases, to win a lawsuit against prison officials for exposing you to infectious diseases, you must prove that: (1) there was a specific and significant risk of infection, and (2) prison officials were aware of that risk but disregarded it. In order to win such a lawsuit, you must show that there is a significant possibility that you will contract the virus or disease. For example, some courts have held that this standard is met when prisoners are housed with people who have known MRSA infections. In order to meet the standard, however, the infected prisoner must have open wounds that are not being adequately covered or cleaned and that are likely to infect other prisoners. You will not win if you only have a general fear of getting the virus.

Additionally, the Prison Litigation Reform Act (PLRA) makes winning money damages even more difficult. Under the PLRA, if you seek money damages, you will have to show you were physically injured, not just mentally or emotionally injured, or placed at an increased risk of being infected.

F. Legal Rights and Confidentiality

Under the U.S. Constitution, you have a right to privacy (a privacy interest) regarding the disclosure of personal matters.

Prisoners with infectious diseases generally have a limited right to keep information about their medical condition confidential. Some courts have held that the right to medical confidentiality also applies to an individual's HIV status. But, other courts have held that there is no constitutional right to privacy regarding HIV status. If you are in federal prison, your HIV test results, if positive, must be disclosed to the prison's employees.

In New York state, your HIV-related information cannot be disclosed to anyone other than you and certain individuals or institutions who are authorized to know by law. Individuals who are authorized to receive your HIV information include health care providers (when knowledge is necessary to provide you with adequate care), employees of the Division of Parole, employees of the Division of Probation and Correctional Alternatives or local probation department, the medical director of the local correctional facility, or an employee or agent of the Commission of Correction. These authorized individuals are allowed to access your HIV information so far as they need the information to carry out their duties and functions.

In New York, prisoners have won lawsuits that found statutory and constitutional rights violations when their HIV status was improperly disclosed. In particular, it is not allowed for a prison official to disclose your HIV status to other prisoners or non-medical personnel. The courts seem to permit disclosure of your HIV status only if such disclosure is reasonably related to legitimate prison interests, like protecting prisoners or corrections officers from infection. But unnecessary disclosure of such information for humor or gossip violates your constitutional rights.

In other jurisdictions, courts are divided about medical privacy. Some courts find that a prisoner's right to medical privacy is not that strong. Other courts protect medical privacy rights for prisoners and people who are arrested. But now that the Prison Litigation Reform Act (PLRA) has been passed, similar cases brought today might turn out differently. For more information on the PLRA. It is important to remember that the PLRA requires a showing of physical injury, not just mental or emotional injury, to recover monetary damages. Thus, to be successful in a lawsuit, you would probably have to prove that the prison official's actions physically injured you. Some courts may require you to show the harm is likely to occur again in order to get injunctions (orders requiring officials to stop or change a policy).

G. Legal Rights and Medical Treatment

1. Right to Medical Treatment

If you are denied medical treatment for an infectious disease, you may have a claim that the prison violated your rights under the Eighth Amendment. The Eighth Amendment protects you from cruel and unusual punishment. To win an Eighth Amendment claim, you must prove that prison officials showed "deliberate indifference" to your serious medical needs. It is important to remember that courts do not think that every claim of inadequate medical care is bad enough to be a constitutional violation. But a few courts have held that a denial of prescribed AIDS or hepatitis C medical treatment does violate a prisoner's constitutional rights

Courts generally do not believe prisoners have a constitutional right to a private doctor or experimental medication. You may still be able to get experimental drugs, but you will probably not have an Eighth Amendment claim against your facility if it does not prescribe them for you. But some prisons have participated in clinical trials for anti-retroviral therapy for AIDS. To take part in such trials, you must first get approval from the Institutional Review Board of the testing site and your prison's medical department.

If you believe that your health is suffering because you are being wrongfully denied medication, you will probably have to show that the medical community agrees that this medication will help your condition. Otherwise, the court may see your claim as a simple disagreement between you and your doctor. If you want to bring a claim about medical treatment or medication that was denied to you sometime in the past, a court may look back to see what the accepted medical practices were at that time.

If you got medical treatment but you think that a prison doctor incorrectly diagnosed your condition, it will be hard to bring a successful case against the prison officials. In the past, courts have dismissed cases for different reasons. The reasons include because the prisoner could not prove that the prison officials had personal involvement. In other cases, the prisoner could not show any physical harm, or the prisoner could not show that his needs were ignored.

If you have hepatitis C and prison officials determine that you should receive a certain treatment for a certain length of time, and you are then denied that treatment, you may have a claim under the Eighth Amendment. The first requirements to bring a claim will be met if you can say that the removal from the prescribed treatment is risking your life by not treating your disease. You do not have to also claim that you have suffered a separate harm in addition to your disease in order to bring your claim. Meeting these requirements allows you to begin your case, but does not mean that you will win. You will still need to show that there was "deliberate indifference" to your medical needs.

This does not change the rule that courts do not like to question doctors' medical decisions. If you have received treatment for hepatitis C but think you should have been given different treatment, or if your doctors said you do not have a condition requiring any treatment, this rule will not allow you to bring suit.

2. Right to Refuse Medical Treatment

Some people, for a variety of reasons, choose to refuse medical treatment. Competent people people who can think and understand well enough to make medical decisions for themselves have the right to refuse treatment, even if it means they will die as a result. However, your right to refuse treatment is limited as a prisoner. Most courts have held that prisons can treat TB-infected prisoners without their consent. Courts balance your interest in refusing treatment with the prison's legitimate penological interest in preventing the spread of disease. Courts will also consider whether the prison's actions are reasonably related to the prison's interests. If you do not have a disease that is transmitted through air, the prison will have a weaker argument for forcing you to take medication than if you have a disease such as TB that is easily spread. See Part C of Chapter 29, Special Issues for Prisoners with Mental Illness.

H. Discriminatory Treatment and Infectious Diseases

1. Constitutional Rights

The Fourteenth Amendment may protect you from being discriminated against for having an infectious disease. For example, your rights under the Equal Protection Clause of the Fourteenth Amendment prohibit discrimination by the state that is not rationally related to a legitimate purpose. The Due Process Clause of the Fourteenth Amendment forbids the prison facility from taking away your life, liberty, or property without due process of law. The Eighth Amendment protects you from cruel and unusual punishment. Keep in mind, however, that the courts balance these constitutional rights against legitimate penological interests, which may allow prison officials to lawfully infringe upon your rights. Prison policies are valid if they are reasonably related to a legitimate penological interest; however, the prison is required to use the least restrictive means of achieving the goals of the policy.

If you bring a suit challenging a prison practice under the Fourteenth Amendment's Due Process Clause, you must prove you were entitled to something the prison took away. Any entitlement must be created by state law. If you think you are entitled to something, you should first determine whether or not a state statute or regulation gives you a right to that entitlement. Also know that prison officials can treat prisoners with infectious diseases differently from other prisoners if they have legitimate penological interests in doing so; however, the reasons must be rational and not purely discriminatory.

The Fourteenth Amendment only applies to the states, but the Fifth Amendment's Due Process Clause protects your rights against the federal government. If you are in a federal prison, you might consider bringing your lawsuit under federal statutes, instead of under the Fifth Amendment.

2. Statutory Rights

Certain laws protect you from forms of discrimination based on disabilities, including HIV status. The Federal Rehabilitation Act of 1973 (FRA) prohibits discrimination, or denial of programs or benefits based on disability, by a federal, state, or local government agency, or any recipient of federal funding. Similarly, the Americans with Disabilities Act (ADA) prohibits public and private entities from discriminating, excluding, or denying services, programs, or activities to a person with a disability. These laws recognize TB and HIV infection as a form of disability because they are physical impairments limiting major life activities. Also, in Brandon v. Abbott, the Supreme

Court clearly stated that under the ADA, HIV infection satisfies the...definition of a physical impairment during every stage of the disease.

Although HIV is viewed as a disability according to the FRA and the ADA, your rights are limited to some extent if: (1) your HIV infection poses a significant risk to the health or safety of others; or (2) it would be an undue hardship on the prison facility to accommodate your needs. Also, the U.S. Supreme Court has decided that individuals cannot recover monetary damages from the state for its failure to comply with the ADA. However, you can still seek injunctive relief, which means that you can file a claim in which you ask the court to require the state to end practices that violate the ADA. If you are suing for violation of your statutory rights, you should cite both the FRA and the ADA, since the remedies, procedures, and rights are the same under both laws. The only difference is the FRA only applies to public (government) entities while the ADA can support a claim against both private and public entities. You should also check the law of your state and city since sometimes states and localities enact additional laws to protect people with communicable diseases, like HIV or hepatitis, from discrimination. In New York State, the Executive Law prohibits discrimination in several settings against people who carry the disease. If you are suing in New York, you should review New York law to see if it applies to your circumstances. Most prison facilities are controlled and financed by federal, state, or local governments, so the ADA and FRA usually apply to prison facilities. Furthermore, the U.S. Supreme Court has stated the ADA and FRA prohibit discrimination in the prison system. This means prison facilities cannot exclude or deny prisoners "benefits of the services, programs, or activities of a public entity" or subject them to discrimination. Benefits include recreational activities, medical services, and educational and vocational programs.

However, when a court evaluates a prison policy, it will consider whether the restriction is reasonably related to a legitimate penological interest. When a prison is defending a policy, it only has to show that the possibility of a risk exists; it does not have to demonstrate that the risk has actually occurred. Examples of interests cited by prison authorities include prison safety and undue financial or administrative burden.

I. Sentencing Persons With Infectious Diseases

If you have an infectious disease and you have been indicted for a crime but not yet sentenced, you may be able to ask the judge to dismiss the indictment or decrease your sentence because of your health condition. Different states have different rules, so be sure to look at your state's statutes and cases.

If your case is in New York State and you have a terminal illness, you may: (1) ask for lower bail, (2) ask to be released on your own recognizance, or (3) make a Clayton motion to have your case dismissed "in the interest of justice" (under New York Criminal Procedure Law § 210.40 and § 210.45). The court will look at the evidence of guilt, the seriousness of the offense, your character, and your criminal record. To support a request for dismissal, try to provide medical documentation that imprisonment would worsen your health.

If you have a terminal disease and are in prison because you violated your parole, you can request to: (1) be returned to parole status, (2) be released to time served or granted conditional release to probation, or (3) have your case adjourned in contemplation of dismissal. The adjournment may be extended indefinitely, which may allow you to live your last days out of prison.

If you are facing sentencing in federal court, judges consider the sentencing guidelines on an advisory basis. The court may impose a lesser sentence (downward departure) if mitigating circumstances exist. The U.S. Sentencing Commission Guidelines Manual states, an extraordinary physical impairment may be a reason to depart downward; e.g., in the case of a seriously infirm defendant, home detention may be as efficient as, and less costly than, imprisonment. Courts usually do not reduce sentences unless the defendant's AIDS is serious enough to be an extraordinary physical impairment. Some courts only consider the defendant's health at the time of sentencing, even if the disease will likely worsen in prison.

Most courts require you to be very sick before dismissing an indictment or reducing your sentence. But one federal district court did grant a downward departure to an HIV-positive defendant in stable condition. The court thought that the defendant believed his good health was a result of his special regimen of strict diet, regular exercise, acupuncture, and a combination of vitamins and natural supplements under the close supervision of a medical professional. In this case the judge was not worried about whether the treatment actually contributed to the defendant's good health. The judge thought that since the defendant believed his regimen was effective, would suffer emotional harm if he had to change treatments in prison.

If you are trying to get your sentence dismissed or reduced because of your health, you have a greater chance of success if you suffer from a very serious illness, like advanced-stage AIDS. You should try to present medical documentation that being in prison will harm your health. Also, keep in mind that courts might not be sympathetic to you if you have a long criminal history. Remember, courts have discretion to grant downward departures. The law does not say exactly what an "extraordinary physical impairment" is, so you may be able to get a reduced sentence or dismissal even if you do not have AIDS but have TB or hepatitis instead.

J. Life After Imprisonment: Planning for Your Release

Chapter 35 of the JLM, Getting Out Early: Conditional & Early Release, contains information about compassionate release and medical parole. If you have been diagnosed with an infectious disease, you should read that Chapter carefully to see whether you might be eligible for either of these options.

If you are about to be paroled or released, you should get a confidential HIV test before leaving prison. Getting a test can be more difficult or expensive outside of prison. If you do have HIV/AIDS or hepatitis, you should continue to be careful to avoid infecting other people. Before release, you should also try to contact local agencies and organizations for help transitioning from prison to community life. You can contact the public health department in your area for free brochures. Appendix A lists other helpful agencies.

K. Conclusion

If you have AIDS, TB, hepatitis B or C, MRSA or another infectious disease, people may treat you differently due to ignorance and fear. Protect yourself by becoming aware of the facts of the disease and your legal rights. As a prisoner, you may find that information and support is not always readily available. But many of the organizations work with prisoners and may be able help you.

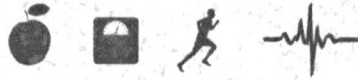

SPECIAL ISSUES FOR PRISONERS WITH MENTAL ILLNESS

A. Introduction

This Chapter will explain your rights as a prisoner with a mental illness. Part A discusses basic information you will need in order to understand how the law applies to prisoners with a mental illness (including the definitions of important terms such as mental illness and treatment). Part B explains your right to receive treatment for a mental illness. Part C explains how and when you can refuse unwanted treatment and transfer, as well as the consequences of transfer for hospitalization. Part D gives details about conditions of confinement, and explains how they overlap with mental health issues. Part E describes things to consider for pretrial detainees with mental illness. Part F explains the resources that are available to help you plan for your release. Part G describes resources available to you as a prisoner.

1. Defining "Mental Illness" and "Treatment"

(a) What Is Mental Illness?

This Chapter is written for prisoners with behavioral or psychological illnesses and diagnosable symptoms or risks. You might have heard people use the terms mental illness, serious mental illness, major mental illness, mental disorder, mental abnormality, mental sickness, serious and persistent mental illness, or mentally retarded. People (including courts and legislatures) use the terms as if they mean the same thing, but they do not. Many people say "mentally ill prisoners" or "prisoners with a mental illness" when they are referring to different groups of people, such as those who are not guilty by reason of insanity (NGIs), those incompetent to stand trial, or those with developmental disabilities (that is, low intellectual function that usually starts at childhood). When you read this Chapter, pay close attention to the way different terms are used to mean different things. The differences between different terms are important for you and any lawsuit you may decide to file.

There are many kinds of mental illness, but some common types include Bipolar Disorder, Borderline Personality Disorder, Major Depression, Obsessive-Compulsive Disorder (OCD), Panic Disorder, Post- Traumatic Stress Disorder (PTSD), and Schizophrenia. Others include Dissociative Disorders, Dual Diagnosis or MICA (Mentally Ill and Chemically Addicted—mental illness with substance abuse), Eating Disorders, Schizoaffective Disorder, Tourette's Syndrome, and Attention-Deficit/Hyperactivity Disorder. This Chapter will not discuss the separate issues of NGIs, sexual offenders, prisoners with developmental disabilities or prisoners with gender-identity issues. For a discussion of matters related to sex offenders.

Many state laws define mental illness to include only behavioral or psychological problems with noticeable symptoms. According to the American Psychiatric Association (APA), a person has a mental disorder if he suffers from a significant disturbance in behavior that reflects a dysfunction in the psychological, biological, or developmental processes underlying mental functioning. Mental disorders are usually associated with significant distress in social, occupational, or other important activities. This definition of a mental disorder does not cover psychological responses to particular events (like the death of a loved one) or certain behaviors (like sexual offenses). Mental illnesses may last for varying periods of time. Some last for a short period and then disappear; others are ongoing. Although courts have recognized that immediate psychological trauma (a sudden event that causes a lot of stress) also deserves mental health treatment, generally serious mental illnesses last longer, affect behavior, and have noticeable symptoms or risks.

To fit within most state law definitions of mental disorder, prisoners must show (1) a behavioral or psychological problem; (2) an accompanying symptom; and (3) a diagnosis of mental illness by a professional. For instance, in New York, mental illness means having a mental disease or mental condition which is expressed as...a disorder or disturbance in behavior, feeling, thinking, or judgment to such an extent that the person afflicted requires care and treatment. Like the APA approach, some state laws specifically exclude sexual offenses, substance abuse, and mental retardation from the definition of mental illness.

(b) What the Law and This Chapter Mean by "Treatment"

The definition of "treatment" under the law generally includes three steps: (1) diagnosis (a finding by a doctor or mental health specialist that there is a mental illness), (2) intervention (a decision to treat the illness with therapy, drugs, or other care), and (3) planning (developing a method to relieve suffering or find a cure).

Whether a particular medical action qualifies as treatment depends on whether it is medically necessary and whether it will substantially help or cure your medical condition. Medical necessity usually involves a serious medical need, which could well result in the deprivation of life itself if untreated. The test to determine whether treatment is necessary is not whether a prisoner suffers from mental illness but instead whether that mental illness requires care and treatment.

The law assumes that doctors are the best people to make medical choices to treat mental illness. Therefore, whether something is an appropriate treatment is a decision that judges and lawmakers leave to medical professionals. Just because a prisoner or a judge prefers a particular course of action to treat mental illness does not mean it is a necessary course of treatment under the law. In New York, the Commissioner of the Department of Correctional Services, in cooperation with the Commissioner of the Office of Mental Health (the head of the department that handles mental illness issues), is responsible for establishing programs in correctional facilities for treatment other than hospitalization. Although programs need only satisfy what the Commissioner of the Department of Correctional Services "deems appropriate" for the treatment of prisoners with mental illness, the law does require that inmates with serious mental illness shall receive therapy and programming in settings that are appropriate to their clinical needs while maintaining the safety and security of the facility. Although adequate medical and health services must always be provided, states require different levels of psychiatric care, as not all types of care are necessary for treatment.

Although you do not have a right to decide your treatment plan, you do have access to the following rights. You have the right to mental health care that meets the standards of the medical profession. Next, you have the right to information about your treatment's risks and alternatives. Finally, you have a limited right to refuse treatment (see Part C of this Chapter). Once a decision to treat your mental illness has been made, you cannot specify which treatment alternatives (such as medication, counseling, or therapy) you should receive. You may, however, be able to protect yourself against unfair medical treatment by arguing that a certain treatment is not necessary.

2. Understanding Treatment Facilities

There are three basic types of psychiatric care that are used to treat prisoners:

    (1) Acute (or crisis) care, which is twenty-four hour care for prisoners whose symptoms of psychosis (losing contact with reality), suicide risk, or dangerousness justify intensive care and forced medication;

    (2) Sub-acute (or intermediate) care, usually outside of a hospital for prisoners suffering from severe and chronic conditions that require intensive care management, psychosocial interventions (treatment that is both social and psychological), crisis management, and psychopharmacology (drugs that affect the mind) in a safe and contained environment; and

    (3) Outpatient care, which is provided to the general population, is for prisoners who can function relatively normally. It can—but does not have to—include medication, psychotherapy (meeting with a psychiatrist or other trained mental health professional), supportive counseling, and other

    (4) Interventions

The most common type of care prisoners receive is outpatient care. If you require more intensive care, you may be treated in a hospital within the prison system or at an off-site hospital set up specifically to treat people with mental illnesses. The severity of mental illness, the types and availability of facilities, and the doctor's medical diagnosis will all factor into your placement.

The Division of Forensic Services at the New York State Office of Mental Health (OMH) runs the New York psychiatric facility system. There are four forensic psychiatric care centers. One of them, Central New York Psychiatric Center, is both a regional forensic unit and the inpatient psychiatric hospital that services all prisoners in the state prisons and operates the many "satellite mental health units" and "mental health units" located within New York State prisons. You should note that administrative segregation, such as solitary confinement or disciplinary segregated confinement in "special housing units" (SHUs) or "keeplock," is not a treatment facility. Many mental health experts, advocates, and clinicians believe that these forms of isolated confinement make mental health conditions worse, and courts have recognized the harm they cause. For more information on isolation and mental health, see Part D(1) of this Chapter.

(a) Treatment Facility Admissions in New York

In New York, whenever the doctor of a prison, jail, or other correctional institution believes you need hospitalization because of mental illness, the doctor must tell the facility superintendent, who will then apply to a judge for a commitment order. The judge will require two other doctors to examine you. In New York City, the two doctors may examine you in your prison or you may be transferred to a county hospital for examination. The doctors must agree that you have a mental illness and need care or treatment in order for you to be hospitalized, but first they must consider other treatment alternatives. They must also consult your previous doctor if they know that you have been treated for mental illness in the past and if it is possible to do so.

If the two doctors agree that you need to be hospitalized to treat a mental illness, the prison superintendent will apply to a judge for permission to commit you. You should receive notice of any court order and have a chance to challenge it. In addition, your wife, husband, father, mother, or nearest relative must also receive notice of the decision to commit you. If you have no known relatives within the state, that notice must be given to any known friend of yours. If you decide to challenge the decision, you have a right to know the hospital's placement procedure. You also have the right to a lawyer, a hearing, an independent medical opinion, and judicial review including a jury trial. However, you do not have a right to a hearing in an emergency, during which two doctors agree that your mental illness is likely to result in serious harm to you or to other prisoners. In that case, you are still entitled to notice, a lawyer, an independent medical opinion, a hearing, and a jury trial, but only after you arrive at a hospital.

B. Your Right to Receive Treatment

This Part explains two doctrines (that is, rules) that relate to your right to psychiatric medical care. Section 1 of this Part discusses whether the prison must provide psychiatric care, and how much care the prison must provide. Section 1 also mentions special considerations for prisoners with substance-related disorders and what medical treatment they should receive. Section 2 addresses your rights if psychiatric medical care is delayed or denied.

1. What to Do if the Psychiatric Medical Care You Receive Is Inadequate

You have a right to adequate medical care and treatment. Under the Eighth Amendment of the Constitution, the government has an obligation to provide medical care to people it is punishing by incarceration. This right includes the regular medical care that is necessary to maintain your health and safety. Many states also have state laws requiring prisons to provide medical care to prisoners.

(a) Your Right to Adequate Psychiatric Care

The provision of mental health care to prisoners is governed in the same way as the provision of physical health care. Most federal circuits have held the right to adequate medical care includes any psychiatric care that is necessary to maintain prisoners' health and safety. In Bowring v. Godwin, an important early decision, the Fourth Circuit Court of Appeals included treatment of mental illnesses as part of the right to medical care. The court noted that there is no underlying distinction between the right of a prisoner to medical care for physical ills and its psychological or psychiatric counterpart.

The Bowring court developed a three-part test to determine whether a prisoner has a right to psychiatric care. Under the test, a prisoner who suffers from a mental illness is likely to have a right to mental health treatment if a health care provider decides that:

(1) the prisoner has the symptoms of a serious disease or injury;

(2) that disease or injury is curable, or can be substantially improved; and

(3) the likelihood of harm to the prisoner (in terms of safety and health, including mental health) is substantial if treatment is delayed or denied.

However, the right to psychiatric treatment is still limited to reasonable medical costs and a reasonable length of time for treatment. Therefore, psychiatric treatment will be given to the prisoner on the basis of what is necessary, not what is desirable.

You should note that the Bowring test is the law only in the Fourth Circuit, which includes Maryland, North Carolina, South Carolina, Virginia, and West Virginia. The only courts that must apply the test are federal courts in these states. However, other courts are likely to consider using the standard in similar cases, especially because no court has issued a disagreeing opinion. You should still cite to Bowring even if you are not bringing a case in the Fourth Circuit, because the court in your circuit might find Bowring persuasive.

The American Psychiatric Association incorporates in its definition of mental illness substance-related disorders, which include illnesses like substance use, abuse, and withdrawal. The law, however, does not always consider such diseases as serious enough to require prison authorities to provide medical care to treat the diseases. However, many courts have found that prisoners have the right to treatment for substance abuse in certain circumstances. The sections below describe these situations.

(i) You Have No Right to Drug and Alcohol Rehabilitation in Prison

As a general rule, you have no right to rehabilitation while in prison. Individual states or corrections departments may decide that rehabilitation is an important goal and may implement programs to achieve that aim, but the Constitution does not require them to do so. One application of this rule is that there is no right to narcotics or alcohol treatment programs in prison. However, courts have at times ordered prisons to implement drug and alcohol treatment programs where the denial of these programs would otherwise lead to conditions that were so bad that they violated prisoners' rights to medical care. Prisoners often raise these issues successfully in the context of broader claims about unconstitutional conditions of confinement. Additionally, at least one court has found that prisoners should be free to attempt rehabilitation or the cultivation of new socially acceptable and useful skills and habits. It might be possible to argue that failure to receive drug treatment violates that freedom.

There is also no right to methadone or to the establishment of methadone maintenance programs in prison. On the other hand, a few courts have found that you do have the right to continue drug treatment with programs in which you already participate. This right primarily protects you pretrial. Pretrial detainees are people who have not been found guilty but still must remain in jail because they cannot afford to post bail or they have been determined to be a flight risk or danger to the community. These individuals cannot be punished beyond detention and the restraint of liberty that comes with it. Courts view forced rehabilitation as a punishment. They also view the pain suffered when methadone is discontinued as a punishment. For more information on your right to treatment as a pretrial detainee, please see Part E(1) of this Chapter.

(ii) Your Right to Avoid Deterioration (Getting More Sick) While Incarcerated

Many courts have held that even if you do not have an absolute constitutional right to treatment for certain illnesses like substance abuse; you do have a right to avoid having your illness get worse while you are in prison. Though some courts have not found a right to avoid getting more sick while incarcerated, several have at least found that where conditions are so bad that serious physical or psychological deterioration is inevitable, you can state an Eighth Amendment claim of cruel and unusual punishment.

So, if your drug or alcohol addiction is likely to worsen your condition, you might be able to make a claim that failure to receive adequate treatment violates your right to avoid getting more sick while in prison. Even though different federal circuits have established differing rules as to the extent of that right, at a minimum, if your deterioration results from the State's intent to cause harm, you can claim the State violated your rights.

(iii) Your Right to Care for Withdrawal from Drugs and Alcohol

Another exception to the general rule that prisons do not need to provide medical care for substance- related disorders is that prisons do need to provide care for withdrawal, which can be excessively painful and dangerous, and is therefore considered a serious medical condition. Because of the seriousness of withdrawal symptoms, you are entitled to treatment. Most of the cases have come up in the context of pretrial detainees going through withdrawal just after arrest, but the courts have not explicitly limited the right to treatment to pretrial detainees. If a convicted prisoner experiences a serious medical need due to withdrawal then he should receive treatment.

2. What to do if Treatment is Denied or Delayed

The above Subsection discussed situations in which a prisoner claims that the medical care he received is inadequate. This Subsection instead focuses on your rights when the treatment you need has been deliberately (purposely) denied or delayed. Although courts do not like second-guessing doctors' decisions, a prison official who denies or delays treatment knowing that you need that treatment might be violating your constitutional right to be free of cruel and unusual punishment under the Eighth Amendment. A court that finds this deliberate denial or delay will step in to help you. Not every delay in medical care is a violation of the Constitution.

A prison official only violates the Eighth Amendment when two requirements are met. The first requirement is that the deprivation of medical care is sufficiently serious. The second requirement is that the prison official must have acted with a culpable (bad) state of mind and ignored your health needs on purpose. To meet this standard you must show that you have actually been deprived of adequate medical care, and that the lack of treatment has caused you harm, or will cause you harm in the future. If care has been denied, the court will look at whether a reasonable doctor or patient would find it important and worthy of comment," whether the condition has significant affects" on your daily activities, and whether it causes chronic and substantial pain. In cases where treatment has been delayed or interrupted, the question of how serious the situation is focuses on the impact of the delay and not on the main medical condition alone. The second requirement for an Eighth Amendment violation is that the prison official acted with deliberate indifference to your medical or mental health needs. These requirements are discussed in more detail below.

(a) You Must Satisfy the Deliberate Indifference Standard

The Supreme Court has decided that a prison official shows deliberate indifference when he knows of and disregards an excessive risk to inmate health or safety. For example, a prisoner might submit evidence that prison officials refused to treat him, ignored his complaints, intentionally treated him incorrectly, or engaged in any similar conduct that would clearly evince a wanton disregard for any serious medical needs.

A prison official can be deliberately indifferent by: (1) taking action (doing something), or (2) refusing to act (not doing something). An example of an act showing deliberate indifference might be knowingly stopping hormone treatments for a prisoner with Gender Identity Disorder. An example of a deliberate omission might be refusing to provide essential or refusing to treat a prisoner's cavity.

Although the deliberate indifference standard has developed in the context of serious medical care, it also applies to medically necessary treatment for mental illnesses. Deliberate indifference to the serious mental health needs of a prisoner violates the Eighth Amendment just as much as deliberate indifference to physical medical needs.

Many deliberate indifference claims about inadequate prison mental health care argue that the facility's mental health staff is too small to meet prisoners' needs or that the staff members are unqualified. Several courts have concluded that the lack of an on-site psychiatrist in a large prison is unconstitutional. The failure to train correctional staff to work with prisoners with mental illness can also constitute deliberate indifference.

Among the deficiencies in prison mental health care that courts have held actionable are the lack of or inadequate mental health screening on intake, the failure to follow up with prisoners who have known or suspected mental disorders, the failure to hospitalize prisoners whose conditions cannot adequately be treated in prison, ross departures from professional standards in treatment, and the failure to separate prisoners with severe mental illness from those without mental illness. Mixing prisoners with mental illness with those who do not have mental illnesses might violate the rights of both groups. Courts have also held that housing prisoners with mental illness under conditions of extreme isolation is unconstitutional. Another recurring situation is stopping psychiatric medications without reason, often with disastrous results.

In a landmark decision in 2011, Brown v. Plata, the Supreme Court held that the mental health care provided in California prisons was inadequate and violated the Eighth Amendment. However, the Supreme Court did not consider whether any particular instance of delay or deficiency in medical treatment would itself violate the Constitution. Instead, the Court looked at the system-wide problems that as a whole subjected prisoners to substantial risk of serious harm. Regardless, the elements considered by the Court included similar factors such as not enough staff, not enough space for the staff to perform their jobs, delays in treatment, and unsafe and unsanitary living conditions that hamper effective delivery of medical care and mental health care.

It is important to remember that the deliberate indifference standard applies to a significant denial or delay of adequate medical care. If you feel that you have been denied mental health treatment, or if you feel that it has been unnecessarily delayed, and you wish to claim deliberate indifference, you must:

> (1) state facts that are sufficient to allege a serious medical need for which medical care has not been provided; and

> (2) assert that a prison official must have been aware of the need for medical care, or at least of facts which might have led the official to believe there was a need for medical care.

(i) You Must Show Serious Medical Need

The first part of your deliberate indifference claim must include facts that show you had a serious medical need for which you did not receive treatment. A medical need is serious when there is a substantial risk that you will suffer serious harm if you do not receive adequate treatment. Courts have also defined a serious medical need as one that a doctor has diagnosed as requiring treatment or one that is so obvious that a non-doctor could easily recognize the need. For example, where a prisoner has attempted suicide, the court has found a serious medical need.

(ii) You Must Show Actual Knowledge of Your Serious Medical Need

For the second part of your deliberate indifference claim, you must show that prison officials actually knew you needed mental health care but still failed to treat you. In Farmer v. Brennan, the Supreme Court explained a prison official knows of a risk when he is not only aware of facts that would lead to the conclusion that the prisoner faces a substantial risk of serious harm but also actually comes to that conclusion. In other words, this part of the deliberate indifference test is subjective (from the point of view of that particular prison official); he must actually believe you will suffer some serious harm before a court will find he had knowledge of the risk. But, if the risk is so obvious, a jury can assume the prison official knew of the risk. For example, the Farmer Court noted that if a plaintiff shows the risk of prisoner attacks was "longstanding, pervasive, well-documented, or expressly noted by prison officials in the past, and the circumstances suggest that the defendant-official being sued had been exposed to information concerning the risk and thus 'must have known' about it," that could be enough to show actual knowledge of the risk.

(b) What Does Not Count as Deliberate Indifference?

Courts will refuse to find deliberate indifference in some situations. The deliberate indifference standard is meant to address unnecessary and wanton infliction of pain. Acts or omissions that are not purposeful, or where the prison officials had no reason to know you might suffer serious harm, will not satisfy the standard. A complaint alleging inadequate psychiatric care because officials did not pursue treatment you would have chosen will not meet the deliberate indifference standard. This is because prison officials have the right to exercise discretion in deciding what treatment is adequate for a serious medical need. In view of this discretion, courts will not find deliberate indifference when prison officials were merely negligent, made a mistake, or had a difference of opinion regarding adequate medical care.

Similarly, a complaint based on malpractice (improper or negligent treatment by a doctor) or misdiagnosis (a medical mistake) will not meet the high deliberate indifference standard. Thus, a complaint that a doctor has been negligent in diagnosing or treating a medical condition does not state a valid claim of medical mistreatment under the Eighth Amendment. You may instead be able to file a medical malpractice claim alleging negligence.

(c) How to Bring a Deliberate Indifference Claim Under Section 1983

If you think your case meets the legal standard, you may bring a claim of deliberate indifference to your personal health and wellbeing under 42 U.S.C. § 1983 (Section 1983). You can use Section 1983 to sue cities and local governments for constitutional violations, including, for instance, the government body controlling the institution where the violation took place. For detailed information on bringing a claim under this law, please read Chapter 16 of the JLM, Using 42 U.S.C. § 1983 and 28 U.S.C. § 1331 to Obtain Relief from Violations of Federal Law. If you plan to file your suit in federal court, you should also read Chapter 14 of the JLM, The Prison Litigation Reform Act.

You can also use Section 1983 to challenge inadequate prison medical care as an Eighth Amendment violation. To prove inadequacy, you must show: (1) you have a mental health need that is serious enough that denial of treatment violates the Constitution; and (2) the prison was "deliberately indifferent" to this serious mental health need. You must show the policy or custom at the prison directly caused the constitutional violation.

In the context of a mental health complaint, you should keep a few things in mind. First, if you believe you suffer from a mental illness and want medical treatment, you should tell prison officials. If you are afraid you will hurt yourself or other people, you should tell prison officials that too. Prison officials can only be held accountable under the deliberate indifference standard if they have actual knowledge of, or some other reason to believe, that you have a mental illness that requires treatment.

C. What to Do if You Receive Unwanted Treatment

While the previous Parts of this Chapter focused on your right to receive medical treatment for your mental illness, this Part discusses treatment that you do not want. You should also look at Part C(5)(a) and (E)(1) of Chapter 23 of the JLM, Your Right to Adequate Medical Care.

1. You Have the Right to Informed Consent

MIKE ENEMIGO

You have a right to receive enough information about a potential medical treatment to make a reasonable decision whether to try the treatment. After you learn about the treatment, you can choose whether or not to give permission for the doctor to treat you. This right is known as informed consent, and it means that you have the right to learn about all treatment options and the risks associated with each option before you allow mental health doctors or other caregivers to treat you. Informed consent is a way of making sure that you understand, before you start the treatment, what a treatment includes, and what effects it may have on you. Informed consent is an important part of your right to refuse treatment. If you do not give your consent, you are refusing treatment; however, informed consent does have some limits. If you pose a danger to yourself or others, the doctor may be able to treat you in a manner that the doctor believes will immediately help and benefit you.

Doctors have a duty to obtain informed consent from patients, including prisoners, before treating them. A doctor must almost always inform you of options and risks when there is penetration of the body (such as with a scalpel, needle, or pill). Also, when the direct side effects of treatment are painful or serious, your informed consent is usually required. Some states specifically require by law that doctors consider alternative forms of care, and inform you of the procedures and risks associated with each. You should research what the law is in your state.

You should carefully consider whether or not to give your consent to receive treatment. State law varies as to whether informed consent for one treatment will extend to all risks associated with a particular procedure or any additional procedures that a doctor believes will help you. In New York, if you have not consented to a previous treatment, doctors cannot imply consent to a separate course of treatment, even in an emergency. The rule in California is that consent to a previous treatment does not mean consent to another course of treatment; there, a court held that a prisoner who consented to shock treatment did not necessarily consent to administration of drugs that produced nightmares.

2. Medication Over Prisoner's Objection

Medication is one form of treatment. Prisoners have a limited right to refuse antipsychotic or psychotropic drugs. Such medications help cure certain symptoms of mental illness but also alter a person's perception, emotions, or behavior. For example, psychotropic drugs can have serious side effects, such as nightmares and muscle tics (sudden movements). The law provides protection against the unwanted use of serious drugs by giving prisoners the right to refuse treatments that interfere to a great degree with the body. However, this right is not absolute—there are some circumstances when medication can be administered, even over your objection.

(a) Your Right to Refuse Medication Under the Due Process Clause

Under the Due Process Clause of the U.S. Constitution, no State shall...deprive any person of life, liberty, or property, without due process of law. Some deprivations are so important that the Constitution requires states to establish processes to ensure that you are not deprived unfairly. For example, in Vitek v. Jones, the Supreme Court found that characterizing a prisoner as mentally ill and moving him to a psychiatric hospital were such serious (grievous) losses that the State was required to have procedural protections in place to make sure that the loss was fair. These losses included the harm to the prisoner's reputation and the change in conditions of confinement.

Similarly, before the State can force you to take medication, it must have procedural protections in place to make sure you are not receiving the medication randomly or unfairly. You must receive procedures, including notice and a hearing, before you can be involuntarily medicated.

260

A decision to treat you with drugs triggers procedural due process protections because drugs can produce serious and irreversible side effects that represent a significant State intrusion into your body.

(b) Your Right to Refuse Medication Based on State Law

Your right to refuse medication may come not only from the Constitution, but also from state laws that specifically require procedural protections (such as notice and a hearing) before you can be forcibly medicated. If your state has such a law, it must follow the procedures set out by the law. If your state wishes to avoid the process that is laid out by state law, it must have a rational reason for doing so, or the avoidance will be considered a due process violation. In other words, your state must show that it has legitimate reasons, reasonably related to its interests, before it may take away an expectation that was granted through its own law.

Unless your state can show both that you have a mental illness and are dangerous, or that your state's rule has so many protections that it is unlikely that you will receive medication unfairly, it cannot force you to take medication without some procedural protections.

(c) Your Right to Refuse Medication Under the Eighth Amendment

In some circumstances, you also have a right to refuse medication under the Eighth Amendment, which prohibits cruel and unusual punishment. Administration of drugs as a means of punishment (rather than as treatment) is unconstitutional.

Forcible treatment with psychotropic medication that causes pain or fright can constitute cruel and unusual punishment, violating the Eighth Amendment. The district court in Souder v. McGuire cited cases in the Eighth and Ninth Circuits that held that treating prisoners with drugs without consent may raise Eighth Amendment claims. In those cases, the courts found that drugs causing pain or fright could invade the body and mental processes to an unconstitutional degree.

While some courts have emphasized that an allegation that you were given a particular kind of medicine is not enough to prove that giving you the drug was cruel and unusual (and thus a violation of the Eighth Amendment), the Supreme Court has held that states may not avoid the obligations of the Eighth Amendment just by calling a medical act a treatment.

(d) Limitations on Your Right to Refuse Medication

The right to refuse medication does not mean that the State can never medicate you against your will. Instead, it means that the State must provide a process (such as a hearing) that reduces the chance that the decision to medicate you will be random or arbitrary.

One important limitation on a prisoner's right to refuse medication is danger or emergency. Prisons may administer psychotropic drugs over a prisoner's objection if the prisoner poses a danger to himself or others. Receiving medication against your will is called medication over objection. In Washington v. Harper, the Supreme Court upheld a policy allowing the state to medicate a prisoner without consent if a licensed psychiatrist found that the prisoner suffered from a mental disorder, and the prisoner was gravely disabled or posed a likelihood of serious harm to himself or others. Therefore, situations in which a prisoner presents a danger to himself or the general prison population are an exception to the right to refuse treatment. A good example is a Kansas prisoner who objected to psychotropic medication but was not allowed to refuse treatment because he had previously destroyed his prison cell and started altercations with other prisoners.

There are a few other limitations on a prisoner's right to refuse treatment. A prisoner may receive medication despite objections or religious beliefs if the State can prove that its interests are legitimate. Also, the State may give drugs to a prisoner over his objections if the court feels that enough procedural protections are in place to ensure that the decision to treat with drugs was reasonable. You should also note that, in some cases, if a doctor finds that medication is necessary and in the prisoner's medical interest, then the State does not have to grant a prisoner's request to stop taking the drugs so that he can prove he can do without them.

A determination of whether the right to refuse is limited in any given case must be defined in the context of the inmate's confinement. This means that the court will review your current prison conditions,

the threat of danger that you pose to yourself or others, and the procedures that the State has in place to protect you from an unfair decision to treat you with drugs.

(e) How Do Courts Decide Whether State Interests Are Legitimate?

To determine whether or not the State may rightfully force a prisoner to take medication due to a situation of danger or emergency, courts apply what is called the Turner v. Safley rational basis test. With this test, the court tries to see if the State's decision to treat a non-consenting prisoner with psychotropic drugs is reasonably related to legitimate penological interests. Legitimate State interests include the health and safety of the public, the prisoner, and the general prison population. The rational basis test presumes that State interests are legitimate. This means that a court will consider the State's choice to medicate a prisoner reasonable unless it does not serve one or more of these legitimate State goals.

There are some common arguments that prisoners use to counter the presumption that the State's actions are the result of a legitimate interest. One challenge to medication over objection is that the decision to medicate is unfair or arbitrary (random or not supported by a reason). In such cases, courts consider a competing risk that the determination of danger will be incorrect and may cause harm to the prisoner's reputation. In order to avoid mistakes in determining if there is a danger, taking the drugs must be in the prisoner's medical interest and can only be for treatment purposes.

In addition, states must provide certain procedural safeguards to ensure that the decision to medicate is not arbitrary or erroneous. Common safeguards include (1) an administrative hearing before an independent decision maker (someone not involved in the prisoner's treatment but who may come from within the institution); (2) written notice; (3) the right to be present at an adversary hearing; and (4) the right to present and cross-examine witnesses. While the State may provide a lawyer to represent the prisoner in administrative hearings, providing a non-attorney adviser may satisfy due process.

3. Challenging Transfers for Treatment

(a) What Is a Treatment Transfer?

Many treatments are available for prisoners and sometimes these treatments must be administered at a site outside of the prison, requiring that the prisoner be transferred from his present location in order to be treated. A prisoner may submit to the transfer or voluntarily agree to various forms of treatment including medication, counseling, therapy, or commitment to a psychiatric center. Or, in some cases, the prisoner may be treated involuntarily. This Section explains when the prison can and cannot transfer you for treatment if you do not consent to the transfer.

Prisoners who suffer from a mental illness may be treated at one of several possible locations. For more details on these facilities, please see Part A(2) above. Please note that if you are transferred to a facility that has a significantly different quality than the normal and typical conditions of prison confinement, this might violate your constitutional rights.

(b) Procedural Safeguards Under the Due Process Clause

Lawful imprisonment may take away some of your rights, but you still have a right to basic protections. In certain circumstances, basic procedures must be in place to protect you from an unfair action of the State. For more information on procedural due process. A hearing and written notice are two common examples of procedures that might be required, often before a prisoner can be involuntarily committed to a psychiatric hospital.

Prison to hospital transfers might mean a significant change in living conditions and type of confinement. A determination of mental illness by a doctor and subsequent transfer does not automatically mean that a prisoner has a mental illness for the purposes of other laws in the state. Still, there is a chance that the prisoner might suffer harm to his reputation. When the risk of physical and/or reputational harm is high, your constitutional right to due process might be triggered.

In addition, if the State tries to avoid the requirements imposed by its own laws, then a law giving you the right to procedures before transfer will also trigger due process protections. Where state regulations require a finding of mental illness before transfer, the State creates an objective expectation in the prisoner that there will be a procedure to determine whether or not a mental illness exists. Without such procedures, the prisoner could suffer a due process violation. In short, you may have a right to due process protections (such as the right to a hearing and the right to receive notice of the hearing) when the State's action creates a high level of harm to you (physical or reputational), or when a state law gives you the expectation that some particular act or process must be followed, and then the State fails to follow this act or process.

The due process protection to which you are entitled is the same, no matter how your liberty interest is implicated.

In Vitek v. Jones, the Supreme Court found that a Nebraska statute requiring a finding of mental illness before transfer to an outside mental facility created an expectation among prisoners that transfer would occur only if they were found to have mental illness.

Under Vitek, the State must adequately protect your liberty interests (if it has created them through state law) in the transfer process by providing:

(1) Written notice that the prison is considering your transfer;

(2) A hearing;

(3) An opportunity to present witness testimony and cross-examine state witnesses at the hearing;

(4) An independent decision maker;

(5) A written statement by the decision maker stating the reasons and evidence relied on for your

(6) Transfer;

(7) Legal assistance from the State if you cannot afford your own; and

(8) Effective and timely notice of rights (1) through (6).

All of these protections are triggered if your liberty interests are implicated and there is a chance that you will suffer a serious loss. Failure to provide them violates your rights.

(i) Are Your Liberty Interests Implicated?

Courts determine whether the State can deprive you of a liberty interest by balancing the interests of the State (for example, prison safety) with your liberty interest in freedom from random deprivations (for example, the right to agree or disagree to medication). If the interest of the prisoner is found to be stronger than the interest of the State, then the individual is entitled to due process protections. Whether or not a prisoner has a state-created liberty interest depends on whether the loss the prisoner faces is serious.

Liberty interests are limited; prisoners are entitled to freedom from restraint only to the extent that restraint cannot exceed the conviction sentence in an unexpected manner. This is true unless there is an atypical and significant hardship on the inmate in relation to the ordinary incidents of prison life. In other words, for due process to apply, you must have both a liberty interest and a deprivation of that liberty that imposes a significant and atypical (unusual) hardship. Only if both of these factors are present are you entitled to due process protections like written notice and a hearing. Transfer from one prison to another within the State's system does not necessarily infringe upon any liberty interest.

The Equal Protection Clause of the Fourteenth Amendment of the Constitution prohibits states from denying any person equal protection of the laws. In other words, state laws must treat each person in the same manner as others in similar conditions and circumstances. In the context of mental health, the equal protection rights of prisoners who are being committed entitle them to substantially the same procedures as those available to free persons subjected to an involuntary commitment proceeding. In United States ex rel. Schuster v. Herold, the Second Circuit found that a New York prisoner who was transferred from prison to an institution for the criminally insane was deprived of equal protection because there was an unlawful difference between procedural protections given to civilians facing involuntary commitment and those given to prisoners. Therefore, to determine the procedural protections that apply in your state, you should review civil commitment laws in addition to laws that govern corrections facilities. We discuss procedural protections and treatment transfers later in this Chapter.

(ii) What is a Serious Loss?

Courts might consider transfers to be a serious loss because of three factors: (1) there is a high risk of stigma associated with a declaration of mental illness; (2) there is an actual change in the type of confinement; and (3) there is actual behavior modification treatment. As with challenges to medication over objection, these changes require that the State provide procedural protections.

The test courts apply to determine if a loss is serious examines whether the loss is significant and atypical. Significant and atypical state actions are those actions not similar to prison conditions or those that substantially alter the environment, duration, or degree of the prison condition. For example, a prisoner who was placed in segregated confinement did not suffer a serious loss that implicated a liberty interest because the segregation was of the same duration and degree as that of his normal prison conditions.

More specifically, under the Vitek standard, significant and atypical means that the loss suffered by the prisoner is different than the loss already suffered as a result of prison confinement. The loss to the prisoner in Vitek was serious enough to require due process protections because he had reasonably developed an objective expectation based on the state law and the risk that mistaken mental illness could damage the prisoner's reputation was great. In another case, a loss of good-time credits was significant because such a loss of credits meant that there was a change in the length of the prison term. Finally, confinement in a psychiatric prison unit might be far more restrictive than prison, and therefore might be considered a serious loss, implicating a liberty interest.

4. When Due Process Procedures Are Not Required For Transfer

The protections discussed in the previous Subsection might not be afforded to the prisoner if the transfer is voluntary or on an emergency basis. Additionally, the Due Process Clause does not protect against every change in the conditions of your imprisonment, even if that change has a negative impact on you. This is true even if the prisoner has a reasonable expectation that state actions will produce a particular result. In some jurisdictions, the law says that the State may not need to have procedures in place for you to participate in clinical evaluations (you are not considered to be under the same great hardship in this case as with commitment). In a few states, procedural protections do not have to occur before transfer, but may instead occur promptly after physical transfer.

As with challenges to medication over objection, there are limits to a transfer challenge. Transfer to a mental health facility without a hearing is generally not a due process violation when a prisoner poses an immediate threat to himself or the general population. These transfers are called emergency commitments. However, a hearing must be held as soon as possible after commitment. If it is determined you will be transferred to a psychiatric hospital or unit, you cannot challenge a transfer back to prison after treatment because no liberty interest existed. For example, in Washington, D.C., prisoners may be moved, with the superintendent's certification, from psychiatric hospitals back to prisons after being restored to health. In New York, administrative transfers from a state hospital to a prison do not violate due process because they are not considered to be punishment. You should check the laws in your state to determine the necessary steps the state must take to transfer you back to prison.

5. If You Are Transferred to a Hospital or Other Treatment Facility

If you are transferred or committed to a psychiatric facility, you maintain many of the same rights you had in prison, including the right to treatment and the right to adequate medical care. Similarly, if you are confined in a hospital or treatment facility prior to serving your criminal sentence in prison, you may be entitled to have your time spent there count toward your sentence.

(a) How Long Will I Be Held?

Generally, the time spent in commitment is left to the judgment of clinical mental health staff and prison officials, but it cannot be longer than your criminal sentence unless you are first granted significant due process protections. Under New York State law, for example, the psychiatric hospital director may apply for a new commitment after your sentence expires. If this happens in a state where there are requirements set up for a civil commitment proceeding, your criminal sentence is not relevant to any post- sentence confinement, and the State must provide the same procedural safeguards before committing or holding you for psychiatric care that it would if you were a non-prisoner. This means that if the State determines you need further commitment and treatment after your prison sentence has ended, you will be treated as a non-prisoner. If the psychiatric hospital director successfully extends commitment past your term sentence, you have the right to another hearing before a jury to determine whether commitment to a civilian mental health facility is appropriate.

(b) What Happens to My Good-Time Credits?

In some states, a prisoner may lose the opportunity to earn good-time credits after a mental illness determination and hospitalization. The reasoning that many courts give for this policy is that the goals of hospitalization differ from the goals of imprisonment. Hospitalization is meant to treat prisoners with mental illness, while incarceration is intended to punish and also rehabilitate. However, the Eighth Circuit found that there is a difference between meritorious credits (credits that are given at the State's discretion) and statutory good-time credits (credits that a state statute specifically grants for particular behavior). Unlike discretionary credits, statutory credits come from state laws. Therefore, a loss of statutory credits based on a mental health assessment could violate your constitutional right to equal protection under the Fourteenth Amendment, which prohibits states from applying the law differently to different citizens in the same condition and circumstances.

Even if the law in your jurisdiction does not permit you to continue to earn credits while you are hospitalized, your existing credits may be held in abeyance (paused) during treatment, meaning that all good-time credits that would have been credited will be restored when you are transferred back to prison. However, if you have existing credits, in many jurisdictions they will not apply until you are restored to health; in other words, you are not entitled to early release if you are still hospitalized on your early release date. Other states, in contrast, do permit you to receive good-time credits even while in the hospital. For example, the Connecticut Supreme Court has found that the language of Connecticut's statute orders the corrections commissioner to apply earned good-time credit to any prisoner's sentence, in keeping with the idea that the law should treat equally prisoners with mental illness confined in hospitals and those incarcerated in prisons. Since the law varies according to the statutes of each jurisdiction, you should check the law in your state, or the United States Code if you are in federal prison, to determine what happens to your credits during transfer to a hospital.

(c) Can I Receive Credit for Pre-Sentence Confinement in a Hospital or Treatment Program?

Though the law varies significantly by state regarding whether you can receive custody or conduct credits for time spent and good behavior in institutions other than prisons, there are a few general rules you can use to determine if you are entitled to custody credit. First, if the facility you are in before you receive your sentence is the functional equivalent of a jail, you might be entitled to credit. Second, some courts make distinctions based on whether the program you are in is voluntary or involuntary. These are general rules, though, so you should make sure to find out how courts have interpreted the law in your state.

6. Credit for Time in a Mental Hospital

If you were housed in a hospital before being sentenced to prison, you might be entitled to custody credit for your time there. State statutes and courts' interpretations of those laws determine whether you can receive custody credits. Several states have found that, because time in these institutions is similar to being in jail, you should receive credit. As one court stated:

The physical place of confinement is not important as the prisoner technically continued to be in jail while held in custody at the hospitals. The prisoner was not free on bail, had no control over his place of custody and was never free to leave the hospitals. For all practical intents and purposes, he was still in jail.

But other courts have found prisoners housed in psychiatric hospitals pre-sentence underwent treatment rather than incarceration and therefore could not receive custody credits for that time. These courts reason the two types of confinement are different in kind: imprisonment punishes, while hospitalization or civil commitment provides treatment. So, some courts have found awarding credits for time in non-penal institutions toward prison sentences does not make sense.

7. Credit for Time in Drug Treatment

The law varies as to whether you may receive credit for time you spent in narcotics or alcohol treatment prior to serving your sentence. Some states permit credit, and some states do not. Additionally, like in the hospitalization context, whether you may count the days in treatment toward your sentence often depends on the nature of the institution and the terms of your confinement there, such as whether or not you will be returned to prison if you fail to complete the program. Typically, the court that sentences you is free to determine whether to award you credit.

(a) How Does Commitment Affect Parole?

Although there is no constitutional right to parole, the State may not use a mental illness as a reason to deny a parole hearing to a prisoner. Even if you have been determined to have a mental illness, you have the right to a parole hearing and the same procedures that prisoners without mental illness have at their hearings. You also should not be denied parole because you have a qualifying mental illness but have not been provided with mental health care by the prison. If state regulations provide for parole and specific conditions of parole, then you may have a constitutionally protected liberty interest in the procedures afforded by the statute. For more information. You should check the laws of your state to determine whether procedural protections apply to parole denial.

D. Conditions of Confinement for Prisoners With Mental Illness

This Part explains how your mental health may be a factor in determining conditions of confinement and in disciplinary proceedings. Section 1 details the rights of prisoners who are subjected to isolation and solitary confinement. This includes an explanation of the steps taken by many states to exclude prisoners with serious mental illness from isolated confinement and to increase mental health services for prisoners held in restrictive settings. Section 2 explains your right to have mental health considered in disciplinary proceedings. Some states require that prison administrators consider a prisoner's mental health when deciding whether and how to sanction prisoners for disciplinary misconduct.

1. Isolation and Solitary Confinement

Courts have recognized that isolating prisoners with mental illness in Special Housing Units (SHUs) or "keep-lock" for various reasons—among them protection or discipline—is a harmful practice. Although isolation of prisoners with mental illness is not unconstitutional as a rule, it is subject to Eighth Amendment limitations. There are certain conditions under which isolating prisoners with mental illness is unconstitutional. When those conditions exist, courts will be more likely to intervene to help prisoners.

For instance, courts will grow more suspicious if prisoners are segregated indefinitely without review or if there is a possibility that a prisoner will experience psychological harm.

Several federal courts have found that, even though segregation does not by itself violate the Constitution, isolation can pose particular risks for those with mental illness or on the verge of developing mental illness. For these groups, isolation can provide extreme stress and worsen their conditions, and therefore violates their rights. However, to succeed on a claim that isolation violated your rights, you will need to show more than mild or generalized psychological pain.

A growing number of states have taken steps to exclude prisoners with serious mental illness from some isolated confinement housing areas and to increase mental health services for prisoners with serious mental illness who are held in restrictive settings. Courts have approved remedies, many in the form of settlement agreements, for prisoners with mental illness in isolation. In New Jersey, prisoners must be released from administrative segregation if they have a mental illness history and it appears that ongoing confinement there would harm them. The Mississippi Department of Correction was ordered to provide yearly assessments and better mental health care for death row prisoners, who were subject to conditions of isolation. In California, Madrid v. Gomez resulted in prisoners with serious mental illness being excluded from the Pelican Bay prison's SHU. In Connecticut, the settlement of Connecticut Office of Protection & Advocacy for Persons with Disabilities v. Choinski called for exclusion of prisoners with serious mental illness from the Northern Correctional Institution. And, in Wisconsin, the settlement in Jones 'El v. Berge excluded prisoners with serious mental illness from super-maximum security housing.

In New York, advocates with the goal of improving mental health treatment in state prisons brought the case Disability Advocates, Inc. v. New York State Office of Mental Health. The suit was brought state- wide and alleged that because of inadequate mental health treatment, prisoners with mental illness were trapped in the disciplinary process and ended up in isolated confinement settings, which caused them to deteriorate psychiatrically. The case resulted in a private settlement agreement that included among its provisions: a minimum of two hours per day of out-of-cell treatment or programming for prisoners with serious mental illness confined in SHU, universal and improved mental health screening of all prisoners upon admission to prison, creation and expansion of residential mental health programs, required and improved suicide prevention assessments upon admission to SHU, and improved treatment and conditions for prisoners in psychiatric crisis in observation cells. A stated goal of this agreement was to treat rather than isolate and punish prisoners with serious mental health needs. This settlement applies only to New York State prisoners. Also, note that because this is a private settlement agreement, it does not create an individual cause of action, and a court did not order its terms. If you intend to bring a lawsuit based on the failure of New York to provide necessary mental health treatment to you in isolation, you must exhaust your administrative remedies and file a separate lawsuit. If you are a prisoner incarcerated in New York State and are concerned you are not receiving services required by the settlement, you may write to the lawyers who are enforcing this agreement. Appendix B contains a list of organizations to contact for help.

In early 2008, the New York Legislature passed and the Governor signed bill S.333/A.4870 into law. This statute amends various sections of the New York Correction Law, expanding on some of the provisions of the settlement agreement and adopting others. Notably, it defines serious mental illness, provides for prisoners with serious mental illness to be diverted or removed from segregated confinement to residential mental health units, and provides them with improved mental health care.

2. Your Right to Have Mental Health Considered in Disciplinary Proceedings

Mental health may be relevant in a prison disciplinary proceeding in three separate but related ways: whether the prisoner is mentally competent to proceed with the hearing; whether the prisoner was responsible for conduct at the time of the incident (or should not be held responsible because of his mental state at the time); and whether the prisoner's mental status should be considered to lessen the penalty or in determining what the penalty should be. When there is a connection between mental illness and disciplinary misconduct, a prisoner with serious mental illness might commit a disciplinary infraction that jeopardizes chances for parole, results in lost good time credits, or results in isolated confinement. Some states recognize the relevance of mental health and require that prison administrators consider a prisoner's mental health during disciplinary proceedings when deciding whether to sanction prisoners and, if so, how to sanction them. In New Jersey, the Department of Correction implemented disciplinary regulations following a lawsuit stating that hearing officers must submit the names of any prisoners facing disciplinary hearings to mental health staff to find out whether mental illness might have played a role in the prisoners' behavior. The hearing officer must take all information available to him into account in deciding whether to request a psychiatric evaluation and in deciding whether to impose punishment or refer the prisoner to a mental health unit instead of disciplining him.

The New York State courts also recognize that evidence of a prisoner's poor mental health at the time of the incident which led to disciplinary charges should be considered at prison disciplinary hearings. The seriousness of the offense or the number of incidents should not interfere with a determination that alleged misconduct was caused by deteriorating mental health. Litigation in New York led to amendment of existing state-wide regulations that govern procedures at prison disciplinary hearings. The amendments contain criteria that establish when a prisoner's mental state must be considered at the hearing. These amendments also establish that the hearing officer must ask the prisoner and other witnesses about the prisoner's condition and interview an Office of Mental Health doctor concerning the prisoner's condition at the time of the incident and the time of the hearing. The amendments also created committees with full-time mental health staff at the maximum security prisons. The committees review SHU prisoners every two weeks and may recommend restoration of privileges, reduction of SHU term, housing reassignment, medication adjustment, or commitment to a psychiatric hospital. Mental illness is taken into consideration in determining whether to dismiss, make a finding of guilt, or lessen any penalty imposed. Recent litigation, Disability Advocates, Inc. v. New York State Office of Mental Health, resulted in a private settlement agreement that provides for additional changes to the disciplinary process including expansion of case management committees to additional prisons, multiple reviews of SHU sentences for prisoners receiving mental health services, restrictions on charging prisoners with serious mental illness for acts of self-harm, and restrictions on punishing prisoners with serious mental illness with the "loaf" (a restricted diet). These changes are contained in a private settlement agreement. They apply only to New York State prisoners. Also, note that the private settlement agreement does not create an individual cause of action and its terms were not ordered by the court. If you intend to bring a lawsuit based on the failure of New York to follow these procedures, you must exhaust your administrative remedies and file a separate lawsuit. If you are a prisoner incarcerated in New York State and are concerned that you are not receiving considerations required by the settlement, you may write to the lawyers who are enforcing this agreement. Appendix B contains a list of organizations to contact for help.

E. Special Considerations for Pretrial Detainees

Pretrial detainees are individuals in custody who have not yet been convicted. Because they are considered innocent until proven guilty, pretrial detainees enjoy many of the rights they would have were they not in jail. Put another way, pretrial detainees, unlike convicted prisoners, may not be punished, and can claim that jail practices subjecting them to punishment violate their due process rights to be found guilty before punishment is inflicted. In Bell v. Wolfish, the Supreme Court declared that the Due Process Clause of the Fourteenth Amendment governs whether conditions of confinement violate prisoners' rights. The Court established in Bell that jail conditions should not be assessed under the Eighth Amendment, which bans cruel and unusual punishment, because pretrial detainees cannot be punished at all. Instead, claims are assessed under the Due Process Clause of the Fourteenth Amendment.

Note that the Supreme Court has also made it clear that losing your liberty by confinement before trial does not violate the Constitution; it is only when your loss of liberty goes beyond what necessarily comes with detention that prisoners may raise claims that their rights have been violated. The Bell rule shapes most of the law surrounding your rights as a pretrial detainee to adequate mental health care and to avoid unwanted treatment.

1. Your Right as a Pretrial Detainee to Psychiatric Medical Care

In City of Revere v. Massachusetts General Hospital, the Supreme Court applied the Bell v. Wolfish rule, that pretrial detainees are entitled to be free of punishment under the Due Process Clause, to the medical care context. In that case, the Court found the Due Process Clause requires the government to provide medical care to pretrial detainees in its custody, and those detainees must receive protections at least as great as the Eighth Amendment protections available to a convicted prisoner. Pretrial detainees' claims that they have been denied adequate medical care are assessed under the Due Process Clause of the Constitution, rather than under the Eighth Amendment. However, many circuit courts have imported Estelle v. Gamble's deliberate indifference test, which is based on the Eighth Amendment, to evaluate pretrial detainees' claims. Some courts have found delaying treatment for pretrial detainees violates due process because delay punishes detainees and shows deliberate indifference to the serious medical needs of the detainees.

The deliberate indifference test is subjective, not objective. This means for an official to be found deliberately indifferent, the official must have been aware there was a substantial risk of serious harm but failed to respond reasonably to the risk. The official's conduct must go beyond mere negligence.

The bottom line is that you, as a pretrial detainee, have at least the same rights that a convicted prisoner has to adequate and timely medical and psychiatric care. Your right comes from the Fourteenth Amendment, and may come from state statutes. So, before filing your complaint, you should find out what the law is in your state.

(a) Your Right to Protection From Self-Harm and to Screening for Mental Illness

One application of the right to mental health care is the right to protection from self-harm and suicide. As a general rule, courts have found that jail staff and administrators have a duty to protect pretrial detainees and/or provide them with adequate psychiatric care. Jail officials are liable for failing to prevent a suicide or a suicide attempt only if they knew or should have known that a prisoner was suicidal. The standard that courts typically apply to determine if the State failed to protect prisoners from themselves or failed to provide mental health care is deliberate indifference, which is outlined in Parts E(1)(a) and B(2) of this Chapter. In a case of self-harm, deliberate indifference requires a strong likelihood that self-infliction of harm will occur.

Similarly, courts have not established a clear rule requiring screening for mental health problems or suicidal tendencies upon arrival at a jail. Some courts have held incoming prisoners must be screened so that they can be provided with mental health care. Other courts have found there is no duty to screen.

(b) Your Right to Continuation of Drug Treatment

Although prisons are not usually required to offer specific types of treatment like methadone maintenance, you do have a protected liberty interest in treatments that you are already receiving at the time you begin your incarceration. Since pretrial detainees retain many of their rights, any unnecessary deprivation of liberty—like withdrawing methadone—violates their due process rights. Additionally, withdrawal pain can be considered punishment, which is not allowed prior to trial or plea. The only limit on this right is if the government can claim that its interest in ensuring, for example, jail security or your presence at trial overrides your interest in liberty. In addition to due process, if you are detained rather than released and are being denied methadone, you may be able to claim that you are not being treated the same as pretrial defendants who are out on pretrial release.

2. Unwanted Treatment as a Pretrial Detainee

Just as you have the right to refuse medication while you are in prison, you have the right to refuse treatment if you are a detainee awaiting trial. However, your right to refuse medication is not absolute. Even though you have more rights as a detainee than as a convicted prisoner, the nature of the government interest in giving you medication is unique in this context. Specifically, the government may give you medication before trial in order to make you competent to stand trial. However, the government may do this only if several conditions are met. Similarly, there are several procedural checks in place to make sure that medicating you is absolutely necessary. If you are a detainee in federal custody, for example, you are entitled to an administrative hearing for which you had prior notice and are provided representation, and at which you may appear, present evidence, cross-examine witnesses, and hear the testimony of your treating mental health professional. You also may appeal a decision that you do not like. The reason that there are so many checks is that you have a strong interest in defining your own treatment as well as in conducting your defense. Thus, courts will be very careful to make sure that your interests are appropriately balanced against the government's interests.

(a) The Sell Test: Conditions the Government Must Meet Before Medicating You

In Sell v. United States, the Supreme Court established the test for when it may be appropriate for the government to forcibly medicate you prior to trial for serious but non-violent crimes, and when it violates your rights to do so. There, the Court required the government to comply with all of the following conditions before medicating the pretrial detainee:

3. Important Government Interests Are at Stake.

The Court has held that determining a defendant's guilt or innocence for a serious crime is an important government interest. However, there is no clear rule defining what serious means, though courts may measure it based on the sentence to which the charged crime exposes you One court, for instance, declined to fix a clear line defining what crimes are serious, but found that one exposing a defendant to a maximum of 10 years of imprisonment was serious. Therefore, the government had an interest in trying the detainee in that case.

4. No Special Circumstances Exist that Lessen the Government's Interest in Prosecution.

If special circumstances exist, the government's interest in trying you will be less important. But, the Sell Court noted that, if the detainee is deemed dangerous to himself or others, the State may medicate him on those grounds instead, and need not reach the question of whether medication is necessary to enable him to stand trial. In such a case, special circumstances might not lessen the government's interest, which would involve safety rather than ensuring a detainee could stand trial. You should note that the burden on the government is lower if it desires to medicate you for dangerousness reasons rather than to stand trial.

5. Involuntary Medication "Significantly Furthers" Government Interests, Making Defendant's Competence to Stand Trial Substantially Likely.

Several courts have tried to define what "substantially likely" means. One court found that a 50% likelihood that the pretrial detainee would regain competency was not enough to justify giving him medication over his objection. Another court held that a 70% success rate among other detainees was enough. Yet another court has stated that an 80% chance was enough. Though it is not clear exactly what counts as "substantially likely," the greater the percentage chance you will be restored to health—a matter about which a psychiatrist will testify at your involuntary medication hearing—the smaller the chance you have of successfully claiming that the government should fail the Sell test. However, because the government must meet all of Sell's conditions, you still might be able to claim that you should not be medicated for other reasons. Furthermore, some courts have been skeptical of the practice of using statistical evidence of how likely a defendant is to regain competence, and so you might be able to argue that the statistics themselves are flawed.

Courts are also concerned that side effects, even if not medically harmful, may alter the detainee in ways that are likely to affect his ability to assist in his defense. Whether this will happen is another factor that courts should consider when deciding whether to allow you to be medicated before trial.

6. Involuntary Medication is Necessary to Further Government Interests, and Less Intrusive Means Are Unlikely to Achieve the Same Result.

The Supreme Court requires the government to explore alternatives before resorting to the very invasive practice of giving you medication over your objection. These means might include non-drug therapies, or a court order to the detainee backed by the court's power to punish him for contempt if he does not comply.

7. Medication is Medically Appropriate (in the Detainee's Best Interest).

If the State is trying to medicate you, the drugs must be in your best interest. If the side effects are too dangerous, for example, a court may deny the government's request to medicate you. Courts have even held that the government must provide evidence as to how the drugs are likely to affect you specifically, rather than people generally

(a) Other Procedural Requirements

The Sell case involves what is called your "substantive due process" right to avoid unwanted intrusions into your personal liberty. The Sell test weighs your interests against the government's interests. You also have the right to certain procedures before your rights are taken away. For example, you are entitled to a hearing before you are forcibly medicated. If the government seeks to medicate you for dangerousness, it must at least give you an administrative hearing. If, however, it is trying to restore your competence to stand trial, you are entitled to a full judicial hearing in a court. In both cases, you have the right to protections like notice (you must be told when and where your hearing will occur), representation by a lawyer, and the ability to present evidence. The precise procedural requirements vary by state.

Another safeguard that courts have established is the burden of proof that the government must meet when trying to forcibly administer medication to pretrial detainees. Though not all federal circuits have decided this question, the general rule is that the government must show medication is necessary by clear and convincing evidence. Although clear and convincing is not as difficult a standard to meet as "beyond a reasonable doubt, which is the standard in criminal cases, it is still very hard to meet. Furthermore, the government may not use conclusory evidence—or evidence that presumes the point it is trying to make—to prove its case Though these protections do not offer you an absolute right to avoid treatment, they make it more difficult for the State to take away your rights.

F. Planning for Your Release

If you are a New York prisoner and are receiving mental health care while in custody, your institution should provide you with some assistance in planning for treatment upon your release. A staff member familiar with your case should complete a written service plan. The plan should at least include a statement of your need for supervision, medication, aftercare services, or assistance in finding employment, as well as a list of organizations and facilities that are available to provide treatment.

G. Where to Go for Help

In most states, there are organizations called Protection and Advocacy (P&A) agencies that protect and advocate for the rights of people with mental illnesses. P&A agencies also investigate reports of abuse and neglect in facilities that care for or treat individuals with mental illnesses. These facilities—which may be public or private—include hospitals, nursing homes, homeless shelters, jails, and prisons. P&As may advocate for prisoners and investigate issues that come up during transportation or admission to such treatment facilities, during residency in them, or within ninety days after discharge from them.

H. Conclusion

This Chapter explains your rights as a prisoner with mental illness. It covers the basic information you will need to understand how the law applies to prisoners with mental illness, your right to receive treatment, and your limited right to refuse unwanted treatment and transfers.

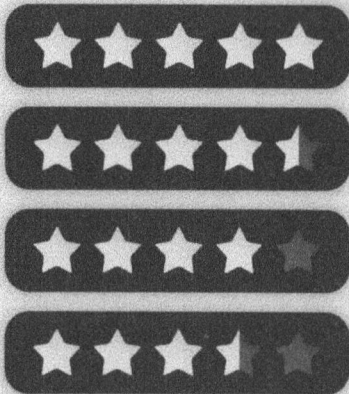

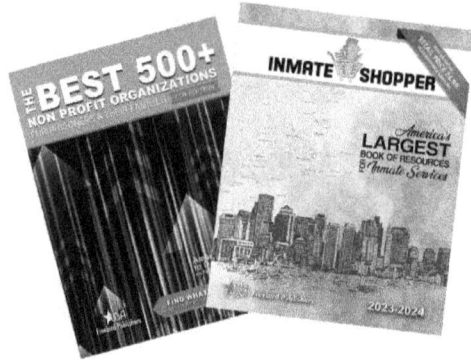

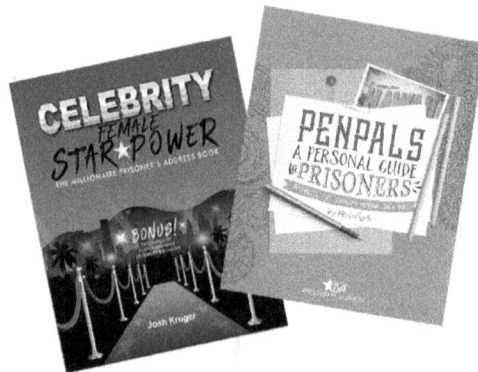

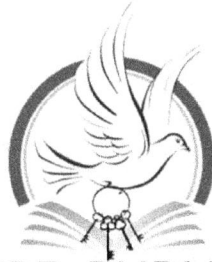

FREEBIRD PUBLISHERS

Thanks for your interest in Freebird Publishers!

We value our customers and would love to hear from you! Reviews are an important part in bringing you quality publications. We love hearing from our readers-rather it's good or bad (though we strive for the best)!

If you could take the time to review/rate any publication you've purchased with Freebird Publishers we would appreciate it!

If your loved one uses Amazon, have them post your review on the books you've read. This will help us tremendously, in providing future publications that are even more useful to our readers and growing our business.

Amazon works off of a 5 star rating system. When having your loved one rate us be sure to give them your chosen star number as well as a written review. Though written reviews aren't required, we truly appreciate hearing from you.

Sample Review Received on Inmate Shopper

poeticsunshine

☆☆☆☆☆ **Truly a guide**
Reviewed in the United States on June 29, 2023
Verified Purchase

This book is a powerhouse of information. My son had to calm/ground himself to prioritize where to start.

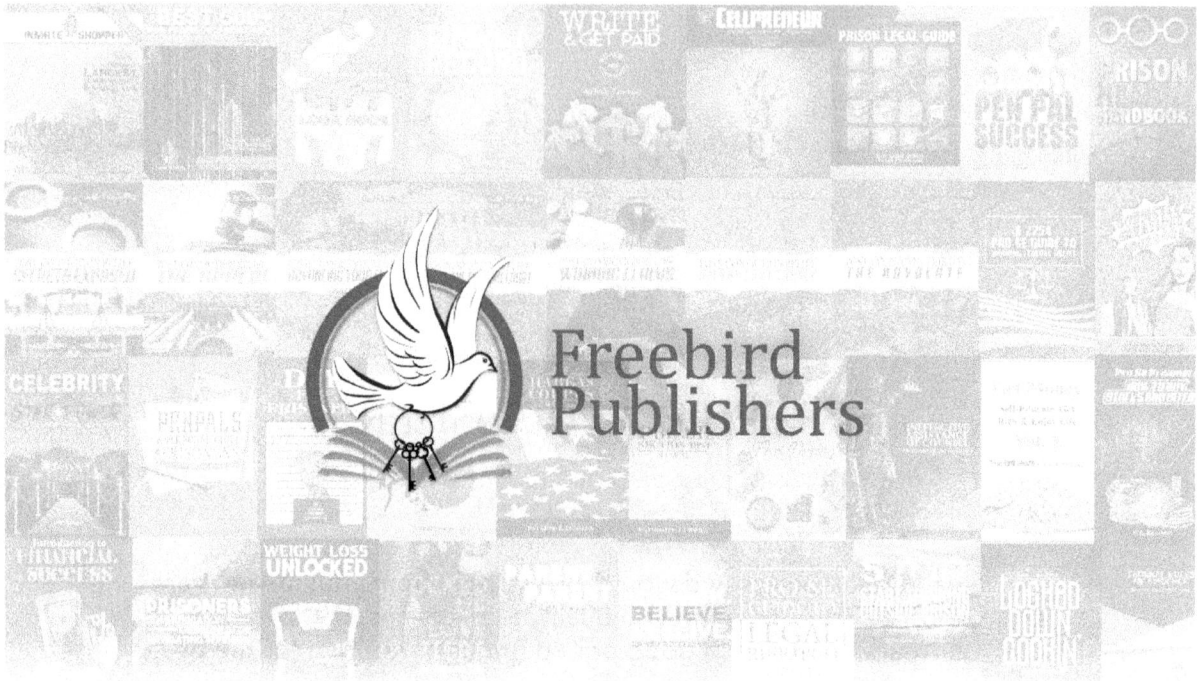

CURRENT FULL COLOR CATALOG

92-Pages filled with books, gifts and services for prisoners

We have created four different versions of our new catalog A: Complete B:No Pen Pal Content C:No Sexy Photo Content D:No Pen Pal and Sexy Content. Available in full Color or B&W (please specify) please make sure you order the correct catalog based on your prison mail room regulations. We are not responsible for rejected or lost in the mail catalogs. Send SASE for info on stamp options.

Freebird Publishers Book Selection Includes:

- Ask. Believe. Receive.: Our Power to Create Our Own Destiny
- Celebrity Female Star Power
- Cell Chef 1 & 2
- Cellpreneur: The Millionaire Prisoner's Guidebook
- Chapter 7 Bankruptcy: Seven Steps to Financial Freedom
- Convicted Creations Cookbook
- Cooking With Hot Water
- DIY for Prisoners
- Federal Rules of Criminal Procedures Pocket Guide
- Federal Rules of Evidence Pocket Guide
- Fine Dining Cookbook 1, 2, 3
- Freebird Publisher's Gift Look Book
- Get Money: Self Educate, Get Rich, & Enjoy Life (3 book series)
- Habeas Corpus Manual
- Hobo Pete and the Ghost Train
- Hot Girl Safari: Non-Nude Photo Book
- How to Write a Good Letter From Prison
- Ineffective Assistance of Counsel
- Inmate Shopper
- Inmate Shopper Censored
- Introduction to Financial Success
- Kitty Kat: Adult Entertainment Resource Book
- Life With a Record
- Locked Down Cookin'
- Locked Up Love Letters: Becoming the Perfect Pen Pal
- Parent to Parent: Raising Children from Prison
- Penacon Presents: The Prisoners Guide to Being a Perfect Pen Pal
- Pen Pal Success: The Ultimate Guide to Getting & Keeping Pen Pals
- Pen Pals: A Personal Guide for Prisoners
- Pillow Talk: Adult Non-Nude Photo Book
- Post-Conviction Relief Series (Books 1-7)
- Prison Health Handbook
- Prison Legal Guide
- Prison Picasso
- Prisoner's Communication Guidelines for Navigating in Prison
- Prisonyland Adult Coloring Book
- Pro Se Guide to Legal Research & Writing
- Pro Se Prisoner: How to Buy Stocks and Bitcoin
- Pro Se Section 1983 Manual
- Section 2254 Pro Se Guide to Winning Federal Relief
- Soft Shots: Adult Non-Nude Photo Book
- The Best 500 Non-Profit Organizations for Prisoners & Their Families
- Weight Loss Unlocked
- Write & Get Paid

CATALOG ONLY $5 - SHIPS BY FIRST CLASS MAIL
ADDITIONAL OPTION: add $5 for Shipping and Handling with Tracking

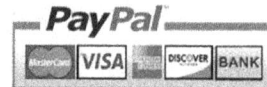

PayPal MasterCard VISA DISCOVER BANK

NO ORDER FORM NEEDED CLEARLY WRITE ON PAPER & SEND PAYMENT TO:
FREEBIRD PUBLISHERS 221 Pearl St., Ste. 541, North Dighton, MA 02764
www.FreebirdPublishers.com Diane@FreebirdPublishers.com Text/Phone: 774-406-8682
We accept all forms of payment. Plus Venmo & CashApp! Venmo: @FreebirdPublishers CashApp: $FreebirdPublishers

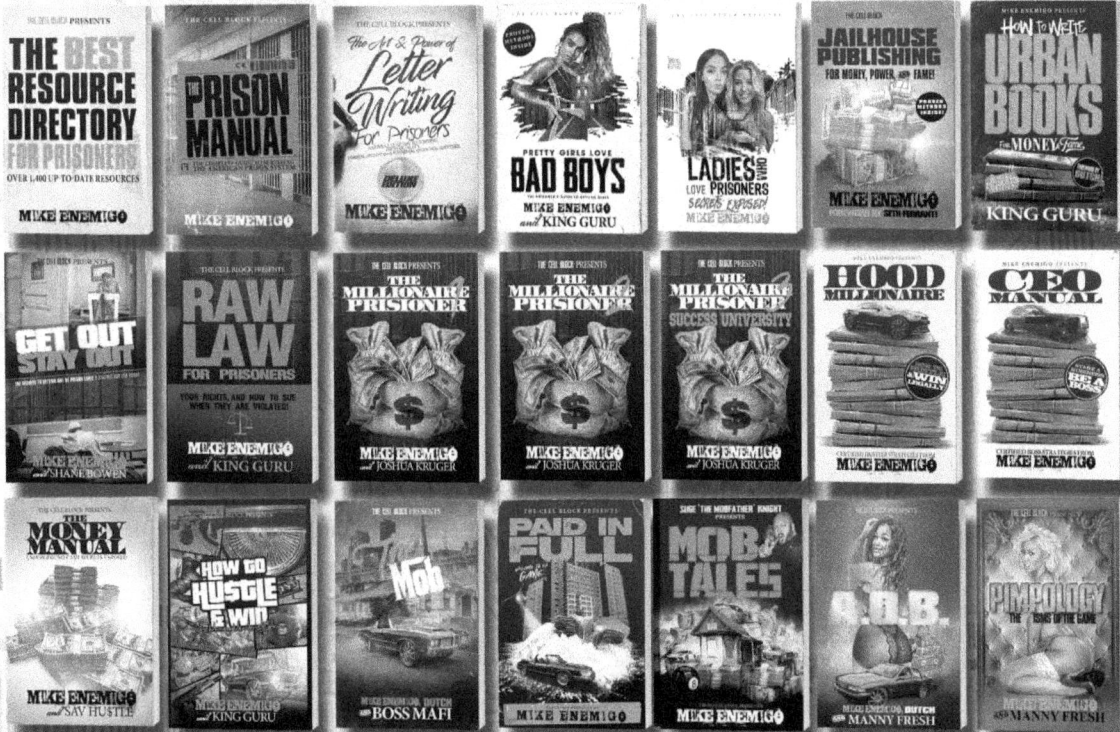

PENACON

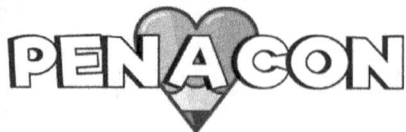

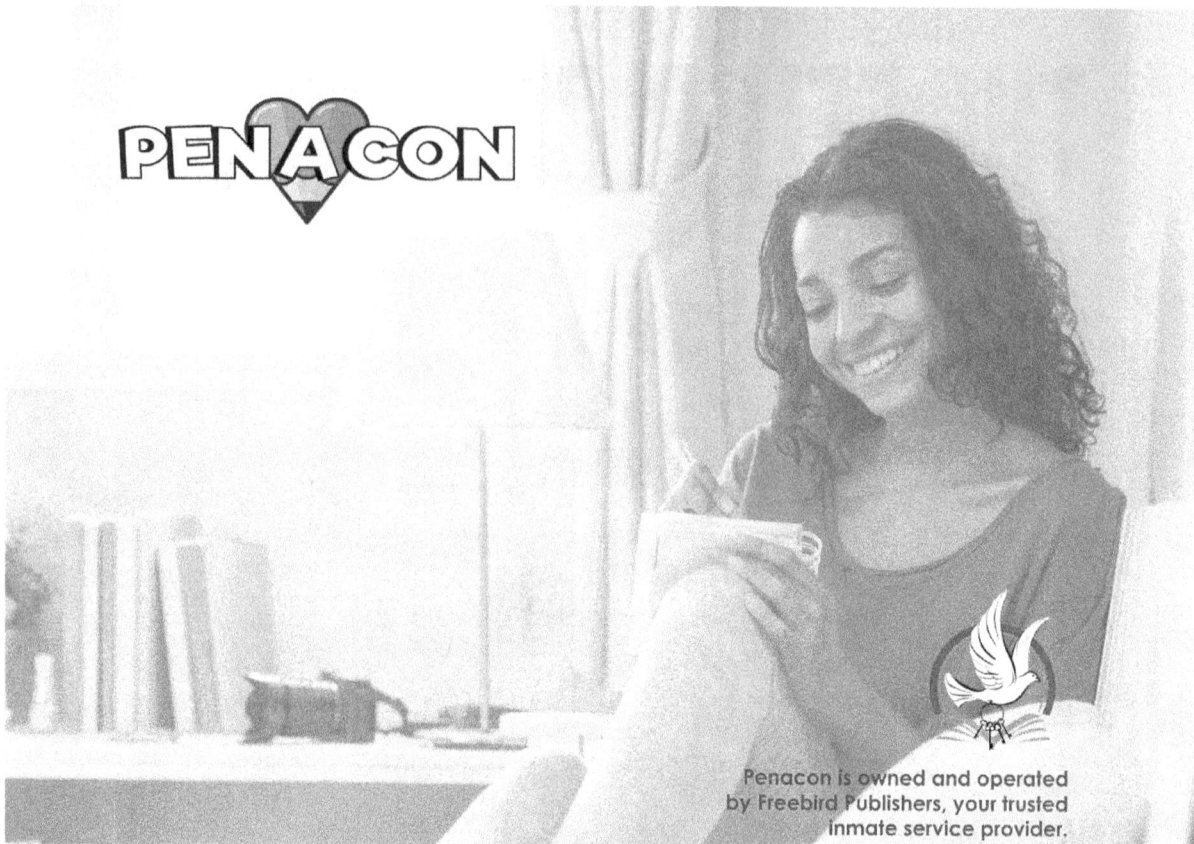

Penacon is owned and operated by Freebird Publishers, your trusted inmate service provider.

Penacon.com dedicated to assisting the imprisoned community find connections of friendship and romance around the world. Your profile will be listed on our user-friendly website. We make sure your profile is seen at the highest visibility rate available by driving traffic to our site by consistent advertising and networking. We know how important it is to have your ad seen by as many people as possible in order to bring you the best service possible. Pen pals can now email their first message through penacon.com! We print and send these messages with return addresses if you get one. We value your business and process profiles promptly.

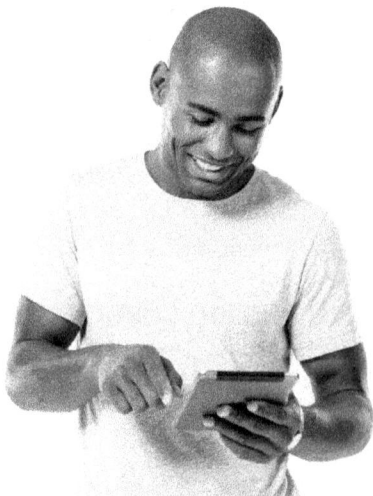

To receive your informational package and application send two stamps to:

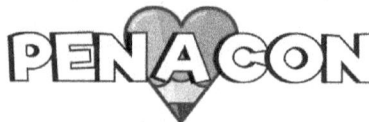

PENACON

221 Pearl St., Ste. 533
North Dighton, MA 02764

Penacon.com
Text 774-406-8682
diane@freebirdpublishers.com